MUSCULOSKELETAL MEDICINE
The Spine

MUSCULOSKELETAL MEDICINE
The Spine

Loïc Burn, BA, MRCS, LRCP, DPhysMed
President of the Fédération Internationale de Médecine Manuelle; Past President of the British Association of Manipulative Medicine; Member Ex-Committee, Scientific Section, British League against Rheumatism; Member, Council of Management, National Back Pain Association

and

John K. Paterson, MB, BS, MRCGP
President of the British Association of Manipulative Medicine; Member of the Scientific Advisory Committee and Chairman of the Terminology Subcommittee of the Fédération Internationale de Médecine Manuelle

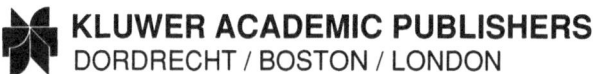

KLUWER ACADEMIC PUBLISHERS
DORDRECHT / BOSTON / LONDON

Distributors

---

for the United States and Canada: Kluwer Academic Publishers, PO Box 358, Accord Station, Hingham, MA 02018-0358, USA
for all other countries: Kluwer Academic Publishers Group, Distribution Center, PO Box 322, 3300 AH Dordrecht, The Netherlands

British Library Cataloguing in Publication Data

Burn, Loïc, *1935 –*
    Musculoskeletal medicine: thw spine
    1. Man. Musculoskeletal diseases. Diseases
    I. Title II. Paterson, John K. (John Kirkpatrick), *1921 –*
    616.7

    ISBN-13:978-94-010-6807-9

Library of Congress Cataloging in Publication Data

Burn, Loïc, 1935–
    Musculoskeletal medicine : the spine / Loïc Burn and John K. Paterson.
        p. cm.
    Includes bibliographical references.
    ISBN-13:978-94-010-6807-9   e-ISBN-13:978-94-009-0715-7
    DOI:10.1007/978-94-009-0715-7

    1. Spine–Diseases. I. Paterson, John K., 1921– . II. Title.
    [DNLM: 1. Backache. 2. Spinal Diseases. 3. Spinal Injuries. WE 725 B963m]
    RD768.B86 1989
    616.7–dc20
    DNLM/DLC
    for Library of Congress   89-24520
                                                   CIP

CONTENTS

ACKNOWLEDGEMENTS

We are very conscious of the fact that we could not have produced this book without substantial help. We wish first to record our gratitude to Dr Peter Clarke for his initial suggestion that we undertake this task and for his forebearance as a publisher. Also we have to thank Mrs Valerie Carpenter for her invaluable help in deciphering tapes and notes and producing many pages of typescript.

We would like to thank Professor Barry Wyke and Dr Mark Mehta for their continued encouragement of our endeavours. We are grateful to the Editor of *Physiotherapy*, for permitting us to use Professor Wyke's illustrations.

In particular we wish to thank Professor John V. Basmajian for vetting our material on muscle function, and to Williams & Wilkins for permitting us to make use of a number of illustrations from *Muscles Alive*. We are also grateful to Professor Basmajian for writing an additional foreword. We are much indebted to Mr Peter French, who was at pains to correct some of our views on surgery and allied therapies. We also acknowledge that, of all the resource material we use, we have drawn most heavily upon the invaluable *Textbook of Pain*, edited by Professors Wall and Melzack.

Finally we have to acknowledge the great help of Dr Ian Haslock, President of the British Society for Rheumatology, who not only looked hard at the whole text, but very kindly consented to write a foreword to this book.

Loïc Burn
John K. Paterson

London, May 1990

FOREWORD

Neck and back pain are common symptoms which vary from the trivial to the incapacitating. Conventional medical textbooks concentrate disproportionately on those causes which have clear-cut diagnostic patterns and pathological features demonstrable by investigations. Discussions of treatment often overemphasize the importance of the tiny minority of patients who proceed to surgery.

Real life is very different. The majority of patients who consult their general practitioners do not suffer from readily categorized diseases, have no diagnostic investigational signs, and often respond to treatment in no other way than that expected from the passage of time. It is not surprising that such a situation has led to the emergence of a number of gurus, both orthodox and unorthodox, who provide diagnostic labels and treatment methods united by only one thing – certainty.

I had expected two such prominent exponents of manipulative techniques as the authors of this book to be among those offering certainty and demanding blind acceptance but I was wrong. This book explores the scientific basis for treatment and evaluates a variety of therapeutic options. It offers an approach to assessment and treatment which is overtly pragmatic but firmly based in conventional clinical medicine. It is a book which invites discussion, comment and criticism in an area where many texts offer little but dogmatism.

Most of us approach back pain narrowly. We are aware that others have different approaches, different techniques, different therapies, yet we tend to base our own treatment within a tiny segment of the available therapeutic spectrum because of the nature of our training, our personalities, our prejudices and the circumstances under which we work. Our patients would benefit from a more eclectic selection of treatments arising out of rational discussion amongst the protagonists of the many different approaches available. If this book does nothing else, its openness of approach and breadth of view should stimulate the sort of dialogue between therapists of different persuasions which is so essential if we are to learn from each other in a way which leads to the greatest possible benefit for all our patients.

Ian Haslock, MB, BS, MD
President of the British Society for Rheumatology

ADDITIONAL FOREWORD

At what point does a promising book turn into a great work of scholarship? I have had the good fortune of seeing that transition occur between the time that Doctors Burn and Paterson let me see their rough draft of this book and when I finally saw its proofs when I was in London. *Musculoskeletal Medicine – the Spine* seemed to start out quite modestly as a helpful and sensible study of the issues, but today it emerges as perhaps the decade's most thoughtful and balanced treatment of the subject. Therefore it is a signal honour and privelege for me to write a foreword for this outstanding work.

What has amazed me most is that these two very busy clinicians have accomplished a miracle; they have balanced logic with hope, commonsense with broad insight, scientific rigour with clinical astuteness, and thorough fairness with gentle scepticism. The reader who seeks a masterly blend of these elements in medical publishing need look no further.

The problems of musculoskeletal pain, particularly in the back, are reviewed with candour and sympathy, and then an excellent scientific groundwork is laid for the clinical realities. Methods of assessment and analysis lead to a systematic review of some thirty major therapies widely used for musculoskeletal problems. In that section of the book the authors demonstrate their special skill in weighing the pros and cons for each class of therapy. That part of the book could stand alone as a major contribution in this otherwise partisan field of medical writing.

The whole book emerges as a model of commonsense combined with a clear knowledge of the whole literature in all its complexity and contentiousness. In short, I believe this book will become the new 'gold standard' in its field.

John V. Basmajian, MD, FRCP(C), FACA, FSBM, FACRM, FABMR
Professor Emeritus of Medicine and Anatomy,
McMaster University, Hamilton, Canada

INTRODUCTION

We present this text of Musculoskeletal Medicine because this is an area much neglected in medical education, worldwide.

Yet the problems are very common. They comprise the largest single group the general practitioner will meet – some 20–25% of his work load.

Further, these problems intrude into many clinical specialities, otorhinolaryngology, cardiology, general medicine and surgery, the many disciplines to be found in the pain clinic, as well as neurosurgery, orthopaedic surgery, neurology and rheumatology. This makes a comprehensive and coherent approach to these matters the more difficult and the more important.

It is important not only because these problems are so common, but because they are likely to fall between the boundaries separating various clinical disciplines.

It has been suggested that Musculoskeletal Medicine constitutes a separate clinical speciality, but we disagree with this opinion. In fact, the Fédération International de Médecine Manuelle, an organization of some 7000 doctors from 23 nations, worldwide, is led in most of its member countries by rheumatologists. This has been facilitated in some cases by the division of rheumatology into one part with an almost exclusive interest in and responsibility for inflammatory disorders, and another part with a greater interest in rehabilitation and mechanical problems of the locomotor system.

If the "proper study of mankind is man", the proper study of the rheumatologist includes musculoskeletal medicine. An alternative title for this book might have been "Rheumatology without the lymphocyte".

This area also contains many widely differing 'schools of thought', medical, paramedical and lay.

The scientific basis of the subject has always appeared weak, no doubt in part a consequence of this confusion and the poor training doctors receive concerning these matters. Many have despaired of the laboratory ever providing them with a rational basis for case analysis and management.

However, the most dramatic advances, most noticeable in physiology and psychology, have taken place in recent years.

We review the literature in an attempt to provide a scientifically based and thereby sound foundation for clinical practice.

The practical clinical consequences of topics addressed in Basic Considerations and in Clinical Presentations are discussed in sequence.

To this end, we present a system of case analysis and make suggestions with regard to management, which are tentative, rather than dogmatic, since they will inevitably be superseded by fresh validated material.

Part I

BASIC CONSIDERATIONS

1
RELEVANT EPIDEMIOLOGY

Introduction
"The epidemiologist attempts to integrate the data necessary for his analysis of a particular disease from diverse disciplines. The need for evaluating the interaction of these factors relative to time, place and persons is the main reason for viewing this frame of reference as primarily an epidemiological concept"[1].

Scale of the problem
The total number of persons afflicted with painful musculoskeletal problems cannot be known for certain. Such figures as are available are limited, and inevitably they are out of date.

1. "It is thought that almost 20% of adults suffer back pain in the course of a fortnight and that approximately 10% will consult their general practitioners."[2]
2. "Out of every 10 000 patients consulting a general practitioner, 600 will be referred to hospital, and most of them will recover whilst waiting to be seen and only 180 approximately will attend."[2]
3. "Of those referred to hospital, 1 in 10 is likely to be admitted, a rate of 19 per 1000 consulting the GP, although only 1 in 12 of those, 1.6 per 1000, consulting will undergo surgical treatment."[3]
4. "In the United Kingdom there are approximately 3.5 million consultations per annum."[3]
5. "3.6% of all sickness absence days in the UK in 1969/70 had a back diagnosis, and the number of sickness absence periods per 1000 person was 11 for women and 22.6 for men."[3]
6. Comparable figures exist for other countries.

Cost
1. "Back pain costs the community about £220 million in lost output, the equivalent of a town of 12 000 people, such as Norwich."[3]
2. "Not all this loss is borne by the sufferers. The Social Security system pays out at least £40 million in sickness and invalidity benefits and disablement

pensions."[3]

3. "In this way, and through lost tax revenue, the whole community bears the economic loss that back pain imposes."[3]

Of course, such figures cannot in the nature of things be precise, and they are affected by a variety of factors, including unemployment rates and inflation. Thus one authority in perhaps less than sanguine mood stated, "personally I have lost interest in 'pop economics'"[4].

Sickness rates
The scale of the problem is great and, sadly, increasing. "Both spells of incapacity and days off work increased between 1961 and 1967, trends that were evident before this period and which in general appear to have continued since then. What is particularly interesting is that the recent increase in days off work reflects not so much longer spells as that more people have been incapacitated, though mainly for shorter periods of time. In other words, illness behaviour has changed, and what this may signify about the alteration of the frequency of occurrence of back pain *per se* is debatable."[3]

Occupation
"An increased sickness absence because of low back symptoms has been found in association with the following six vocational factors:
1. Physically heavy work.
2. Static work postures.
3. Frequent bending and twisting.
4. Lifting and forceful movements.
5. Repetitive work.
6. Vibration.

These factors are all similar and they all increase the load on the spine. They are often present at the same time, so that the association with any single vocational factor is difficult to establish"[5]. We may interpret this as meaning that it is impossible!

Physically heavy work
Comparison between heavy and light occupations from the point of view of back pain is not straightforward. "Most studies define heavy physical work as jobs with high energy demand and contrast these with jobs with low energy demands. This can be entirely misleading and reflects different loading conditions of the spine. Manual work, for example, involves dynamic loading, office work static loading"[5].

2

1. Nachemson's work on changes in intradiscal pressure in the third lumbar disc in various positions in living subjects reveals some quite surprising results. The highest intradiscal pressure was in fact recorded from people lifting whilst sitting. The consequences therefore for telephonists lifting telephone directories while seated is clear[6].

2. In a comparison of low back disability in heavy and light occupations, it was found that low back pain was experienced by 53% of the workers in light occupations and 64% of the workers in heavy occupations. A difference of only 11%. On the other hand, low back disability in the heavy occupations was twice that in the light occupations[7].

3. A more recent study showed no difference in the incidence of back pain amongst office and manual workers. However, manual workers had a longer period of disability both during the initial episode of back pain and in recurring episodes[8].

4. An interesting study comparing the incidence of low back pain in nurses and teachers revealed little difference between these two occupations in the overall incidence. However, low back pain came earlier in nurses, and was largely precipitated by factors at work, whereas in teachers the incidence of low back pain gradually increased with time, and was not generally related to their occupation[9].

"These studies suggest that the setting of acceptable workloads will have little impact on the incidence of low back pain, but significant effect on low back pain disability and compensation."[10]

Static work postures
Several studies indicate an increased risk of low back pain in subjects with predominantly sitting postures, although other studies differ. Therefore the issue remains unclear[11]. People who spend more than half their working day in a car have a threefold increase in risk of disc herniation, in comparison with non-drivers[12].

Frequent bending and twisting
This combination has been identified as being the most frequent cause of back injuries in England[13]. However, lifting is usually also involved, and dissociation of these factors is difficult.

Lifting and forceful movement
It has been established that back pain can be triggered by lifting, but

estimates of the frequency of circumstances in which lifting is a factor vary between 15% and 64% in these studies[8]. Nevertheless, a direct association between the occurrence of low back pain and frequent lifting has been clearly identified[14].

Repetitive work
This increases sickness absence in all occupations, and low back pain does not differ in this respect from other categories of invalidity[5].

Vibration
Many studies suggest an increased risk in drivers of tractors[15,16], trucks[12,17] and aeroplanes[18,19]. It has been found that truck driving increases the risk of disc herniation by a factor of four, while tractor driving and car commuting of more than 20 miles per day increase the risk by a factor of 2^{12}. It will be remembered, however, that proven disc herniation reflects but a small minority of cases of low back pain.

General factors
A number of general features have been proposed as possible causes of low back pain.

Genetic
HLA-B27 has been identified as a marker for ankylosing spondylitis, "however, as far as every day accounts of back pain is concerned, we know virtually nothing of the genetical aspects, which is scarcely surprising in view of the unsatisfactory . . . classification of these complaints."[3]

Evolutionary
Evolution has been cited, in particular the adoption by man of the erect posture and bipedal locomotion. However, it is known that hominids were walking upright as long ago as nearly 4 million years. "Moreover, in the process of adopting the erect posture man had sufficient time to undergo appreciable evolutionary changes in other aspects of his physical structure, notably his dentition."[3]

Cultural
A cultural theory that has been proposed is that in preneolithic times the hunter/gatherer undertook probably 50 lifts a day, whereas in the postindustrial revolution era, workers can undertake up to 5000 lifts a day. "This is altogether too simplistic a concept." For example, "The increased lifting stress would appear to apply to all of us, whereas back pain, frequent a scourge though it is, is by no means universal"[3].

4

Individual factors
"Data on the association between individual factors and low back pain are quite confusing."[5]

Age
Low back pain is most frequent between the ages of 35 and 55, as has been universally demonstrated. This is of great clinical importance because there is an almost ingrained tendency amongst clinicians to associate low back pain with degenerative spinal changes, particularly when the latter have been demonstrated radiographically. However, it has now been shown unequivocally that after the age of 55 the incidence of low back pain decreases[20].

Gender
This seems to be unimportant, save that disc surgery is twice as common in males as in females[21,22]. It has also been shown that sickness absence is much more common in women doing heavy physical labour than in men[23].

Posture
Scoliosis, kyphosis, hypo- or hyperlordosis and leg length discrepancy do not seem to predispose to low back pain, though they may be concomitant[7,24-28]. Scoliosis has been particularly suggested, but no hard evidence of a true association with low back pain has so far been established[29-31]. The same is true of body build, there being no correlation between height or weight and low back pain, save in the very tall and very obese[32-35].

These matters are of importance because all of them have been postulated at some time or another as being major contenders for back pain aetiology. In no case has this been confirmed.

Muscular strength and physical fitness
The evidence here is again conflicting.

1. Weakness has been identified by some investigators as being associated with pain,while others have found no such association. "Difficulties in measuring back and abdominal muscle strength and the subject selection make assessment of possible correlations difficult."[32]

2. Some have found insufficient physical exercise and some sports (e.g. baseball, golf and bowling) to be associated with the development of prolapsed lumbar intervertebral discs, but others have indicated that training methods rather than the sport itself may be responsible for the injuries. For example, "men practising Olympic weight lifting for many

years do not show any differential affection when compared with light workers, and in parachutists, despite the frequency of spinal trauma, disc degeneration and serious disability with pain are uncommon"[3].

3. It has been shown by using pre-employment strength testing procedures, that the risk of back injury increases threefold when employment demands exceed the strength capability of an isometric simulation of the work[36].

4. A study from Los Angeles has shown that physical fitness and conditioning have a significant preventative effect on the occurrence of back injury. However, it was also found that those who were physically fit differed from others in several respects, for example smoking and drinking was less prevalent, and those who had an enthusiasm for leisure activities tended to have different types of occupation[37]. "No studies to present have considered mobility as a factor in the causation of back pain."[5]

Radiological factors
Degenerative changes
1. "The relationship between the occurrence of disc degeneration and low back pain is controversial. It is obvious from many different studies that disc degeneration per se is not symptomatic and is part of a general age process."[5]

2. Back pain does seem to be more prevalent in the presence of severe degenerative changes, but in the presence of moderate or light degeneration there is no correlation[33,38–44].

There is an important clinical point here, in that since we know that the incidence of low back pain decreases after the age of 55, the common clinical practice of ascribing such pain to degenerative changes revealed on X-ray is clearly a clinical error. Yet, despite all the evidence to the contrary, this practice remains widespread.

Skeletal defects
These seldom give rise to pain. In spondylolisthesis, Scheuermann's disease and severe lumbar scoliosis, an increased risk has often been claimed. Such an association has never been established in any of these conditions[28,45–49]. This is also the case in sacralisation or the presence of a lumbar transitional vertebra, as with other abnormalities[50,51].

Ergonomics
This is a contentious subject.

1. "There is little evidence based on prospective epidemiological studies to prove the value of training, but there is no doubt that a well-planned programme can have satisfactory results, even if one of the mechanisms is the Hawthorn effect, i.e. the initial improvement in performance which tends to follow any change in management"[3].

2. "There is little convincing evidence that the incidence and duration of low back pain have been influenced by instruction in manual handling and lifting"[52].

3. ". . . efforts . . . are handicapped by the generally unsatisfactory state of present knowledge . . . For instance, instruction in manual handling and lifting is fairly widely believed to have prophylactic value, although there is no scientific evidence that this is in fact effective in reducing the frequency or severity of back pain"[53].

Conclusion
Ergonomic considerations are not currently of practical value to the clinician.

Difficulties with back pain data
Several problems present:
1. Investigators tend to have their own definitions of back pain.
2. Much of the information will depend upon patient recall, itself frequently inaccurate (see Chapter 3, Relevant Physiology).
3. The factors affecting working capacity are bound to be complex in an industrial society.
4. The most important factor, however, in making the survey of back pain difficult is the problem of diagnosis.

In discussing back pain, one author writes, "this field is perhaps richer than any other in what can be described as the syndrome phenomenon. The situation arises from the fact that practitioners specializing in low back pain form the opinion over a long period of observation and therapy that when a specific group of symptoms and signs are found to coexist then treatment along certain lines is associated with a high degree of recovery. The details of the syndrome are seldom tested in terms of inter- or intra-observer error, nor is the therapy likely to be the subject of a randomly controlled trial. After all, it has taken years of careful observation to evolve the syndrome, so neither disciple can ever achieve the same diagnostic expertise as the originating master, and if the treatment is 'obviously successful' it would be unethical to withhold it from the sufferer."[54]

"The range of labels used in connection with back pain is a fair reflection of medical ignorance and factional interest. Furthermore it is virtually impossible to classify statistical data on sickness absence in a meaningful way, . . . specific surveys are difficult to compare in the absence of agreed semantics."[55] This fundamental problem of musculoskeletal medicine is still not widely enough appreciated as a reality by many clinicians. For the epidemiologist this means that he has to rely on the "diagnostic quiddities of faceless doctors"[56]. To quote a hostile observer on the role of Lindeman, a scientific adviser to Churchill, "you can't blame the lion for the quality of the carrion brought to it by its jackal." The consequences of these diagnostic difficulties for the management of low back pain are ominous and inevitable. "In the absence of a valid diagnosis controlled therapy is not possible and all treatment becomes an exercise in therapeutic empiricism."[57]

Clinical conclusions to relevant epidemiology

1. Clinically important features of epidemiology in musculoskeletal medicine are that there is no positive correlation between pain and:
   a. Skeletal defect,
   b. Degenerative changes demonstrated radiographically,
   c. Postural deformity.

2. Available back pain data reveal that diagnosis, and thereby management, suffer equally from insufficient validated evidence.

3. With regard to posture, what is clinically good or bad is a matter for speculation. It follows that advice to patients should be what the clinician finds useful, provided it is harmless.

4. With regard to prophylaxis and ergonomics, these again are subjects for speculation, and the same considerations are valid. Therefore the scientific realities truncate a good deal of agonizing, since there is no current certitude in this field.

5. We have chosen Relevant Epidemiology as an introduction to this book because it provides a comprehensive 'tour d'horizon' of the whole of musculoskeletal medicine. It is therefore neither arcane nor academic, because it relates directly, if banefully, to the problems the clinician meets in case analysis and management.

References

1. Lilienfeld (1976). Selected epidemiological concepts of disease. In *Foundations of Epidemiology*, Chapter 3. (New York: Oxford University Press)
2. Jayson (1982). Rheumatology. In *Proceedings of the International Symposium organised by the Back Pain Association, 1982, London*
3. Wood (1980). The epidemiology of back pain. In Jayson (ed.) *The Lumbar Spine and Low Back Pain*. 2nd Edn. (London: Pitman Medical)
4. Wood (1982). Towards an appreciation of the social impact of back pain. In Colt Symposium (London: National Back Pain Association)
5. Andersson (1982). Occupational aspects of low back pain. In Colt Symposium, op. cit.
6. Nachemson (1980). Lumbar intradiscal pressure. In Jayson (ed.) op. cit.
7. Hult (1954). The Munkfors investigation. *Acta Orthop. Scand.* (Supp.) 16
8. Bergquist-Ullman and Larsson (1977). Acute low back pain in industry. *Acta Orthop. Scand.* (Supp.) 170
9. Cust *et al.* (1972). The prevalence of low back pain in nurses. *Int. Nurse. Rev.*, **19**, 169–179
10. Snook (1982). Workloads. In Colt Symposium, op. cit.
11. Andersson (1982). In *Proceedings of the International Symposium organised by the Back Pain Association*, op. cit.
12. Kelsey and Hardy (1975). Driving of motor vehicles as a risk factor for acute herniated lumbar intevertebral disc. *Am. J. Epidemiol.*, **102**, 63–73
13. Troup *et al.* (1970). Survey of cases of lumbar spinal disability. A study. Med. Officers Broad Sheet. (London: National Coal Board)
14. Chaffin and Park (1973). A longitidunal study of low back pain as associated with occupational weight lifting factors. *Am. Ind. Hyd. Assoc. J.*, **34**, 531–525
15. Rosegger and Rosegger (1960). Arbeitsmedizinische Erkenntmiss beim Schlepperfahren. *Arch. Landtechn.*, **2**, 365
16. Dupuis and Christ (1972). *Untersuchung der moglichkeit von Gesundheits-schadig-ungen im Bereich der Wirbelsaule bei schlepperfarhen.* (Bad Kreuznach: Max Planck Institute) A. 72/2
17. Wilder *et al.* (1982). Vibration and the human spine. *Spine*, **7**, 243–254
18. Fitzgerald and Crotty (1972). The incidence of back ache among air crew and ground crew in the RAF. (London: Ministry of Defence, Flying Personnel Research Committee) FPRC/1313
19. Schult-Wintrop and Knoche (1978). Back ache in the UH/ID helicopter crews. (Lodon: Advisory Group for Aeronautical Research and Development) AGARD CP 255
20. Hay (1974). The incidence of low back pain in Busselton. In Twomey (ed.), *Symposium: Low Back Pain.* (Perth: Western Australian Institute of Technology) 7
21. Braun (1969). Ursachen de lumbalen bandscheiber falls. In *Die Wirbelsanle in Vorschung und Praxis*, 43
22. Spangfort (1972). The lumbar disc herniation. A computer aided analysis of 2504 operations. *Acta Orthop. Scand.*, (Supp.) 142
23. Magora (1970). Investigation of the relation between low back pain and occupations. 1. Age, sex, community, education and other factors. *Ind. Med. Surg.*, **39**, 465–471
24. Horal (1969). The clinical appearance of low back pain in disorders in the city of Gottenborg, Sweden. *Acta Orthop. Scand.*, (Supp.) 118
25. Rowe (1969). Low back pain in industry. A position paper. *J. Occup. Med.*, **11**, 161–169
26. Hodgson *et al.* (1974). The prevention of spinal disorders in dock workers. (London: National Dock Labour Board)
27. Magora (1975). Investigation of the relation between low back pain and occupation. 7. Neurologic and orthopaedic conditions. *Scand. J. Rehabil. Med.*, **7**, 146–151
28. Sorensson (1964). Scheurmann's juvenile kyphosis. Thesis. (Copenhagen: Munksgaard)
29. Nilsonne and Lundgren (1968). Long term prognosis in ideopathic scoliosis. *Acta Orthop. Scand.*, **39**, 456–465
30. Nachemson (1968). Back problems in childhood and adolescence. *Lakartidningen*, **65**, 2831–2843

31. Collis and Ponsetti (1969). Long term follow-up of patients with idiopathic scoliosis not treated surgically. *J. Bone Joint Surg.*, **51A**, 424–455
32. Kelsey (1975). An epidemiological study of acute herniated lumbar intervertebral discs. *Rheumatol. Rehabil.*, **14**, 144–155
33. Lawrence (1955). Rheumatism in coalminers. Part 3. Occupation factors. *Br. J. Ind. Med.*, **12**, 249–261
34. Tauber (1970). An unorthodox look at back aches. *J. Occup. Med.*, **12**, 128–130
35. Ikata (1965). Statistical and dynamic studies of lesions due to overloading on the spine. *Shikoku Acta Med.*, **40**, 262–286
36. Keyserling *et al.* (1980). Isometric strength testing as a means of controlling medical incidents in strenuous jobs. *J. Occup. Med.*, **22**, 332–336
37. Cady *et al.* (1979). Strength and fitness and subsequent back injuries in firefighters. *J. Occup. Med.*, **21**, 269–272
38. Bistrom (1954). Congenital anomalies of the lumbar spine in persons with painless backs. *An. Chir. Gynaecol. Fenn.*, **43**, 102–115
39. Caplan *et al.* (1966). Degenerative joint disease of the lumbar spine in coal miners. A clinical and X-ray study. *Arthritis Rheum.*, **9**, 693–702
40. Hult (1954). Cervical, dorsal and lumbar spinal syndromes. *Acta. Orthop. Scand.*, (Supp.) 17
41. Magora and Schwartz (1976). Relation between the low back syndrome and X-ray findings. 1. Degenerative osteoarthritis. *Scand. J. Rehabil. Med.*, **8**, 115–125
42. Rowe (1963). Preliminary statistical study of low back pain. *J. Occup. Med.*, **5**, 336–341
43. Torgerson and Dotter (1976). Comparative X-ray study of the asymptomatic and symptomatic lumbar spine. *J. Bone Joint Surg.*, **58A**, 850–853
44. Wiikeri *et al.* (1978). Radiological detectable lumbar disc degeneration in reinforcement workers. *Scand. J. Work Environ. Health*, (Supp. 1) **4**, 47–53
45. Fischer *et al.* (1958). X-ray abnormalities in soldiers with low back pain. A comparative study. *Am. J. Roentgenol.*, **79**, 673–676
46. Kettelkamp and Wright (1971). Spondylithesis in the Alaskan eskimo. *J. Bone Joint Surg.*, **53A**, 563
47. Wiltse (1971). The effect of the common anomalies of the lumbar spine on disc degeneration and low back pain. *Onthop. Clin. North Am.*, **2**, 569–582
48. La Rocca and Macnab (1969). Value of pre-employment radiographic assessment of the lumbar spine. *Can. Med. Assoc. J.*, **101**, 49–54
49. Rowe (1965). Disc surgery and chronic low back pain. *J. Occup. Med.*, **7**, 196–202
50. Paillas *et al.* (1979). Role des malformations lombo-sacrees dans les sciatiques et les lombalgies. Etude de 1500 dossiers radiocliniques dont 500 hernies discal verifiées. *Presse Med.*, **77**, 853
51. Tilley (1976). Is sacralization a significant factor in lumbar pain? **70**, 238–241
52. Glover (1971). Occupational health research and the problem of back pain. *Trans. Occup. Med.*, **21**, 2
53. Troup (1979). Biomechanics of the vertebral column. *Physio*, **65**, 238
54. Anderson (1976). Back pain in industry. In *The Lumbar Spine and Back Pain*. (London: Sector Publishing)
55. Anderson (1977). Problems of classification of low back pain. *Rheum. Rehabil.*, **16**, 34
56. Black (1968). The nature of disease. In *The Logic of Medicine*, Chapter 2. (London and Edinburgh: Oliver and Boyd)
57. Wyke (1983). In *Seventh Congress of Federation of International Manual Medicine*, Zurich. (Unpublished)

2
RELEVANT ANATOMY

Introduction
The material presented here is not intended to be a comprehensive review of the anatomy of the vertebral column; this can be found in other texts. It is a summary of those anatomical features which are of particular interest and significance in musculoskeletal medicine.

The cervical spine

Functional anatomy
The cervical spine is relatively mobile for the following reasons:
1. The discal height, relative to that of the vertebral body, is 1:3, as against 1:6 in the thoracic spine and 1:3 in the lumbar spine.
2. The AP diameter of the vertebral body relative to the height is small.
3. The sagittal facet angle of approximately 45° permits movement in every direction, particularly flexion and extension.
4. The anatomy peculiar to C1 and C2, the atlas and axis. (See below.)

The atlas
This has four functionally significant features:
1. The posterior tubercle is small, permitting considerable extension.
2. The transverse processes extend a considerable distance laterally, affording great leverage for rotation.
3. As a consequence of this, however, the vertebral artery has to kink laterally to reach the foramen transversarium, and then back again to enter the foramen magnum.
4. The vertebral canal is large in diameter at the level of the atlas (the most mobile part of the vertebral column) thus keeping to a minimum the chances of cord compression.

The axis
This has two significant features:
1. The dens, gripped to the anterior arch of the atlas by the transverse

ligament, and with its own articular facets anteriorly and posteriorly, clearly facilitates rotation.
2. The massive spinous process provides insertion for the long extensors of the neck.

The occipito-atlanto-axial joints

There are six joints in the occipito-atlanto-axial complex, the facets for the dens, two between the atlas and occiput and two between the atlas and axis. These are so shaped as to permit a marked AP rocking movement at the cranio-vertebral junction and substantial rotational movement at the atlanto-axial junction. These are known in German as the "Ja sager" and the "Nein sager".

The joints of Luschka are formed between the elevated lateral edges of the upper surfaces of vertebral bodies C3 to C7, and the lower, lateral border of the vertebral body above. Their clinical significance lies in their being very prone to osteophytosis, which may involve neighbouring structures.

The intervertebral discs

There are no intervertebral discs between the atlanto-occipital and the atlanto-axial levels.

The zygoapophyseal joints

These are of great importance in mobility and, being to some extent weight-bearing, are subject to osteophyte formation. The spinous processes are difficult to palpate, with the exception of C6 and C7.

The ligaments

Most of the ligaments in the cranio-vertebral region are loose and weak, permitting considerable movements to take place at this level. There are two ligaments of particular clinical significance:
1. The transverse ligament, to hold the dens to the anterior arch of the atlas.
2. The alar ligament, from the dens to the occipital condyles, to check rotation and, to a lesser extent, sidebending.

The spinal canal

The sagittal diameter of the spinal canal at this level is about 17 mm, and that of the cervical cord about 10 mm. Fielding *et al.*, in 1971, showed that, if the transverse ligaments were sectioned, the arch of the atlas was displaced forwards by about 7 mm, and by about a further 3 mm if the alar ligaments were also severed[1].

The muscles

The trapezius and splenius are both primarily extensors, the two recti and two obliques are primarily rotators. These latter muscles have a higher innervation ratio, in that the number of muscle fibres per motor neurone is small, being approximately 3–5. This compares with the sacrospinalis muscles, in which the ratio is about 3000 muscle fibres per motor neurone. The significance of this is that these smaller muscles, which have an innervation ratio as high as that of the external ocular muscles, are capable of very rapid and delicate activity.

Blood supply
The vertebral arteries

These run through the foramina transversaria of the first six cervical vertebrae, before entering the foramen magnum, where they unite to form the basilar artery, which subsequently divides to form the two posterior cerebral arteries. The vertebral artery is therefore at risk of compression:
1. From congenital anomaly,
2. From degenerative changes,
3. From postural causes.

The consequences of this may be enhanced in the presence of atheroma of the vertebral artery.

Blood supply to the cervical spinal cord

This is provided by the anterior spinal arteries, derived from the vertebral arteries, and the posterior spinal arteries, derived from the posterior inferior cerebellar arteries. The anastomoses are inadequate, and these structures provide a complex and very variable system. Therefore, compression or interference with the vertebral arteries or the anterior or posterior spinal arteries may produce clinical consequences which are both unpredictable and widespread, depending on the pattern of supply in any given situation.

For example, "The terminal distribution of arterial supply accounts for many apparent anomalies in the level of the lesion relative to the cause, e.g. compression at the foramen magnum can cause wasting of the hands by interruption of the downward flow in the anterior spinal artery"[2].

Nerve supply
The paravertebral plexus

The nerve supply to spinal structures is derived from the paravertebral plexus. A relevant comment is, "this system of very fine nerves is much too fine for medical students to see in the dissecting room, and accordingly is not well known in the medical profession. It belongs to that enormous field of anatomy which is never really learned in the medical course, and in fact is not at all well known, and yet in which a great deal more research work is needed."[3]

The zygoapophyseal innervation
"Each cervical apophyseal joint is innervated not only through articular branches of its own segmentally related spinal nerve, but also by articular nerves which descend to it from the nerve root rostral to it and ascend to it from the caudally related nerve root."[4] The clinical consequence of this is that it is now generally accepted that injections of the zygoapophyseal joints (in order to be effective) should be given at at least 3 levels. There are plentiful connections between the anterior and posterior primary rami and the autonomic nervous system, and the sinuvertebral nerves derived from these re-enter the spinal canal to supply structures therein. They usually consist of two or more branches, ascending and descending to varying and unpredictable levels and supplying the ligaments, periosteum and other structures associated with the zygoapophyseal joints.

Innervation of the posterior cranial fossa
Mixed nerves from the upper three cervical segments also supply the periosteum of the posterior cranial fossa, with the clinical implications this has with regard to possible headache[5].

Autonomic nerve supply
This is also extremely complex and widespread. For example, pain afferents from the face can pass, via the cervical sympathetic chain to the spinal cord, as far caudal as the upper thoracic levels. The plexus surrounding the vertebral artery enters the posterior cranial fossa and supplies other intracranial structures[6].

The trigeminal nucleus
The nucleus of the 5th cranial nerve descends from the pons to the 3rd or 4th cervical segment, and receives inputs from the 5th, 7th, 9th and 10th cranial nerves as well as from the 1st, 2nd and 3rd cervical dorsal nerve roots. It can be seen that, given the intricacy of innervation of the cervical spine, lesions (for example ischaemic) may produce consequences far removed from the actual site of pathology[7].

Anatomical anomalies
Bony
"Asymmetry of the cranio-vertebral bony and ligamentous structures is almost the rule, rather than the exception."[8] Major malformations, such as:

14

1. Defective fusions of the arch of the atlas,
2. Fusion of separate bony elements, near to or united with the foramen magnum, or
3. A third occipital condyle,

are not uncommon[8].

Much more common are minor asymmetries; for example one occipital condyle being smaller than the other. The superior facets of the atlas are frequently asymmetrical in shape and size. Cleavage of the cervical spinous processes is common, as is asymmetry of the normally bifid spine. With regard to the canal, the normal dimensions have been given, but minor anatomical variations and projections are very common. These abnormalities are, of course, all likely to be compounded by degenerative changes.

The relevance of this to clinicians using palpatory examination techniques and believing in positional diagnosis is obvious; because congenital variation is common and acquired changes are universal with increasing age.

Nervous

The patterns of root and plexus formation vary commonly. With regard to the brachial plexus, about 11% are prefixed (i.e. they receive contributions from C4) and similarly 11% are postfixed (receiving contributions from T2)[9]. Anomalous innervation of the hand is present in 20% of patients.

Vascular

The vertebral arteries are equal in calibre in less than 25% of the population.

That these anomalies of bones, nerves and blood vessels are so common may surprise many clinicians in musculoskeletal medicine; they should surely be borne in mind in case analysis. This illustrates, as will be shown later, that physical signs should be interpreted with a degree of caution.

Movements of the cervical spine

Flexion/extension

The approximate ranges are as follows:

1. At the atlanto-occipital joint, 20° flexion and 30° extension.
2. The other joints, in sequence, take part in this movement, giving a rough total in flexion of 20° ± 10°, and in extension 25° ± 10°.

Side-bending

The approximate ranges are as follows:

1. At the atlanto-occipital joint, 15–20° , restricted by the lateral ligaments.
2. Between atlas and axis, only 5°. This movement is associated with contralateral rotation.

3. The remainder give 45° ± 10° each side, associated with ipsilateral rotation.

Rotation

The atlas rotates on the axis 30°–35° to each side, (approximately half of the overall rotation of the cervical spine.)

It must be remembered that all these figures have been derived from radiological studies, and that they have limited clinical significance (see Mobility Testing, p.26). These figures are both approximate and represent-ative of movements of the greatest complexity. There is much confusion in the literature as to precisely what movements take place, and the degree to which this happens. For example, with regard to the cranio-vertebral junction, one authority states that the range of rotation is 8°–10°[10], other authors state that no rotation takes place at all[11,12]! Again, with regard to side-bending at this level, one author states, "lateral tilting of the head does not alter the atlanto-odontoid relationship unless there is undue relaxation of the ligaments"[3]. Another says, "there is no movement at the atlanto-axial joint"[10].

What is obvious, however, is that there are wide variations of movement. "With reference to the probable lack of movement stereotype, Jirout, attempted to explain the varying positions taken up by cervical vertebrae in side flexion."[13] In 168 films of this movement he observed three separate categories:
1. In which flexion was added to the combined side flexion rotation (237 examples), the more cranial the segment the greater its degree.
2. In which extension was added to the normal combination of of movements (118 examples).
3. In which no forward or backward tilt was added.

His analysis of the cause of these idiosyncrasies did not take into account all of the soft tissues which would be having a 'guy rope effect', although his findings confirm the presence of individual differences in the nature of vertebral movements. Further, he reminded his readers that, "if the vertebral structures then showed pathological changes, their dynamics were altered, and the nature of the added movement was different".

"However, the range of normal movement of the cervical motor segments shows wide variation."

It is clear to us that:
1. The movements of the cervical spine are complex.
2. Many authorities disagree with one another.
3. These movements are not fully understood at the present time.

The clinical consequences of these observations will be considered later (see p.26).

The thoracic spine

Functional anatomy
This is the least mobile region of the spinal column:
1. Because of the attachments of the rib cage,
2. Because the discs are thin, comprising only one seventh of the vertical height of the vertebral bodies

Vertebral bodies
Twelve in number, these are short, diminishing in vertical height from T1 to T3, then increasing to T12, which shares the same mass and general shape as the lumbar vertebrae.

Joints
Costo-vertebral
The head of the rib is inserted into a concavity formed by the segmentally related vertebral body and that rostral to it, and the disc between. It is secured by a fibrous capsule and the fan-shaped radiate ligament.

Costo-transverse
The typical rib, half way between head and angle, articulates with the anterior aspect of the transverse process of the numerically corresponding vertebra. The joint has a capsule and three costo-transverse ligaments, and it is important in restricting thoracic movement.

Zygoapophyseal
These are practically vertical in a near coronal plane.

Thoracolumbar
At a variable level (T10/T11, T11/T12 or T12/L1) the zygoapophyseal joints change from the thoracic to the lumbar type. This results in the upper joints of the particular vertebra being thoracic, the lower lumbar, in type[14]. The fact is that the stereotype many clinicians have in mind with regard to typical cervical, thoracic and lumbar vertebrae does not of necessity reflect reality!

Ligaments
These are the same as elsewhere in the spinal column, anterior and posterior longitudinal ligaments, interspinous and supraspinous ligaments,

17

intertransverse ligaments and the ligamentum flavum. Thicker than in the cervical spine, they are less dense than in the lumbar spine.

Blood vessels
These form extraordinarily complicated anastomoses. From T4 to T9 the spinal canal is at its narrowest, and the blood supply to the cord is at its poorest[15]. Therefore, any patient who has lower mid-thoracic problems is a potential manipulative hazard.

Nerve supply
Complexity
As elsewhere in the spinal column, the nerve supply in the thoracic region is extremely complex, and its 'activation' has far-reaching effects. For example, stimulation of the capsules of the costo-vertebral joints not only produces powerful, unco-ordinated spasm of thoracic musculature, but also respiratory, cardiovascular and hormonal consequences[16].

The autonomic supply
Sympathetic neurones may be involved in the somatic innervation of the upper limb from as far distant as T8[17]. Similarly, T12 is often involved in the lumbar plexus.

Cord length
The disproportion between cord and column length means that the upper thoracic roots have to travel only 3 cm caudally to reach their respective exits, while at the thoracolumbar junction this disparity is as great as 7 cm[18].

Anomalies
1. Thoracic spinous processes are frequently laterally asymmetrical by up to 5 mm; therefore positional diagnosis is particularly likely to prove misleading in this region.
2. The obliquity of the spinous processes may lead to difficulty in the identification of precise anatomical levels.

Movements of the thoracic spine
As already mentioned, this is the least mobile region of the spinal column.

Flexion/extension
Movements are limited, figures given being T9 to T12, 1–2°. A total range of between 2 and 6° will take place sagittally, of which 30–40% is extension, the remainder flexion[19].

Side-bending
This is least at T5; the figure of approximately 2° is given[19].

Rotation
Thoracic vertebral movement does not always depend upon facet plane orientation[20]. This is, of course, significant, because many clinicians give great emphasis to the orientation of zygoapophyseal joint planes as being the major factor in determining spinal movements. It is clearly but one factor amongst many (see Lumbar spine, below).

The lumbar spine

Functional anatomy
Vertebral bodies
These are five in number, as a group presenting an anterior convexity in a neutral posture.

Zygoapophyseal joints
These, like those more rostral to them, are true synovial joints, virtually anteroposterior in a vertical plane. They have joint capsules, supported by substantial ligaments.

Intervertebral discs
These account for one third of the height of the lumbar spine in the healthy, young adult. Their component parts are described individually, but together they form the core of the mobile segment, taking the stresses of weight-bearing as well as of various distortions, and permitting a strictly limited mobility of the whole.

The annulus fibrosus
This is in the form of a fibrocartilaginous ring, which has no intrinsic nerve supply. A report in 1980 that the outer part has a rich sensory innervation has not, to our knowledge, since been confirmed[21]. However, the outer fibres of its posterior surface are closely associated with the posterior longitudinal ligament, which has, of course, a lavish nociceptor system. For this reason, events at this site can give rise to pain. The annulus is constructed of layers of fibroelastic tissue, the fibres running obliquely in alternate directions between the vertebral bodies above and below, the attachments being very strong. In conjunction with the cartilaginous end plates of the vertebral bodies, it encloses the nucleus pulposus.

The nucleus pulposus

This is a semi-fluid gel, comprising about 40% of the intervertebral disc. Contained within the annulus fibrosus, it is separated from the cancellous bone of the vertebral bodies above and below by the hyaline cartilage plates. Being a semi-fluid, it does not change volume on changes in pressure, but is readily deformed on movement.

The hyaline cartilaginous plates

These are the growth centres for much of the vertebral bodies. They help to anchor the the fibres of the annulus fibrosus peripherally and transmit any compression force between the vertebral bodies, at the same time separating the nucleus from the vascular spongiosa.

Thus the intervertebral disc is in effect a self-contained, semi-hydraulic shock-absorbing coupling, permitting movement in shear, in rotation, in tilt and (by distending the annulus fibrosus) in compression. Under load it changes shape, the force applied between vertebral bodies being transmitted equally in all directions by the nucleus pulposus. The effect of this application of hydraulic pressure is to deform the nucleus and to distort the annulus asymmetrically, depending upon its local strength and the prestressing of its fibres by positional factors.

The posterior portion of the annulus fibrosus is a site of potential weakness because:

1. The fibres are relatively thin posteriorly.
2. The posterior longitudinal ligament is thinner as it passes over the disc than it is over the vertebral body.
3. In flexion, and under load of a lifting strain, the nucleus pulposus is forced posteriorly against the overstretched posterior fibres of the annulus, thereby increasing the stress put upon them to a sometimes unacceptable level.

Ligaments

These are generally thicker and stronger than elsewhere in the spine. The same pattern as is found rostrally is largely followed in the lumbar spine, with one or two important differences. Heylings, in 1978, has shown that below the spinous process of L5 there is no true interspinous or supraspinous ligament; instead there are decussating fibres of the lumbar fascia[22]. The importance of this is that some clinicians, often injecting the soft tissues between L5 and the sacrum with benefit, assume that they are injecting a ligament. This is clearly not the case.

The iliolumbar ligaments attach the L5 spinous and transverse processes to the posterior iliac crests.

Blood vessels
These form an extremely complex system of arterial and venous anastomoses.

The nerve supply
This again is very intricate. For example, a recurrent branch from the segment at the L2 level can descend as far as the vertebral body of L5. Therefore, involvement at this level can have widespread clinical consequences[23].

The innervation of ligaments
This is densest in the posterior longitudinal ligament, less in the sacroiliac and other longitudinal ligaments, and least in the ligamentum flavum.

Spinal roots
Because the spinal cord terminates at the level of L1, these have a considerable distance to travel within the vertebral canal before reaching their respective intervertebral foramina, at least 9 cm, the lower as much as 16 cm[18]. They are intimately related to the posterior aspects of the discs, and the possibility this offers for root involvement in both disc abnormalities and disease is clear.

Anomalies
These are common.

Asymmetry
1. Asymmetry of the lumbosacral joints is present in approximately one quarter of the population[24].
2. In a series of 3000 pre-employment X-rays, taken over a two-year period, many asymptomatic conditions, including degenerative and developmental anomalies, were demonstrated[25].
3. A further series of X-rays on patients admitted to hospital for conditions other than back pain, showed many minor congenital abnormalities, particularly at the lumbosacral junction[26].
4. Schmorl describes the junctional regions of the spine as being, "ontogenetically restless", and, discussing the lumbosacral angle, writes, "critical evaluation of all available investigative results makes it difficult to diagnose an abnormal lumbosacral angle, and it is even more difficult to consider it as a cause of pain."[27]

Spinal stenosis

First described as long ago as 1900, this has now become a matter of intense clinical interest[28]. The ultrasound studies of Porter *et al.* show that patients with disc symptoms and neurogenic claudication may have narrow or trefoil canals, the latter feature increasing from L1 to L5[29]. Again, it must be emphasized that a large but unknown number of people with these anomalies do not have symptoms.

Soft-tissue abnormalities

As in the cervical region, these are frequently found.

1. Many anastomoses between nerve fibres have been described, as have inter-radicular connections[30].
2. The common dural origin of two nerve roots, as well as the common exit of two nerve roots by the same intravertebral foramen are also often found[31].

The movements of the lumbar spine

In the cadaver

Nachemson showed in fresh cadavers:

1. If the normal physiological motions were applied, together with anterior, posterior and lateral shears, whilst differences were observed, these were seldom marked.
2. "There was, however, a pronounced scatter in the behaviour of individual segments, and this overshadowed the class differences.
3. Age appeared to have no consistent effect on mechanical behaviour of adult segments.
4. Disc levels seldom had a marked effect on response.
5. In the six grossly degenerated specimens of this series of 42, no relative disc space narrowing was observed."[32]

This last finding is of interest, since it reveals yet another variable which may surprise some readers, who have been led to assume that disc narrowing is an integral part of degenerative change. This is not necessarily the case.

In an analysis of 103 postmortem specimens of the lower spine, Hilton showed:

1. "At each disc level in both sexes there is a wide scatter of mobility values, but the mean mobility falls progressively from L5."
2. "However, the small fall shown by the mean is misleading, since the mobility in most individuals is to a varying degree irregularly distributed."
3. "Only 9 females and 7 males conformed to the mean mobility pattern, and of these 13 were aged less than 50 years."
4. "The irregularity in mobility pattern occurs irrespective of age and sex, and can be due to either reduction or increase in mobility at any level."

5. "These irregularities are often unpredictable on straight X-rays, and do not necessarily reflect gross pathology, since they can occur in relatively healthy specimens."[33]

Comment

The objection that these findings might not be applicable in the living must be considered in the light of the fact that postmortem changes in mobility are likely to occur at much the same rate at all spinal levels. Hilton's work indicates that variations in segmental mobility are extremely common.

In vivo

Global movements

Moll and Wright observed spinal mobility *in vivo*. They found:
1. In normal subjects there was a marked decrease in spinal mobility with age, and also a sex difference.
2. The scatter not only varied between decades, but was considerable within each age group.
3. This wide range of variation in normal mobility was observed in flexion, extension and side-bending[34].

Comment

Yet again, this work shows movements of the lumbar spine to be wholly unforeseeable.

Flexion/extension

1. In general, the total flexion/extension range of the five lumbar segments is of the order of 50° to 70°, side-bending being rather less[20].
2. Anomalies are common in the lower lumbar spine, and "the lumbosacral angle varies greatly, making the establishing of a generalised movement pattern very difficult". For the clinical significance of this finding, see below[27].

Rotation

1. This is about 12° standing and 3° when sitting at the lumbosacral joint[20].
2. It has been shown that, "rotation ranges are not influenced by the orientation of the lumbar sacral facets"[35]. This finding is of importance because many clinicians believe that facet joint orientation is the dominant and determining factor in spinal mobility.
3. Again, "no correlation was found between: (a) variations of rotation and build, (b) height, age or weight, (c) rotation and the presence of Schmorl's nodes, (d) disc narrowing, (e) sclerosis of a facet, (f) laminar defects, (g) spina bifida, (h) asymmetrical facet planes." With regard to

23

thoracic and lumbar rotation, considerable differences between individuals have been demonstrated[35].

4. In another series of radiographically observed flexion/extension ranges, it was found that:
   a. In healthy pain-free individuals the greatest lumbar movement occurs in the lower vertebrae and gradually becomes less in the upper segments.
   b. In some the greatest movement is at the L4 segment, in some at L5 and in others the amplitudes of movement are equal at the two segments.
   c. Anterior spur formation on vertebral bodies was noted at or after middle age and was always associated with movement limitation of the segment concerned.
   d. In 4 young patients who had acute back pain without bony abnormality, there was a general restriction of movement not confined to a particular segment[36].

This material demonstrates beyond any doubt that the movements of the lumbar spine in the symptom-free population vary greatly and unpredictably. The clinical significance of this will be discussed shortly (see p.26).

The sacroiliac joint

Functional anatomy
The structure of this joint is complex.
1. Both the sacral and the iliac surfaces vary greatly in size, shape and contour, and between individuals.
2. The surfaces are unpredictably and markedly irregular.
3. The surfaces do not mirror one another.

Therefore each joint has at least two surfaces angled to one another, and often three, and these are frequently dissimilar within the same individual. In 30 sacra it was found that variations in width of the lateral part existed in 25 cases, the left lateral being wider in 19 and the right in 6, and only in 5 cases were the two sides similar[37].

Variations are common in the following:
1. The height of the sacral body and ilea.
2. The tilting of the upper surface of the sacrum.
3. Trapezoidal 5th lumbar vertebrae.
4. Iliac horns.
5. Calcified iliolumbar ligaments.

6. Asymmetrical facets.
7. Spina bifida of the upper sacral segments.
8. In 30% accessory sacroiliac articulations exist between the lateral sacral crest and the ilia[27].

Wide anatomical variations are thus seen to be normal, and the consequences of this for clinicians using palpatory diagnostic techniques are clear.

Movements of the sacroiliac joint
These were originally described as being about two axes (1878)[38] and others described the motion as being slight and consisting of an up and down gliding and slight sagittal movement.

Radiological studies
It has been shown:
1. "The axis of movement lies about 10 cm below the sacral promontory and varies by about 5 cm."
2. "The axis tends to be higher in puerperal women."
3. "Differences in the degree and nature of the movement cannot be correlated with height, weight, sacral curve index or sex."[39]

Another study concluded:
1. There is certainly movement, but it is usually small and varies greatly with the individual; shifts of 5 mm were recorded between iliac spines.
2. There is evidence that both angular and parallel movements take place, rather than rotational motion.
3. The authors find it difficult to accept previous authors' impressions that movements occur around a fixed mechanical axis.
4. Colachis and Warden also noted a great variation in movement between individuals[40].

More recent work on a cadaver showed:
1. "The movements between points on the sacrum and ilium ranged up to 12 mm with an average of 2.7 mm."
2. "Between the ilia themselves ranges were up to 15.5 mm."[41]

In a male subject:
1. "Ranges were considerably larger than those observed in the cadaver."
2. "Movements of the ilia relative to the sacrum for example ranged up to 26 mm, a little over an inch, with tortional and flexing movements of the same order."[41]

Another study showed:

1. "In the standing position all motions of the trunk, with the exception of flexion and extension, normally are associated with unpaired and antagonistic movements of the ilia."
2. "Rotation and lateral bending of the sacrum do not occur alone, but constitute a correlated motion that is coincidental to antagonistic movements of the ilia."
3. "Positions of the ilia in normal stance as well as their relative mobility are affected by the dominant eye and hand."[42]

Clinical significance of sacroiliac mobility

This material is of note because, world-wide, many clinicians have devised systems of diagnosis based on the supposed movements of these joints.

1. As can be seen, their structural complexity is considerable, and their actual movements, though usually slight, are shown to be extraordinarily complex.
2. These movements can and do vary greatly, not only in range, but also in axis and above all in direction.
3. For this reason, the idea that movements of these joints can be 'systematized' to produce methods of case analysis and treatment that have clinical application should, perhaps, be regarded with some caution.
4. As so often within this field, increasing knowledge seems to counsel prudence, rather than certainty.

Clinical assessment of spinal mobility

1. This is of great clinical importance because all over the world many different systems of clinical analysis and treatment have been evolved for the assessment of mobility.
2. These have been based upon the idea that there is such a thing as a normal range of movement which can be assessed, so that limitations of that range or excessive movements can be accurately detected.
3. Thereafter various treatments may be directed to correcting these findings, not only relieving symptoms, but restoring what are regarded as normal ranges of movements.

There are certain reservations to be expressed concerning these hypotheses.

1. Such methods of assessment are wholly subjective. Therefore it is impossible to convince a third party, if he or she remains sceptical.
2. The material presented here shows beyond reasonable doubt that these movements are complex, and that they are as yet not fully understood.
3. Variation is the rule, rather than the exception, and authors frequently disagree.

4. If one adds to these complexities and difficulties the very common incidence of structural anomaly and the unpredictable consequences of degenerative change, it is clear that the range of what may be termed normal must vary greatly.

It is for these reasons that we do not use mobility assessment clinically. Nonetheless, we appreciate that many clinicians in many countries find it of great value (see Notes to Case Analysis, p.160).

Biomechanics

Many workers in this field have been interested in and impressed by the publications of White and Panjabi[43], in particular by the excellent illustrations to their text. However, before drawing clinical conclusions, it is the authors themselves who have written:

1. "The experimental techniques for precise, no-risk, *in vivo* measurement in the human are yet to be developed."
2. "The physiological muscle forces have not been simulated."
3. "The characteristics of the force vectors that cause *in vivo* physiological motion are not known."
4. "Studies are done to simulate vertebral motion, but it is not known whether the motion experimentally produced is the same as that which is physiologically produced *in vivo*."
5. "The vectors that should represent the existing physiological preloads are not known."
6. "At present we are not aware of published studies of kinematics that take them into consideration."[43]

More succinctly, in 1986, at the 8th International Congress of the Fédération Internationale de Médecine Manuelle in Madrid, Professor Panjabi stated, "I cannot see the relevance of this material to the work you do." This happy blend of expertise, candour and common sense should be an example and encouragement to us all.

Clinical conclusions to relevant anatomy

1. The complexities of spinal structure, innervation and blood supply have been emphasized.
2. It is worth stressing how frequently congenital abnormality is found in the asymptomatic.
3. It is plain that, on anatomical grounds alone, these factors make accurate diagnosis difficult.
4. We do not use mobility testing (see p.26).
5. Biomechanics can have but limited clinical relevance.

References

1. Fielding *et al.* (1971). Fixed atlanto-axial rotary subluxation. *J Bone Joint Surg.*, **53a**, 1031
2. Leading article (1967). Infarction of the spinal cord. *Lancet*,11, 143
3. Scott Charlton and Roebuck (1972). The significance of posterior primary divisions of spinal nerves in pain syndrome. *Med. J. Aust.*, **2**, 945
4. Wyke (1979). Neurology of the cervical spinal joints. *Physiotherapy*, **65**, 72
5. Kimmel (1961). Innervation of the spinal dura mater and dura mater of the posterior cranial fossa. *Neurology*, **11**, 800
6. Jackson (1966). *The Cervical Syndrome.* 3rd Edn. (Springfield, Illinois: Thomas)
7. Keuter (1970). Vascular origin of cranial sensory disturbances caused by pathology of the lower cervical spine. *Acta Neurol.*, **23**, 229
8. Dalseth (1974). Anatomical studies of the osseous cranio vertebral joints. *Man. Med.*, **6**, 130
9. Seddon (1954). *Peripheral nerve injuries. MRC report.* (London: HMSO)
10. Kapandji (1974). *The Physiology of Joints. 3. The Trunk and Vertebral Column.* (London: Churchill Livingstone)
11. Penning (1968). *Functional Pathology of the Cervical Spine.* (Amsterdam: Excerpta Med. Foundation)
12. Gray (1973) *Anatomy*, 35th Edn. (London: Longman)
13. Jirout (1971). Pattern of changes in the cervical spine in lateroflexation. *Neurol. Radiol.*, **2**, 164
14. Davis (1955). The thoraco-lumbar mortice joint. *J. Anat.*, **89**, 370
15. Dommisse (1974). The blood supply of the spinal cord. *J. Bone Joint Surg.*, **56b**, 225
16. Vrettos and Wyke (1974). Articular reflexogenic systems in the costovertebral joints. *J. Bone Joint Surg.*, **56b**, 382
17. Keele and Neil (1971). In Samson and Wright (eds.) *Applied Physiology.* 12th Edition. (London: Oxford University Press)
18. Hewitt (1970). The intervertebral foramen. *Physiotherapy*, **56**, 332
19. White (1969). Analysis of the mechanics of the thoracic spine in man. *Acta Orthop. Scand.* (Supp.) 127
20. Gregersen and Lucas (1967). An in vivo study of axial rotation of the human thoraco-lumbar spine. *J. Bone Joint Surg.*, **49a**, 24
21. Yoshizawa *et al.* (1980). The neuropathology of intervertebral discs removed for low back pain. *J. Pathol.*, **132**, 95–104
22. Heylings (1978). Supraspinous and interspinous ligaments of the human lumbar spine. *J. Anat.*, 125–127
23. Wyke (1980). The neurology of low back pain. In Jayson (ed.) *The Lumbar Spine and Low Back Pain.* 2nd Edn. (London: Pitman Medical)
24. Keith (1948). *Human Embryology and Morphology.* (London: Edward Arnold)
25. La Rocca and McNab (1969). Value of pre-employment radiographic assessment of the lumbar spine. *Can. Med. Assoc.*, **101**, 383
26. Epstein (1969). *The Spine. A Radiological Text and Atlas.* 3rd Edn. (Philadelphia: Lea and Febiger)
27. Schmorl and Junghaas (1971). *The Human Spine in Health and Disease.* 2nd American Edn. (New York: Grune and Stratton)
28. Sachs and Fraenkel (1900). Progressive and ankylotic rigidity of the spine. *J. Nerve Ment. Dis.*, **27**, 1
29. Porter *et al.* (1980). The shape and size of the lumbar canal. In *Proceedings of the Conference on Engineering Aspects of the Spine.* (London: Mechanical Engineering Publications)
30. Pallie and Manuel (1968). Intersegmental anastomoses between dorsal spinal rootlets in some vertebrates. *Acta Anat.*, **70**, 341
31. Agnoli (1976). Anomalies in the pattern of lumbo-sacral nerve roots and its clinical significance. *J. Neurol.*, **211**, 217

32. Nachemson (1979). Mechanical problems of human lumbar spine motion segments. Influence of age, sex, disc level and degeneration. *Spine*, **41**
33. Hilton (1980). Systematic studies of spinal mobility and Schmorl's nodes. In Jayson (ed.) *The Lumbar Spine and Low Back Pain*. 2nd Edn. (London: Pitman Medical)
34. Moll and Wright (1980). Measurement of spinal movement. In Jayson (ed.) *The Lumbar Spine and Low Back Pain*. 2nd Edn. (London: Pitman Medical)
35. Lumsden and Morris. An in vivo study of axial rotation and immobilisation of the lumbo sacral joint. *J. Bone Joint Surg.*, **50a**, 1591
36. Allbrook (1957). Movements of the lumbar spinal column. *J. Bone Joint Surg.*, **39b**, 339
37. Solonen (1957). The sacro-iliac joint in the light of anatomical X-ray and clinical studies. *Acta Authop. Scand.*, **26.**
38. Meyer (1878). Der Mechanismus der symphysis sacroiliaca. *Archive für Anatomie und Physiologie* (Liepzig), 11
39. Weisl (1955). The movements of the sacro-iliac joint. *Acta Anatomica*, **23**, 80
40. Colachis and Warden (1963). Movement of the sacro-iliac joint in the adult male. *Arch. Phys. Med. Rehab.*, **44**, 490
41. Frigerio *et al.* (1974). Movement of the sacro-iliac joint. *Clin. Ortho. Rel. Res.*, **100**, 370
42. Pitkin and Pheasant (1936). Sacrarthrogenetic telalgia. *J. Bone Joint Surg.*, **18**, 365
43. White and Panjabi (1978). The basic kinematics of the human spine. *Spine*, **3**, 12

3
RELEVANT PHYSIOLOGY

Introduction – why physiology matters

For many years clinicians working in the field of musculoskeletal medicine have felt that the laboratory had little to offer them in their day-to-day practice. However, "neurophysiology has made tremendous strides, and modern methods by neuroanatomists which depend upon active transport retrograde or antegrade have demonstrated the wealth of connectivity"[1]. The complexity and connectivity of neurophysiology can be illustrated by the fact that it was recently postulated that, ". . .even before entering the central nervous system, for an explanation of the dysaesthesia and pain associated with injury of a peripheral nerve, at least 12 sorts of physiological abnormalities must be taken into consideration"[1].

Many years ago Lewit wrote, ". . .since symptoms are usually the result of several factors:

1. "We have to single out each time the factor or lesion which we think the most important at the moment, while we have the patient before us.
2. "Which lesion we think is the most accessible for treatment.
3. "If we succeed in our intentions a different therapeutic approach will probably be needed when we next see the patient.
4. "Our aim is not to promote one type of therapy but to improve symptoms by the most adequate and efficient method."[2]

This reveals an insight with which many clinicians would agree. However, it remained an impression for many years, but:

1. "It is now possible to record the firing of first order central cells in the trigeminal system of alert behaving monkeys."[3]
2. "Here one sees the remarkable subtlety of the brain. With an abrupt, isolated stimulus to a naive animal, the first central cells respond in a classical and predictable way, whether the animal is awake or even anaesthetized.
3. "However, the response changes radically if other events are in progress. For example, some cells 'learn' to respond not only to the stimulus, but also to the alerting signal which tells the animal that a noxious test stimulus will follow.

30

4. "Facts such as these show us that the signalling of injury even by the first sensory cells is dependent not only on the arrival of nociceptive afferent impulses, but on the signalling of other peripheral events and on the setting of excitability by central nervous system mechanisms."[4]

Comment
This must justify the clinical approach described. However, it is reasonable to point out that it is the latter which validates the former. For this reason a review of up-to-date material relating to this field is clearly necessary. The remainder of this chapter covers in logical sequence those features of applied physiology which offer a scientific background to musculoskeletal practice.

Mechanoreceptor nerve endings and their behaviour
Anatomy
The nerve endings in joints are internationally classified as Types I–IV. Types I, II and III are corpuscular in type; that is they are nerve terminals enclosed in capsules with a varying number of layers. These are the mechanoreceptors, converting mechanical forces applied to the nerve endings into electrical impulses discharged into the central nervous system. Their response varies with the amplitude, velocity and direction of the forces applied to them, including those forces applied in therapeutic manipulation.

Types I and II
These are embedded in the joint capsules and are, in fact, the only joint capsule mechanoreceptors. Type I mechanoreceptors are situated principally in the superficial layers, Type II deeper. Neither type is present in synovial membrane, there being no nerve endings in that tissue.

Type III
These are found only in ligaments; but in all ligaments.

Behaviour
Types I and II
The behaviour of any mechanoreceptor, in whatever tissue it may be situated, is related to the thickness of its capsule. This determines the way in which it responds in terms of both time and resilience, to movement, active or passive, to traction or to the application of external forces such as manipulation. The following characteristics are important.

Adaptation: This is defined as the length of time for which a mechanoreceptor will continue to discharge nerve impulses, when exposed to a mechanical force of constant intensity. Type I mechanoreceptors are slowly

31

adapting, Type II fast. Type I have thin capsules, Type II thicker, the general rule being that the thinner the capsule the more slowly the adaptation will take place.

Static and dynamic discharge: A further significant difference between these two nerve ending types is the way in which they behave at rest or when they are moved, actively or passively. Type I receptors fire constantly at rest in the neutral position of the joint at about 15 Hz, whereas Type II do not fire at all at rest. Thus Type I have a static or tonic postural discharge. However, the character of these discharges varies on movement according to the amplitude, direction and velocity of the forces applied to them. It follows that Type I receptors exhibit both static and tonic discharges.

Threshold: Types I and II have a feature in common, in that they have a low threshold, being very easily stimulated. An applied force of approximately 3 g is sufficient to stimulate a Type I mechanoreceptor.

Since the resting neutral tension in the joint is greater than 3 g, there is a static discharge from these particular mechanoreceptors. On the other hand, although the Type II mechanoreceptors also have a low threshold, they do not exhibit a static discharge because their discharge is velocity dependent. This means that, in order to recruit them, movements, active or passive, have to be rapid; this is why they are referred to as acceleration mechanoreceptors.

Type III
These are the ligament mechanoreceptors. They have thin capsules, which means that they are slow adaptors. But they differ from Types I and II in that they have a high threshold. This has implications of importance.

In order to induce them to discharge, forces of kilograms, rather than grams, need to be applied; therefore they have no static discharge.

They will only fire at the limits of range of movement of a joint, either active or passive, or on powerful traction, (such as may be produced on forceful manipulation.)

It must be emphasised here that these nerve endings in the spinal joints and the peripheral joints are identical.

It will be shown later that peripheral joint mechanoreceptor input is an integral part of the functioning of the musculoskeletal system, and should not be considered in isolation (see Control Systems, p.82).

Nociceptor endings and behaviour
Nociception
In this and subsequent sections we lean heavily of the chapters by Lynn[5], Fitzgerald[27], Wall[12], Willis and also Fields and Basbaum[119], in Wall and Melzack's *Textbook of Pain*.

The term nociception has been used since the time of Sherrington. "Whilst we cannot be sure of the sensations experienced by the experimental animal, it has become usual to refer to afferent systems involved in the detection of tissue injury as nociceptive and the receptors as nociceptors rather than pain receptors."[5]

Skin nociception
There are two nociceptive units that are to be found in skin[5]. These are the high-threshold mechanoreceptor units with A-δ axons and the polynodal nociceptor units with C axons[6].
1. "High threshold mechanoreceptor units appear to be specialised for detecting dangerous mechanical stresses and for triggering rapid protective responses."[7]
2. "Polynodal nociceptor units also respond to strong mechanical stimulus. Thus, as well as reinforcing the immediate response of high threshold mechnoceptor units to mechanical stress, they can also signal presence of damaged or inflamed tissue areas."[5]

Musculoskeletal nociception
Type IV nerve endings are quite different from the mechanoreceptors, in that they are non-capsulated. They are subdivided into two types: *Type IVa* are plexiform and are found in the joint capsules and fat pads; *Type IVb* are free nerve endings, found in ligaments and tendons.

Nociceptor behaviour
These units, by comparison with mechanoreceptors, are described as high threshold, in that they only respond to certain chemical irritants or to comparatively strong mechanical forces[5]. While "there is no doubt that many of them have a high threshold, before they are activated low threshold receptors must have come into action"[8].

It is now evident that afferent units which signal tissue injury and inflammation also signal events that only threaten such damage, and that, while nociceptors specialize in responding to tissue injury and inflammation[1], mechanoreceptors in general are not able to signal the difference between noxious and innocuous events[6].

If lightly stimulated, mechanoreceptors rapidly return to their resting threshold. This is not the case with nociceptors, which change their

33

properties when activated, some becoming less sensitive, others more sensitive to succeeding stimulation, even at times firing without additional stimuli[5,9].

Even neighbouring nociceptors which were not initially excited may become sensitive[10]. This results in tenderness and prolonged hyperalgesia, although the cause is unknown[11]. It has been suggested that initial stimuli could alter the structure of the terminals and thereby their reaction to stimuli. Tissue breakdown products may be present, but none responsible for sensitization have so far been identified[12]. There may be substances emitted from the stimulated nerves, although none has been identified as yet[13].

Comment
Therefore consideration of mechanoreceptor and nociceptor behaviour alone reveals a complicated and unpredictable situation.

Chemistry of peripheral pain
Substances capable of irritating these receptors include potassium ions, 5-hydroxytryptamine, lactic acid and other polypeptides, histamine and prostaglandin-E^{14}. Their role in the production of pain under these circumstances is at present unknown.

This is of great practical importance since, if the chemistry of pain is not understood, it is impossible to design specific analgesics.

Distribution of nociceptor nerve endings
The only two spinal tissues in which nociceptive receptors do not exist are the synovial membrane and the intervertebral disc. The latter is a matter of some controversy, since Yoshizawa *et al.* (1980) claimed to find that the outer half of the annulus fibrosus has a rich sensory innervation[15]. So far as we know, this is the only claim of this kind that has been made of recent years.

Clinical consequences
Because these endings are present in so many tissues, and since symptoms from them, singly or together, can cause muscle spasm which may or may not of itself be painful, the accurate localization of its source at any given time is in the great majority of cases very difficult. Together with the problems of referred pain, this is one of the principal causes of diagnostic uncertainty in pain of vertebral origin.

Nerve fibres
Nerve fibres are divided into three groups, A, B and C. Both A and B fibres are myelinated, and the greater their diameter, the greater their conduction velocity[16].

A-δ and C fibres

As long ago as 1933 it was shown that nociceptive input was conducted along small, myelinated A-δ and unmyelinated C axons[17].

These small fibres are relatively insensitive to mechanical stimulation, which is of therapeutic importance to the use of transcutaneous nerve stimulation, as will be discussed later. On the other hand, they are sensitive to blockade by local anaesthetics[18].

While there is no doubt that the majority of A-δ and C fibres are nociceptive, C fibres may have additional roles. The reasons to doubt their only function being related to pain are summarized by Wall:

1. Their number. Since 70% of all dorsal root afferent fibres are unmyelinated, this vast number suggests that they have additional functions[19].
2. The A-δ and C fibres both signal many of the same aspects of tissue damage, and it is reasonable to enquire as to why the duplicate system should be necessary. It has been shown in rats that if 95% of all C fibres are destroyed by capsaicin they appear normal on many tests of reaction to injury, although their response to chemical irritants is decreased, but not abolished[20].
3. About 20% of the fibres in ventral roots are unmyelinated afferents, and there is no evidence that they evoke pain[19].
4. C fibres contain four peptides and an enzyme, and this chemical diversity raises the issue as to whether there is also a functional diversity[21].

A-β fibres

These large, myelinated fibres, while primarily involved in mechanoreceptor input, can relate to pain in four ways.

1. "Afferent barrages in these fibres inhibit the response of cord cells to noci-stimuli and decrease pain"[22]. This observation was one of the major leads to the 'gate control' theory[23,24].
2. "If the electrical stimulus is raised to include the smaller fibres in this group, the inhibition of painful sensation and of the flexor reflex to noxious inputs is replaced by a facilitation[25].
3. In pathological states, such as trigeminal neuralgia, pain may be evoked by stimulation of A-β afferents[26].
4. In areas to which pain is referred and in tender areas distant from injury, light mechanical stimuli may evoke pain, and there is no good reason yet to question that the A-β fibres contribute to the tenderness"[1].

Summary

The primary afferent terminals receive an input which is dependent: upon stimulus, on the background traffic, on the response to a nociceptive stimulus to both large and small fibres, on further modification by the unpredictable post-stimulation behaviour of high-threshold receptors, and on similar unpredictable behaviour of neighbouring high-threshold receptors. Thus the barrage received is already modified by a variety of factors.

The causes of nerve pain are shown in the following table:

Spontaneous discharges from neuroma and dorsal root ganglia
Ectopic foci along nerve (chronic compression, ischaemia)
Cross talk – ephaptic foci
Excess C fibres
Lack of Ab fibres to inhibit C fibre activity
Slower conduction   )
Fewer fibres   )   altered profile to CNS
Abnormal activity   )
Abnormal sensitivity to noradrenalin (leakage from sympathetic fibres)
Central effects –   sprouting
                                unmasking of deafferented cells
                                spontaneous firing

Conclusion
"The eventual outcome of the localisation and subsequent correct identification of the focus must depend upon the total afferent spectrum which travels centrally."[1]

Afferent terminations
The complexities of the input reaching the cord have already been described, including the fact that in the course of time it is bound, of itself, to alter. It is also of great interest to consider the termination of the primary afferent fibres. This is because:
1. The exact site and distribution of afferent terminals will determine the nature of information received by different groups of second-order neurones in the CNS.
2. Cells in the vicinity of the afferent terminals have the opportunity for fast, efficient, monosynaptic transmission, while those at some distance from the terminals do not.
3. Distant cells may still receive information via distal dendrites, one or more interneurones, or possibly by chemical messengers.
4. Consequently, the pattern and timing of their response will be very different from that of the nearby cells.
5. Cells in the vicinity of the terminals may be the first link in the chain of

information flow, and may be involved in local and descending or ascending control of afferent input to the CNS[27].

Technological advances

Of particular interest here are recent technological advances which have made the study of termination of the afferents much easier, and indeed have permitted some insight into 'dorsal horn circuitry'.

"Neurophysiology has made tremendous strides, and modern methods of staining by neuroanatomists which depend on active transport, retrograde and anterograde, have demonstrated the wealth of connectivity."[1]

"Horseradish peroxidase (HRP) can be crushed into dorsal roots, and it is taken up by the damaged axones and transported orthogradely to the central terminals, where its presence can be detected histologically by both light and the electron microscope."[28-30]

"It can also be crushed into peripheral nerves and transported transganglionically into the central nerve terminals."[31-34]

"Single afferent fibres can be impaled and intracellular recordings made with microelectrodes filled with HRP. The great advantage of this technique is that the physiological properties of the afferent can be established (modality, receptive field, etc.) and then the fibres filled with HRP by passing current through the electrode. HRP is transported to the central terminal, and the anatomical distribution of a single afferent can be determined."[35]

As yet, this technique is limited to A fibres, C fibres being too small to penetrate[27]. This restricts the study of nociception, but, for example, Jankowska and Lundberg[36], "have used these techniques on circuits related to muscle afferents and shown that it is now technically feasible to unravel cell links"[12].

A-β fibre terminations

This remains a matter of some dispute. However, whatever their superficial level of termination, the large part of their arborations are in laminae 3, 4 and 5 (see The Dorsal Horn, p.40)[37-39].

A-δ fibre terminations

These terminate primarily in the superficial levels of laminae 1 and 2, although some collaterals have been detected in the deeper layers, 4 to 6[40].

C fibre terminations

These appear to take place exclusively in the superficial layers of the horn. This has been repeatedly demonstrated, using many different methods[28-30,41-43]. However, the exact site of termination within these superficial levels is a subject of continuing controversy[30-34].

Segmental distribution

Dorsal root afferents issue most collaterals in their segment of entry, but the rostrocaudal spread is very large. Upper cervical roots spread six segments, and the lower ones fourteen (six above and seven below the segment of entry) in the cat, and L3 to S3 roots all show some projection in all of these segments, the most dense being their own segment[45-48].

There is generally very little contralateral projection of dorsal roots[49].

Practical clinical consequences

The clinical significance of this to people interested in musculoskeletal medicine is (perhaps surprisingly to clinicians involved primarily in other fields,) of great importance. For many decades debate has continued, sometimes with almost theological intensity as to the existence of the 'facilitated cord segment' (see p.136). To continue to believe in this concept in the light of the evidence now available requires something of an act of faith, since the distribution of these afferents is unequivocally plurisegmental.

"In the last decade our understanding of the primary afferent terminations in the CNS has increased enormously."[27]

"It is hoped that over the next decade controversies will be settled and the gaps in our knowledge filled, for until we have a complete understanding of the distribution of primary sensory input to the CNS, we cannot hope to understand the pathways involved in pain."[27]

The gate

In 1965, Melzack and Wall proposed the gate theory of pain control[50]. In 1978 this was redefined by Wall, as follows[51]:

1. (a) "Information about the presence of injury is transmitted to the central nervous system by peripheral nerves."
   (b) "Certain small-diameter fibres (A-δ and C) respond only to injury, while others with lower thresholds increase their discharge frequency if the stimulus reaches noxious levels."
2. "Cells in the spinal cord or fifth nerve nucleus which are excited by these injury signals are also facilitated or inhibited by other peripheral nerve fibres which carry information about innocuous events."
3. "Descending control systems originating in the brain modulate the excitability of the cells which transmit information about injury."
4. "Therefore the brain receives messages about injury by way of a gate control system which is influenced by:
   (a) injury signals,
   (b) other types of afferent impulse, and
   (c) descending control."

However, in 1978 Wall wrote further:
1. "All the work since 1965 shows that cord cells responding to injury are subject to inhibitions of peripheral origin, but the mechanism remains obscure."
2. "That the gate control exists is no longer open to doubt, but its functional role and its detailed mechanism remain open to speculation and for experiment."

This relatively simple idea has remained extremely popular ever since, although, as might be expected, it has been criticized. Such criticism has been aimed at the diagrammatic representation used, on the grounds that it was too simplistic. "The mechanisms are so complicated that it is useless to attempt to represent them in a simple diagram. The diagram should be abandoned, but there is every reason to retain the term 'gate'."[1]

Practical clinical consequences of the gate control theory
1. It emphasizes the daunting complexity of the problems and the difficulties of diagnosis and management.
2. It provides one of the themes for the world-wide flowering of pain clinics, with its emphasis on a multidisciplinary approach towards pain problems.
3. It provides a banner under which all clinicians interested in the subject (or whose work involves the treatment and management of pain) may enlist.
4. With regard to management, it justifies the use of mechanoreceptor stimulation to inhibit pain; (for example in massage, manipulation, TNS and vibration) (see The Dorsal Horn, p.40).
5. It provides a scientific basis for employing TNS, which is now used world-wide (see Management: TNS, p.223).
6. It also raises the issue of the use of other therapies which must, of necessity, at least in part, operate on this basis; for example, massage and manipulation (see Management under these headings, pp. 214, 215).

Comment
We accept that many doctors interested in this work, particularly those with chiropractic or osteopathic sympathies, will be unhappy with this explanation of the effects of the manipulative procedures they use. Some will feel that this will greatly (and sadly) diminish the standing of these therapies, revealing them as being in reality rather prosaic. However, if these matters are to be interpreted logically, on the basis of the available evidence, these factors are indisputably relevant.

But there is another side to the coin. As TNS is so widely used, other treatments operating the same mechanisms should also be considered. On this premise it would seem reasonable to suggest that any clinician involved in the treatment of pain of musculoskeletal origin should have a working knowledge of manipulative techniques, their indications, contraindications and dangers.

None of us involved in the management of these problems is so successful that we can afford to be ignorant of any form of treatment which may, in safety, be of service to our patients. Nevertheless, it must be stressed that the material here presented does not afford a complete explanation of the mode of action of massage and manipulation (see Management: TNS, p.223).

The dorsal horn

Consequences of acute nociceptive input
Excitatory links
CNS cells have a multiplicity of functions, and frequently the same cell will subserve different functions under different circumstances[52,53]. A classification is convenient, using Rexed's division of these cells into laminae 1 to 6, but these divisions are imprecise[54].

Lamina 1
This lamina has received particular attention in relation to nociception, because it is a specialized region for the termination of nociceptive afferents and because it contains cells which respond only to noxious stimuli[55].

While both these statements are true, many types of cell response are to be found[56-59].

The area of the receptive fields of the majority of cells is restricted to some fraction of their dermatome, but some extend to include as much as a whole leg[60]. This further complexity is relevant to the use of the dermatome as a diagnostic tool (see Relevant Pathology: General considerations, p.130). There are three characeristics of these cells which are shared with lamina 2 and which make them particularly interesting:
1. Some cells exhibit such striking habituation to the stimulated fraction of their receptive field that they may be considered as novelty detectors. Habituation is defined as a rapid fading of response to repeated stimuli[12].
2. Some cells produce very prolonged responses after brief stimuli.
3. Finally, many cells show amoeboid changes in the receptive fields they subserve[61].

Lamina 2
The cells of lamina 2 have excitatory receptor fields (RFs) and their properties do not differ qualitatively from those of lamina 1[57,59,62,63].

Quantitatively the gradient continues so that the ventral region, 2(i), contains a predominance of units responding only to light brush, whilst the dorsal part has a majority responding to light and heavy mechanical stimuli and to noxious heat and chemicals, while some are specialized nociceptive cells[60].

Lamina 3
Its function is currently unknown.

Lamina 4
No clear function has yet been established.

Lamina 5
Many of these cells send axons to the brain. With the lamina 1 cells, they are the major candidates for informing the brain of the existence of injury.

While, as we have seen, all groups of cells may contribute to pain, the lamina 5 cells may be particularly important[64,65].

Lamina 6
This layer has a convergent input from muscle, skin and viscera, and it is under descending control[66].

Excitatory links – the cascade theory
Jankowska and Lundberg[36] showed that it is now possible to unravel cell-links relating to muscle. However, work on cells subserving nociception remains in relative infancy, because of soluble but difficult problems due to the small size of cells and fibres, and to their variable physiology and close packing[12].

We know regrettably little about the undoubtedly crucial polysynaptic systems.

Many anatomical possibilities for interconnection exist (see review by Wall[12]) but the overall picture fits a general flow of excitation from dorsal to ventral in a cascade fashion.

From lamina 3 to lamina 6 the response of cells becomes increasingly complex, each lamina being excited by more and more inputs.

Some of the excitation can best be explained by the cells in each lamina being excited by the cells immediately dorsal to them.

In addition to this overall plan for segmental circuitry, each successive dorsal to ventral stage from lamina 3 sends axones to the brain. The brain is therefore informed of the excitation of each of the stages. This leads to the proposal that the function of lamina 1 is to inform the brain of the excitatory state of lamina 2. A complete cascade would then be formed, starting with the linked complex of lamina 1 and lamina 2, extending to lamina 6, in which each lamina receives and computes additional information in part from its dorsal neighbour and projects to the brain and to its ventral neighbour[12].

The complexity and connectivity of these links is self-evident.

Inhibitory links

These are of great practical interest in relation to the gate control theory:
1. With regard to the use of A on C inhibitions in management.
2. With regard to interactions within the dorsal horn.
3. With regard to descending controls, the endogenous pain control systems.

Presynaptic controls

The location of the cells which project onto the afferent terminals remains uncertain, but lamina 2 is the most likely origin[67].

The depolarizing effect of afferent volleys on the terminals of large myelinated afferents and the association of this with inhibition are well established[23,68,69].

Only recently has it become clear that C fibre terminals are also affected[70,71].

It is still not certain if presynaptic facilitation can be achieved either (a) by removal of inhibition or (b) by active hyperpolarization.

Similarly, the mechanism of presynaptic control remains in doubt, since it could be achieved (a) by the blockade of afferent impulses in the terminal arbour[23,72], and/or (b) by modulation of the amount of transmitter released[67].

Postsynaptic controls

It is clearly established that afferents may produce postsynaptic inhibition[73]. It is possible that pre- and postsynaptic mechanisms could be in operation, sometimes simultaneously and sometimes independently.

Inhibition of high-threshold input, while leaving low-threshold input excitation unaffected, has been reported frequently. This could be achieved (a) by presynaptic control of afferent terminals and/or (b) by postsynaptic control of excitatory interneurones.

Yet again, both pre- and postsynaptic inhibitions are seen to be inextricably complex.

Clinical relevance of dorsal horn inhibition

The importance of spatial origin is where there is excitatory summation of small-diameter afferents from viscera with large-diameter afferents from the skin[74].

If the receptive field of a lamina 5 cell responding only to skin is

42

examined, it is found that the receptive field excited by brush or touch is surrounded by a much larger inhibitory area activated by the same stimuli.

If the stimulus intensity is now increased to include nociceptors, the excitatory field is found to be much larger than that produced by light stimuli, which means that the inhibitory surround to light stimuli overlies some of the excitatory field of the high-threshold afferents.

If the intense input is applied beyond the edge of the high-intensity excitatory receptive field, a high-intensity inhibitory surround is revealed.

This conflict is the basis of the immediate effect of massage and manipulation[24].

Chemistry

We do not know the identity of the transmitters released by afferent fibres, although there are a number of strong possibilities.

Two groups of compounds, the amino acids and the peptides, have been proposed as different transmitters.

Amino acids

The firm evidence for their action comes largely from isolated preparations, whose simple anatomy differs from the many structures surrounding afferent terminals.

These compounds are present in all cells and play a part in many aspects of metabolism, including protein synthesis. This means that there are inevitably multiple receptors and points sensitive to the availability of these compounds.

This in turn means that the crucial discovery of antagonists which affect only one of their many actions is immensely difficult.

These problems together define the reasons for the inability to put one of the many suspects 'on trial'. These difficulties have baneful effects on pharmacology.

Peptides

The peptides have some of the same and some different problems. Four have been identified, but many more are probably in existence. Substance-P and cholecystokinin coexist in the same afferents[75]. This coexistence of active compounds has now been found in a number of terminals. It therefore seems likely that the nerve terminals may emit a series of compounds under different circumstances, and we may no longer expect to find a single neurotransmitter[76,77].

This, together with peripheral and central 'pain chemistry', presents the clinical pharmacologist with intractable problems.

43

Consequences of chronic nociceptive input

All these facts, taken together and excluding the effects of peripheral events on transmission and descending controls, reveal a complexity and wealth of connectivity in the reaction to acute nociceptive input within the dorsal horn itself. Reactions to chronic pain taking place within the cord reveal additional phenomena, quite different in nature and of great clinical significance.

Habituation

Some cells in both lamina 1 and lamina 2 respond for seconds or minutes after brief stimuli only[59].

Others habituate, so that slow repeated stimuli evoke an initial response which rapidly fades with repetition. This novelty detection property means that these cells fail to respond to a train of identical stimuli, and remain non-responsive for as long as the intermittent stimulus is continued, and do not again respond for seconds or minutes after the train of stimuli has stopped.

This property is highly specific in space, so that, if one part of the reactive field habituates, movement of the stilumus to a fresh site within that field immediately evokes a response[61].

The mobility of receptive fields

It has been shown that, if an injury is placed on the skin outside the normal receptive field, the field slowly moves so as to include the part damaged and holds there.

If local anaesthetic is injected into the area of injury, then the receptive field slowly returns to its previous location. The injury acts as a magnet, attracting cells to move their receptive fields into the area of injury, and this process can be reversed.

In referred pain, the area to which pain is referred, which itself is not involved in the disease process, becomes tender. A prolonged afferent barrage from one source has changed the way in which the central nervous system handles an impulse from another[78].

There is clear evidence that some at least of these phenomena must be attributed to spinal cord processes, rather than to tissue changes.

Inhibitions

The use of large-fibre inhibition has already been mentioned from a therapeutic point of view.

In their most beneficial form, these inhibitions appear to adjust excessive sensitivities towards the norm, without affecting other aspects of sensation. This is a clinically useful phenomenon[79].

There are mechanisms which may be long lasting, which control excitability, and a part of the pathology of pain is the setting of these mechanisms at incorrect levels of excitability.

The effect of diminished input on receptive fields

If dorsal roots are cut, after a period of time cells which have lost their input begin to respond to intact afferents[80-82].

Similar changes take place if a peripheral nerve is cut[83,84].

Therefore new connections have come about. These are are currently thought to be created by the unmasking of existing afferents which are normally held ineffective by the action of interneurones.

The trigger for these changes in connection is not degeneration, nor is it the absence of nerve impulses, since they are not produced by prolonged impulse blockade[85].

Inhibitions are also affected in the presence of a decreased input. After deafferentation, the cord reacts to increase the remaining input by diminishing inhibition, and this is part of the homoeostatic mechanism[86,87].

Whatever the mechanism, it is evident that slowly-acting mechanisms exist which control the connection of afferents into spinal cord cells, and presumably control interconnections within the cord.

Summary

1. a. Technology has afforded us an insight into the physiology of the dorsal horn not previously available.
    b. While we do not at present have so detailed a knowledge of other parts of the CNS, there seems no reason to assume that their complexity will prove less.
    c. The consequences to the clinician of the relatively recent 'insights' will be discussed shortly (see p.47).
2. The pain chemistry of the dorsal horn, as is the case with central and peripheral pain chemistry, is so complex as to make identifiable specific pharmacological interventions unlikely in the foreseeable future.
3. In acute pain: (a) not only do individual horn cells have multiple functions, but (b) their excitatory and inhibitory properties, both pre- and postsynaptic, vary constantly.
4. In chronic pain, there are in addition the features of (a) habituation, (b) mobility of receptive fields, (c) long-term inhibition and (d) the effects of diminished input.

This emphasizes that chronic pain differs physiologically from acute pain, and every clinician should bear this in mind. The following two diagrams (Figures 3.1 and 3.2) illustrate some of these difficulties.

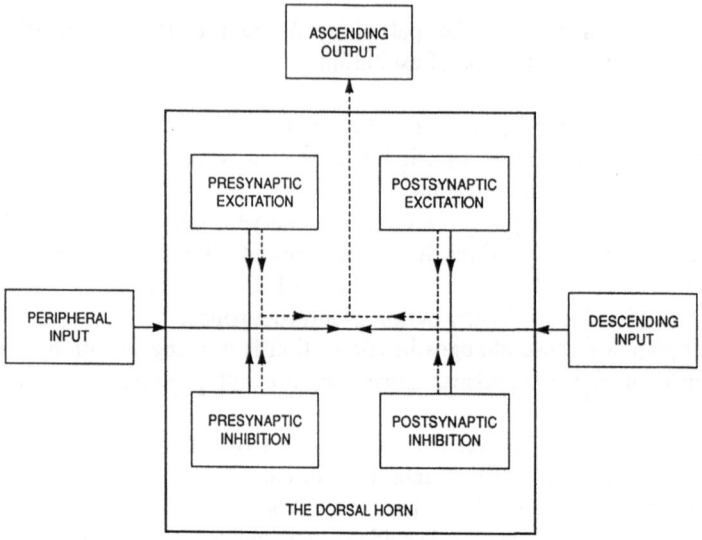

Figure 3.1 Acute pain mechanisms

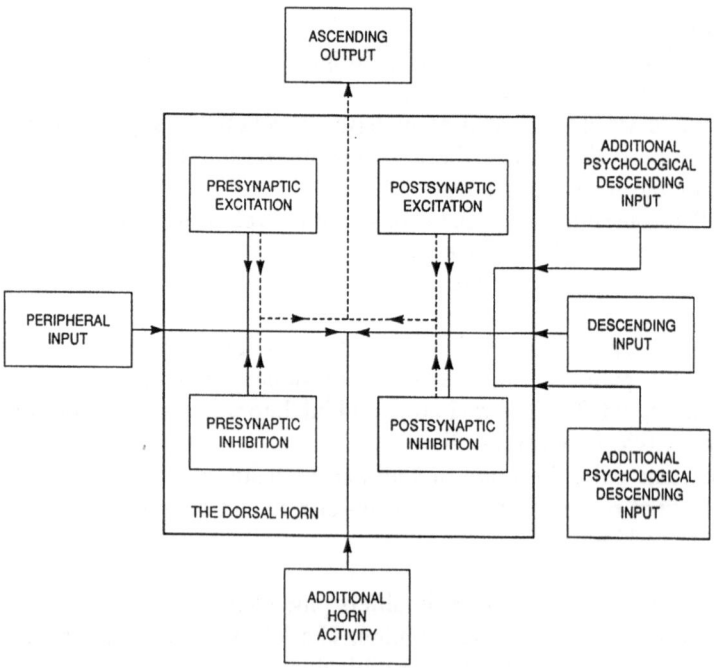

Figure 3.2 Chronic pain mechanisms

Practical clinical consequences

Case analysis

Clinical history has less significance than some would wish, as the physiology of the dorsal horn, in both acute and chronic pain, is ever 'on the move'. If the physiology is subject to continuous subtle changes, pain description has of necessity limitations as a tool for making a specific diagnosis. It is also, for different reasons, unreliable psychologically as a diagnostic tool (see p.105 *et seq.*).

Physical examination is based on phenomena which may be transient and,inter alia, subject to multiple continuous changes in dorsal horn activity. It is thus seen that horn phenomena alone present diagnostic difficulties, both in history and examination.

In the great majority of cases of pain of vertebral origin (PVO), accurate diagnosis remains beyond our reach. To a considerable extent this may be explained by the complexity of dorsal horn physiology.

Management

The A on C inhibition that has been described is clearly of the greatest significance to the clinician. (For its relevance to massage, manipulation and TNS, see the appropriate sections in Management, pp. 214, 215, 224.)

Recent laboratory work on the horn is seen to intervene in the consulting room, in respect of both case analysis and management.

The complexities revealed must be a strong argument in favour of empiricism. The 'ideal' clinician is one with access to a variety of treatments.

Transmission pathways

Introduction

As Willis points out, the somatosensory system includes a number of parallel ascending pathways, having what appear to be overlapping functions. Short polysynaptic systems may be important.

Cord pathways

Nociceptive information is transmitted from the spinal cord to the brain over several different pathways, including the spinothalamic, spinoreticular, mesencephalic, spinocervical and second-order dorsal column tracts[19,88].

In addition, nociceptive information may ascend through a multisynaptic system of propriospinal neurones[89].

The distinctions between these various pathways tend to blur somewhat when it is realised that in many instances a given neurone sends collateral projections to several different target nuclei. For example, some spino-thalamic neurones projecting on the ventrobasal complex of the thalamus appear to give off collaterals to the lateral periaqueduct grey and the adjacent midbrain reticular formation[90]. Thus some spinothalamic and some spino-mesocephalic projections are from the same neurones.

Supraspinal mechanisms
Data concerning supraspinal mechanisms are still very incomplete, and it must be especially noted that the electrophysiological data on neurone responses to noxious stimuli are completely missing in respect of most strucures, in particular in respect of those which do not receive spinothalamic or spinoreticular projections[91].

Functions of the ascending nociceptive tracts
These include:
1. Signalling not only of the sensory discriminatory aspects of pain, but also of the motivational affective components.
2. They trigger motor and autonomic adjustments as well perhaps as activating descending analgesia systems. The detailed operations of this complex sensory motor system are far from clear at the present time[92].

The existing state of knowledge with regard to these transmission pathways does not currently provide much practical help for the clinician.

Supraspinal mechanisms
Despite contradictory results in the past, much work is now going on, but there are certain experimental difficulties.

There are experimental ethical problems, related to the fact that experiments have to be performed on intact animals and therefore with anaesthetic preparations. These produce very varied responses.

Interspecies differences are often important, and results may therefore be difficult to compare.

The nomenclature in this field is particularly varied and confusing.

Most important, besides these problems it should be noted that the multiplicity of pathways which can reach a given nucleus, and the likely existence of various modulatory systems at a supraspinal level create further obstacles for experimenters.

In conclusion, data concerning supraspinal mechanisms of nociception and pain are still very incomplete, and it must be especially noted that electrophysiological data on neurone responses to noxious stimuli are completely missing for most structures, in particular for those which do not receive spinothalamic or spinoreticular thalamic projections.

Practical clinical consequences
The present state of knowledge with regard to transmission pathways is of little practical clinical value.

Endogenous pain control mechanisms

Introduction

Although the concept of a specific pain control system is a recent development, as early as 1911 Head and Holmes explicitly postulated modulatory influences on pain[93]. Again the thalamus appeared to be implicated. Clearcut examples of centrifugal control of sensory transmissions was subsequently described. Hagbarth, Kerr and Khan provided the first direct evidence that supraspinal brain cells could control ascending presumably sensory pathways[94], and Carpenter *et al.* demonstrated descending control of sensory inputs to ascending pathways[95].

Gate theory[50].

Evidence of descending control was limited to start with, but in 1967 Wall reported that the cells in lamina 5 of the dorsal horns of decerebrate cats were more responsive to noxious stimuli when the spinal cord was cold blocked, thus showing that structures in the brain stem inhibit putative pain transmission cells in the spinal cord[52]. The hypothesis that the descending systems contribute to pain modulation was strongly supported by the discovery of the phenomenon of stimulation-produced analgesia, SPA[96,97]. SPA is a highly specific suppression of pain-related behaviour produced by electrical stimulation of certain discrete brain sites. Thus SPA is both powerful and highly selective. Electrical stimulation in analogous brain nuclei in patients with persistent pain produces a similar phenomenon: pain subsides with no other consistent changes. The specificity of analgesic effect, coupled with the fact that it is consistently elicited from discrete homologous brain sites in a variety of species is powerful evidence in favour of a specific pain modulating system.

A parallel and equally significant breakthrough in the study of pain modulating systems is the discovery of the endogenous opioid peptides or endorphins. Although there are probably several CNS networks that modulate pain, we know most about one that has endorphin links[98].

Endogenous opioid agonists and their receptors

Endorphins

The characterization of CNS opiate binding sites stimulated intense hunts for endogenous opiate ligans, which may be generically termed endorphins[99]. There are at least three distinct populations of endorphin-containing cells[100,101]; all presumably release peptides with opium like activity at their terminals, but differ in their distribution within the brain.

Opiate receptors
There is now evidence for at least two and probably three biologically significant binding sites. The two best characterised binding sites, μ and δ, are defined primarily by differences in rank order of potency of various opiates to displace a high-affinity labelled ligand from one or other binding site[102].

The existence of a κ receptor was originally proposed by Martin *et al.* in 1976[103], and confirmation that the κ and μ receptors are distinct has recently been provided by studies demonstrating high-affinity selective binding sites[104]. Perhaps the most fascinating aspect of the κ agonists is that they may have a distinctly higher analgesic potency on tests for nociception than those that use mechanical stimuli[105,106]. This raises the possibility that pain arising from the activation of different classes of primary afferents could be susceptible to different drugs.

Descending systems for the modulation of pain
Sites and connections
The endorphin-mediated analgesia system (EMAS) has well-established components in the midbrain, periaqueduct grey (PAG) the rostral ventro-medial medulla (RVM) and the superficial layers of the dorsal horn[107,108]. Both PAG and RVM contain opioid peptides and produce analgesia when stimulated[109,110]. Thus pain modulation is subserved by an especially extensive system; it is distributed along the entire neuraxis, and it includes neocortical, limbic, brainstem and spinal components.

Distribution of transmitters and their role in descending pain modulation
It is clear that the endorphins are closely associated with the analgesic system at several levels and, given the naloxone sensitivity of this system, the endorphins must be critical to its operation. The cellular mechanism of action of opiates is not known[111–114].

Biogenic amines
This multiplicity of transmitters in apparently parallel descending neurones presents methodological problems for functional analysis. The use of any single pharmacological antagonist would be insufficient to block completely any analgesia evoked by electrical stimulation to the region[115,116].

Activation of endorphin-mediated analgesia systems
Information on the normal functioning of these tissues is less certain. For example, we are not sure when these analgesia systems are called into play.

Experimental work

The majority of cells in either the PAG or the RVM are activated by noxious stimuli, though a significant minority are inhibited by these same stimuli.

Some PAG cells also increase their discharge with cortical arousal. Mayer *et al.* suggested that perhaps attentional as well as sensory factors control EMAS[117].

The peripheral receptive fields of the raphe spinal neurones frequently include the entire body. In the cat, both noxious stimuli and light tapping of the skin consistently excite many raphe spinal cells[118].

"Recently we recorded from cells in the RBM while monitoring the tail flick reflex produced by noxious heat. In addition, we used microstimulations through the recording electrodes to map low-threshold sites for stimulation produced analgesia (SPA). Using this approach, we found two classes of cell in low-threshold SPA sites: those which discharged just prior to the occurrence of a tail flick (on cells) and those which shut off just prior to a tail flick occurrence (off cells). On cells are consistently excited by noxious stimulation over a large part of the body. Most off cells are inhibited by noxious stimuli."[119]

This leads to the hypothesis that cells in the RVM are most consistently affected by noxious stimuli, suggesting that the major element in the analgesia system is a negative feedback loop for nociception, i.e. noxious stimuli activate the system, and it in turn suppresses pain transmission[119].

This suggests some testable predictions. Since pain modulating cells can be activated by noxious stimuli from over most of the body surface, it follows that pains from different parts of the body should inhibit one another. In fact, acupuncture and many other pain therapies based on counter-irritation may work in this manner. Thus, biting ones lip, banging ones head against the wall, mustard plasters, cupping, moxibustion, trephination and other manipulations would be expected indeed partially and temporarily to relieve pain anywhere in the body.

Lewis *et al.* raise several important points[120].
1. Not all analgesic actions in the CNS are mediated by endorphins.
2. Under certain conditions, pain duration or stress, instead of or in addition to pain intensity, are important factors in activating pain modulating systems.
3. Activation of different analgesia producing networks involves complex environmental attention and conditional factors, which may make straightforward pharmacological studies difficult to interpret.

Practical clinical consequences

The EMAS are capable of being activated by a wide variety of factors, including counter-irritation, stress and suggestion. This activation is, however, unpredictable.

With regard to diagnosis, the fact that these systems may or may not be operating during case analysis at any given time must further attenuate diagnostic certainty.

With regard to management, this means that NOT to consider a spectrum of possible therapies is physiologically unrealistic.

In practical terms, this further means that the more therapies that are available to the clinician, provided by himself or by referral, the greater must be the potential advantage to the patient.

Those who question the relevance of psychological factors to musculo-skeletal practice will find here a close correlation between stress and attentional factors and proven physiological consequences. Surely a fascinating and unexpected interface.

Therefore, for the clinician to ignore suggestion and placebo factors, the latter currently common in practice (see Management: Placebo, p.249), would seem sadly remiss on scientific grounds.

"Thus future research on pain modulating systems holds promise not only for greater understanding of the variability of the pain experience, but for significant advances in pain management as well."[119]

Input delivery in the CNS

As Wyke shows[141], the mechanoreceptor input succeeds in activating the thalamic nuclei and a number of effects are produced.

1. If the input reaches the frontal lobes, it will be appreciated as pleasant or unpleasant[121–127].
2. If it is projected to the hippocampus, it will involve the memory component[127–134].
3. If it reaches the hypothalamic nuclei, it will produce visceral, nervous and hormonal responses via the anterior and posterior hypothalamic nuclei, which influence the sympathetic and parasympathetic outflow, and it will therefore have cardiovascular and gastrointestinal effects, amongst others[125,135–138].
4. The visceral responses are primarily hypothalamic and not spinal at all, which fact has consequences for the concept of the facilitated cord segment (see p.136).
5. Input to the anterior pituitary via the hypothalamic nuclei affects the entire hormonal status, and therefore mechanoreceptor input (normal or abnormal) inevitably modifies visceral, nervous and hormonal status[127,139–140].

6. It may activate respiratory neurones in the brain stem[8].
7. Such input will also involve the reticular system nuclei in the caudal end of the brain stem, with effects on the fusimotor muscle loop system and motor unit activity, both static and dynamic[8].

Practical clinical consequences

It is thus apparent that all input, mechanoreceptive and nociceptive, produces a complex array of responses which are inevitably plurisegmental in nature, and far-reaching in an unpredictable manner.

The activity of the autonomic nervous system is inextricably entwined with any input delivery (mechanoreceptor and/or nociceptive) into the central nervous system (see p.135). In view of the motor unit activity mentioned above, this seems an appropriate stage at which to consider muscular function.

Clinical conclusions to relevant physiology

1. The clinical problems presented by dorsal horn physiology in both case analysis and management are reviewed on pp. 47. These are mirrored with regard to input to the central nervous system, muscular activity and control of the musculoskeletal system.
2. This evidence must cast grave doubt upon any system based on the supposed predictability of musculoskeletal function (see p. 56).
3. In the light of this evidence, any 'school of thought', medical or non-medical, which makes such assumptions should perhaps be reviewed.
4. The whole of relevant physiology demonstrates conclusively that the clinician is an empiricist, diagnostic and therapeutic, like it or not.

References

1. Noordenbos (1983). Prologue. In Wall and Melzack (eds.) *Textbook of Pain*. (London: Churchill Livingstone)
2. Lewit (1985). *Manipulative Therapies in Rehabilitation of the Motor System*. (London: Butterworth)
3. Dubner *et al.* (1981). Neuronal activity in medullar dorsal horn of awake monkeys trained in a thermal discrimination task. Task related responses and their functional role. *J. Neurophysiol.*, **46**, 444–464
4. Wall and Melzak (1983). The detection of injury and tissue damage. In Wall and Melzack (eds.) *Textbook of Pain*. (London: Churchill Livingstone)
5. Lynn (1983). The detection of injury and tissue damage. In Wall and Melzack (eds.) *Textbook of Pain*. (London: Churchill Livingstone)
6. Burgess and Perl (1973). Cutaneous mechano receptors and nociceptors. In Iggo (ed.) *Handbook of Sensory Physiology*. pp. 2978 (Berlin: Springer Verlag)
7. Burgess and Perl (1967). Myelinated afferent fibres responding specifically to noxious stimulation of the skin. *J. Physiol.*, **190**, 541–562
8. Wyke (1983). In *Seventh Congress of International Federation of Manual Medicine*, Zurich. (Unpublished)

9. Campbell *et al.* (1979). Sensitization of myelinated nociceptive afferents that innervate monkey hand. *J. Neurosurg.*, **42**, 1669–1680
10. Lamotte *et al.* (1982). Peripheral neural mechanisms in cutaneous hyperalgesia following mild injury by heat. *J. Neurosci.*, **2**, 765–781
11. Fitzgerald (1979). The spread of sensitization of polymodal nociceptors in the rabbit from nearby injury and by antidromic nerve stimulation. *J. Physiol.*, **297**, 207–216
12. Wall (1983). Introduction. In Wall and Melzack (eds.) *Textbook of Pain*. (London: Churchill Livingstone)
13. Perl *et al.* (1976). Sensitization of high threshold receptors of unmyelinated afferent fibres. *Prog. Brain Res.*, **43**, 263–277
14. Keele and Armstrong (1964). *Substances Producing Pain and Itch*. (London: Edward Arnold)
15. Yoshizawa *et al.* (1980). The neuropathology of intervertebral discs removed for low back pain. *J. Pathol.*, **132**, 95–104
16. Gasser (1935). Conduction in nerves in relation to fibre types. *Res. Publ. Assoc. Nerve Ment. Disc.*, **15**, 35
17. Heinbecker *et al.* (1933). Pain and touch fibres in peripheral nerves. *Arch. Neurol. Psychiatr.*, **29**, 771–789
18. Natham *et al.* (1963) Susceptibility of nerve fibres to analgesics. *Anaesthesia*, **18**, 467
19. Willis and Coggeshall (1978). *Sensory Mechanisms of the Spinal Cord*. (New York: Wiley)
20. Fitzgerald (1983). Capsaicin. Action on peripheral nerves. A review. *Pain*, **15**, 109–130
21. Hokfelt *et al.* (1982). Immunohistochemical evidence for separate populations of somatostatin containing and substance P containing primary afferent neurones in the rat. *Neuroscience*, **1**, 13–16
22. Wall and Cronly-Dillon (1960). Pain, itch and vibration. *Arch. Neurol.*, **2**, 365–375
23. Wall (1964). Presynaptic control of impulses at the first central synapse of cutaneous pathway. *Prog. Brain Res.*, **12**, 92–118
24. Wall and Sweet (1967). Temporary abolition of pain in man. *Science*, **155**, 108–109
25. Willer *et al.* (1980). Human nociceptive reactions. Effects of spatial summation of afferent input from relatively large diameter fibres. *Brain Res.*, **201**, 465–470
26. Kugelberg and Lindblom (1959). The mechanism of the pain in trigeminal neuralgia. *J. Neurosurg. Psychiatr.*, **22**, 36–43
27. FitzGerald (1983). Primary afferents. In Wall and Melzack (eds.) *Textbook of Pain*. (London: Churchill Livingstone)
28. Proshansky and Egger (1977). Staining of the dorsal root projection to cat's dorsal horn by antegrade movement of horse radish peroxidase. *Neurosci. Lett.*, **5**, 103–110
29. Light and Perl (1979). Spinal termination of functionally identified primary afferent neurones with slowly conducting myelinated fibres. *J. Comp. Neurol.*, **186**, 133–150
30. Gobel *et al.* 1981. Morphology and synaptic connection of ultrafine primary axons in laminar 1 of the spinal dorsal horn. Candidates for the terminal axonal arbors of primary neurones with unmyelinated C axons. *J. Neurosci.*, **1**, 1163–1179
31. Mesulam and Brushart (1979). Transganglionic and anterograde transport of HRP across dorsal root ganglia. A tetramethylbenzidine method for tracing the central sensory connections of muscles and peripheral nerves. *Neuroscience*, **4**, 1107–1117
32. Grant *et al.* (1979). Transganglionic transport of HRP in primary sensory neurones. *Neurosci. Lett.*, **12**, 23–28
33. Koerber and Brown (1980). Projection of two hindlimb cutaneous nerves to cat dorsal horn. *J. Neurophysiol.*, **44**, 259–269
34. Morgan *et al.* (1981). The distribution of visceral primary afferents from the pelvic nerve to Lissauer's tract and the spinal grey matter and its relationship to the sacral parasympathetic nucleus. *J. Comp. Neurol.*, **201**, 415–440
35. Brown (1981). *Organisation in the Spinal Cord*. (New York: Springer Verlag)
36. Jankowska and Lundberg (1981). Interneurones in the spinal cord. *Trends Neurosci.*, (Sept), 230–233
37. Scheibel and Scheibel (1968). Terminal axonal patterns in the cat's spinal cord. The dorsal horn. *Brain Res.*, **9**, 32–58

38. Beal (1979). Reconstruction of Ramon y Cajal large primary afferent complexes in laminae 2 and 3 of the adult monkey spinal cord. A golgi study. *Brain Res.*, 166, 161–165
39. Beal *et al.* (1977). Spinal cord potentials evoked by cutaneous afferents in the monkey. *J. Neurophysiol.*, 40, 199–211
40. Hamano *et al.* (1978). Reconstruction of trajectory of primary afferent collaterals in the dorsal horn of the cat's spinal cord using golgi stain serial sections. *J. Comp. Neurol.*, 181, 116
41. Rethely (1981). Geometry of the dorsal horn. In Brown *et al.* (eds.) *Spinal Cord Sensations*. (Edinburgh: Scottish Academic Press)
42. Lamotte (1977). Distribution of the tract of Lissaue and the dorsal root fibres in the primate spinal cord. *J. Comp. Neurol.*, 172, 529–562
43. Ralston and Daly Ralston (1979). The distribution of dorsal root axons in laminae 1, 2 and 3 on the macaque spinal cord. A quantitative electronmicroscope study. *J. Comp. Neurol.*, 184, 643–684
44. Beal *et al.* (1981). Primary afferent distribution pattern in the marginal zone (laminar 1) of adult monkey and cat lumbo-sacral spinal cord. *J. Comp. Neurol.*, 202, 255–263
45. Sterling and Kuypers (1967). Anatomical organisation of the brachial spinal cord of the cat. 1. The distribution of dorsal fibres. *Brain Res.*, 4, 115
46. Imai and Kusama (1969). Distribution of the dorsal root fibres in the cat. An experimental study with the Nauta method. *Brain Res.*, 13, 338–359
47. Wall and Werman (1976). The physiology and anatomy of long ranging afferent fibres within the spinal cord. *J. Physiol.*, 255, 321–334
48. Brown and Culberson (1981). Somatotopic organisation of hind limb cutaneous dorsal root projections in the cat's dorsal horn. *J. Neurophysiol.*, 45, 137–143
49. Culberson *et al.* (1979). Contralateral projection of primary afferent fibres to mamalian spinal cords. *Exp. Neurol.*, 64, 83–97
50. Melzack and Wall (1965). Pain mechanisms. A new theory. *Science*, 150, 971
51. Wall (1978). The gate control theory of pain mechanisms. A re-examination of statements. *Brain*, 101, 1
52. Wall (1967). The laminar organisation of the dorsal horn and effects of descending impulses. *J. Physiol.*, 188, 403–423
53. Wall *et al.* (1967). Dorsal horn cells in spinal and in freely moving rats. *Exp. Neurol.*, 19, 519–529
54. Rexed (1952). The cyto-architectonic organisation of the spinal cord in the cat. *J. Comp. Neurol.*, 96, 415–495
55. Perl (1980). Afferent bases of nociception and pain. In Bonica (ed.) *Pain*. (New York: Raven Press)
56. Handwerker *et al.* (1975). Segmental and supraspinal actions on dorsal horn neurones responding to noxious and non-noxious skin stimulation. *Pain*, 1, 147–166
57. Price *et al.* (1979). Functional relationships between neurones of marginal and substantial gelatinosa layers of primate dorsal horn. *J. Neurophysiol.*, 42, 1590–1608
58. Menetry *et al.* (1982). Neurones at the origin of the spino-mesancephalic tract in the rat. An anatomical study using the retrograde transport of HRP. *J. Comp. Neurol.*, 206, 193
59. Wall *et al.* (1979). Responses to single units in laminae 2 and 3 of cat spinal cord. *Brain Res.*, 160, 245–260
60. FitzGerald (1981). A study of the cutaneous afferent input to substantiate gelatinosa. *Neuroscience*, 6, 2229–2237
61. Dubuisson *et al.* (1979). Amoeboid receptive fields of cells in laminae 1, 2 and 3. *Brain Res.*, 177, 376–378
62. Kumazawa and Perl (1978). Excitation of marginal and substantia gelatinosa neurones in the spinal cord in the primate. *Comp. Neurol.*, 177, 417–434
63. Bennett *et al.* (1980). Physiology and morphology of substantia gelatinosa neurones intracellularly stained with HRP. *J. Comp. Neurol.*, 194, 809–827
64. Mayer *et al.* (1975). Neurophysiological characterization of the antero-lateral spinal cord neurones contributing to pain perception. *Pain*, 1, 51–58

66. Wall (1967). The laminar organisation of dorsal horn and effects of descending impulses. *J. Physiology*, **188**, 403–423
67. Wall (1980). The role of substantia gelatinosa as a gate control. In Bonica (ed.) *Pain* (New York: Raven Press)
68. Eccles (1964). *The Physiology of Synapses*. (Berlin: Springer Verlag)
69. Schmidt (1971). Presynaptic inhibition in the vertebrate central nervous system. *Ergebnisse Physiol.*, **63**, 20–104
70. Hentall and Fields (1979). Segmental and descending influences on intra-spinal thresholds of single C fibres. *J. Neurophysiol.*, **42**, 1527–1537
71. Fitzgerald and Woolfe (1981). Effects of cutaneous nerve and intra-spinal conditioning on C fibres afferent terminal excitability in decerebrate spinal rats. *J. Physiol.*, **318**, 25–39
72. Howland *et al.* (1955). Reflex inhibition by dorsal root interaction. *J. Neurophysiol.*, **18**, 117
73. Hongo *et al.* (1968). Post-synaptic excitation and inhibition from primary afferents and neurones in the spino-cervical tract. *J. Physiol.*, **199**, 569–592
74. Pomeranz *et al.* (1968). Cord cells responding to fine mylenated afferents from viscera, muscle and skin. *J. Physiol.*, **199**, 511–532
75. Dulsgaard *et al.* (1982). Immunohistochemical evidence for coexistence of cholcystokinin and substance P-like peptides in primary sensory neurones. *Neurosci. Abstr.*, **8**, 474
76. Brown (1982). Peptidergic transmission in ganglia. *Friends Neurosci.*, **5**, 30–35
77. Jan and Jan (1982). Peptidergic transmission in sympathetic ganglia of the frog. *J. Physiol.*, **327**, 219–246
78. McMahon and Wall (1983). Plasticity in the nucleus gracilis of the rat. *Exp. Neurol.*, **80**, 195–207
79. Lindblom and Mayerson (1975). Influence on touch vibration and cutaneous pain of dorsal stimulation in man. *Pain*, **1**, 257–270
80. Basbaum and Wall (1970). Chronic changes in the response of cells in adult cat dorsal horn following partial de-afferentiation. *Brain Res.*, **116**, 181–204
81. Millar *et al.* (1976). Restructuring of the somatotopic map and appearance of abnormal neuronal activity in the gracile nucleus after partial deafferentiation. *Exp. Neurol.*, **50**, 658–672
82. Mendell *et al.* (1978). Properties of synaptic linkage from long ranging afferents onto dorsal horn neurones in normal and deafferented cats. *J. Physiol.*, **285**, 299–310
83. Devor and Wall (1981). The effect of peripheral nerve injury on receptive fields of cells in the cat spinal cord. *J. Comp. Neurol.*, **199**, 277–291
84. Lisny (1982). Receptive fields of spinal cord horn neurones in cats shortly after peripheral nerve section. *J. Physiol.*, **325**, 76b
85. Wall *et al.* (1982). Chronic blockade of sciatic nerve transmission by tetrodotoxin does not produce central changes in the dorsal horn of the spinal cord of the rat. *Neurosci. Lett.*, **30**, 315–320
86. Wall and Devor (1981). The effect of peripheral nerve injury on receptive fields of cells in the cat spinal cord. *J. Comp. Neurol.*, **199**, 277–291
87. Woolf and Wall (1982). Chronic peripheral nerve section diminishes the primary different A fibre mediate inhibition of rat dorsal horn neurone. *Brain Res.*, **242**, 77–85
88. Dennis and Melzack (1977). Pain signalling systems in the dorsal and ventral spinal cord. *Pain*, **4**, 97–132
89. Basbaum (1973). Conduction of the effects of noxious stimulation by short fibre multisynaptic systems of the spinal cord in the rat. *Exp. Neurol.*, **40**, 699–716
90. Mehler (1969). Some neurological species differences. *A. Posteriori Ann. N. York Acad. Sci.*, **167**, 424–468
91. Guilbaud *et al.* (1983). Experimental data related to nociception and pain at the supraspinal level. In Wall and Melzack (eds.) *Treatment of Pain*. (London: Churchill Livingstone)
92. Willis (1983). Transmission pathways. In Wall and Melzack (eds.) op. cit.
93. Head and Holmes (1911). Sensory disturbances from cerebral lesions. *Brain*, **34**, 102–254
94. Hagbarth, Kerr and Kahn (1954). Central influences on spinal afferent conduction. *J. Neurophysiol.*, **17**, 295–307

95. Carpenter *et al.* (1965). Differential supraspinal control of inhibitory and excitatory actions from the FRA to ascending spinal pathways. *Acta Physiol. Scand.*, **63**, 103–110
96. Reynolds (1969). Surgery in the rat during electrical analgesia induced by focal brain stimulation. *Science*, **164**, 444–445
97. Mayer and Liebeskind (1974). Pain reduction by focal electrical stimulation of the brain. An anatomical and behavioural analysis. *Brain Res.*, **68**, 73–93
98. Fields (1981). An endorphin mediated analgesia system. Experimental and clinical observations. In Martin Reichlin and Bick (eds.) *Neurosecretion and Brain Peptides. Implications for Pain Function and Neurological Disease.* (New York: Raven Press)
99. Hughes *et al.* (1975). Identification of two related pentapeptides from the brain with potent opiate agonist activity. *Nature*, **258**, 577–579
100. Goldstein *et al.* (1979). Dynorphin (113). An extraordinarily potent opioid peptide. *Proc. Natl. Acad. Sci. USA*, **76**, 6666–6670
101. Weber (1981). Co-localization of alpha neo endorphin and dynorphin immunoreactivity in hypothalamic neurones. *Biochem. Biophys. Res. Commun.*, **103**, 951–958
102. Chang and Cuatrecasas (1979). Multiple opiate receptors. Enkephalins and morphine bind to receptors of different specificity. *J. Biol. Chem.*, **254**, 2610–2618
103. Martin *et al.* (1976). The effects of morphine and nalorphine like drugs in the non dependent and morphine dependent chronic spinal dog. *J. Pharmacol. Exp. Ther.*, **196**, 517–532
104. Kosterlitz and Patterson (1980). Characteristics of opioide receptors in nervous tissue. *Proc. R. Soc. London*, Series B, **210**, 113–122
105. Upton *et al.* (1982). Differentiation of potent and K opiate agonists (using heat and pressure antinociceptive profiles and combined potency analysis. *Eur. J. Pharmacol.*, **78**, 421–429
106. Tyers (1980). Classification of opiate receptors that mediate antinociception in animals. *Br. J. Pharmacol.*, **69**, 503–512
107. Basbaum and Fields (1978). Endogenous pain control mechanisms. Review and hypothesis. *Ann. Neurol.*, **4**, 451–462
108. Mayer and Price (1976). Central nervous system mechanisms of analgesia. *Pain*, **2**, 379–404
109. Fields *et al.* (1977). Nucleus raphe magnus inhibition of spinal cord dorsal horn neurones. *Brain Res.*, **126**, 441–453
110. Willis *et al.* (1977). Inhibition of spinothalamic tract cells and interneurones by brain stem stimulation in the monkey. *J. Neurophysiol.*, **40**, 968–981
111. Hosobuchi *et al.* (1979). Stimulation of human periaqueductal ductal grey for pain relief increases immunoreactive beta endorphin in ventricular fluid. *Science*, **203**, 278–281
112. Azami *et al.* (1982). The contribution of nucleus reticularis paragigantocellularis and nucleus raphe magnus to the analgesia produced by systematically administered morphine, investigated with the micro-injection technique. *Pain*, **12**, 229–246
113. Takagi *et al.* (1977). The nucleus reticularis gigantiocellularis of the medulla oblongata is a highly sensitive site in the production of morphine analgesia in the rat. *Eur. J. Pharmacol.*, **45**, 91–92
114. Glazer and Basbaum (1981). Immunohistochemical localization of leucine enkephalin in the spinal cord of the cat. Enkephalin containing marginal neurones and pain modulation. *J. Comp. Neurol.*, **196**, 377–389
115. Bowker *et al.* (1981). Origins of serotogenic projections to the spinal cord in rats. An immunocytochemical retrograde transport study. *Brain Res.*, **226**, 187–199
116. Gilbert *et al.* (1982). The effects of monoamine neurotoxins on peptides in the rats spinal cord. *Neuroscience*, **7**, 69–87
117. Mayer *et al.* (1982). Periaqueductal grey neuronal activity. Correlation with EEG arousal evoked by noxious stimulation in the rat. *Neurosci. Lett.*, **28**, 297–301
118. Fields and Anderson (1978). Evidence that raphe spinal neurones mediate opiate and mid-brain stimulation produced analgesias. *Pain*, **5**, 333–349
119. Fields and Basbaum (1983). Endogenous pain control mechanisms. In Wall and Melzack (eds.) *Textbook of Pain*, p.148 (London: Churchill Livingstone)

120. Lewis *et al.* (1980). Opioid and non-opioid mechanisms of stress analgesia. *Science*, **28**, 623–625
121. Walker (1938). *The Primate Thalamus.* (Chicago: University of Chicago Press)
122. Le Gros Clarke (1948). The connections of the frontal lobes of the brain. *Lancet*, **254**, 353
123. Kaada (1960). Cingulate, posterior orbital, anterior insular and temporal pole cortex. In Field, McGune and Hall (eds.) *Handbook of Physiology, Section 1. Neurophysiology*, pp. 42, 1345. (Washington, DC: American Physiological Society)
124. Purpura and Yahr (1966). *The Thalamus.* (New York: Columbia University Press)
125. Brodal (1969). *Neurological Anatomy in Relation to Clinical Medicine.* 2nd Edn. (London: Oxford University Press)
126. Wyke (1969). *Principles of General Neurology.* (Amsterdam and London: Elsevier)
127. Wyke (1979). Neurological mechanisms in the experience of pain. *Acupuncture Electrother. Res. J.*, **4**, 27
128. Penfield and Jasper (1954). *Epilepsy and the Functional Anatomy of the Human Brain.* (London: Churchill Livingstone)
129. Penfield (1958). The role of the temporal cortex in recall of past experience. An interpretation of the present. In Wolstenholme and O'Connor (eds.) *The Neurological Basis of Behaviour*, p. 149. (London: Churchill Livingstone)
130. Wyke (1958). Surgical considerations of the temporal lobes. *Ann. R. Coll. Surg. Eng.*, **22**, 117
131. Barbizet (1963). Defect of memorizing of hypocampal-mamiliary origin. A review. *J. Neurol. Neurosurg. Psychiatr.*, **26**, 127
132. Kimble (1965). *Anatomy of Memory.* (Palo Alto, Cal.: Science and Behaviour Books)
133. Pribram and Broadbent (1970). *Biology of Memory.* (New York: Academic Press)
134. Newcombe (1972). Memory. In Critchley, O'Leary and Jennett (eds.) *Scientific Foundations of Neurology*, p. 205. (London: Heinemann)
135. Fulton *et al.* (1940). *The Hypothalamus and Central Levels of Autonomic Functions.* (Baltimore: Williams and Wilkins)
136. Miller (1942). *Central Autonomic Regulation in Health and Disease.* (New York: Grune and Stratton)
137. Haymaker *et al.* (1969). *The Hypothalamus.* (Springfield, Ill.: Thomas)
138. Martini *et al.* (1971). *The Hypothalamus.* (New York: Academic Press)
139. Engel (1959). Some physiological correlates of hunger and pain. *J. Exp. Psychol.*, **57**, 389
140. Black (1970). *Physiological Correlates of Emotion.* (New York: Academic Press)
141. Wyke (1980). The neurology of low back pain. In Jayson (ed.) *The Lumbar Spine and Back Pain* (London: Pitman Medical)

4
MUSCULAR ACTIVITY

Introduction
In this section we rely heavily upon the work of Basmajian and DeLuca's *Muscles Alive*[77].

In any text on musculoskeletal medicine, consideration of muscle activity and its control are fundamental. This is because there are numerous hypotheses, world-wide, relating to this subject, which heavily influence case analysis and management. For this reason it is relevant to review the realities, in so far as they are currently understood.

The motor unit
This is the nerve cell body and the long axon running down the motor nerve, together with its terminal branches and all the muscle fibres attached to it.

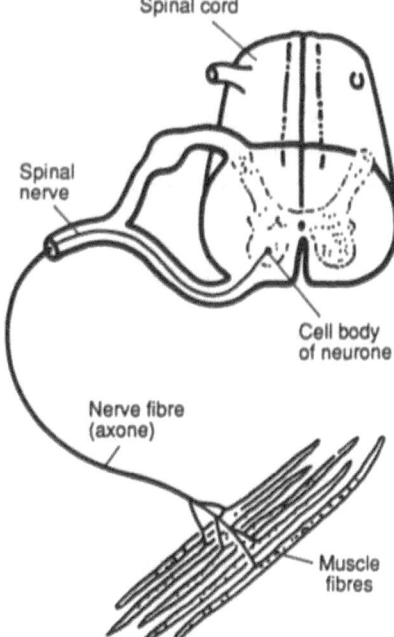

Figure 4.1 Scheme of a motor unit

This is the functional unit of striated muscle, since a nerve inpulse descending the motor neurone causes all the muscle fibres in one motor unit to contract almost simultaneously. Any slight disparity may be due to either or both of two causes:

1. Variable delay introduced by the length and diameter of the individual axon branches.
2. Random discharge of acetyl choline packets, known, (because it is random) as a 'jitter'[1].

The axon terminates at the endplate region of the muscle fibre.

The number of muscle fibres served by one axon varies, and (in general) in small muscles this is few, while in large muscles it is many.

Small motor units are served by small α motor neurones and are excited earlier in a contraction requiring progressively increasing force. Larger motor units are served by larger α motor neurones and become activated at progressively higher force levels.

As a rule of thumb, the motor unit territory occupies approximately one third of the cross-sectional area of the muscle[2].

Muscle fibre type

The physical and biochemical qualities of a muscle fibre are a continuum. In animals, the typing distinction appears to be clearer than in man.

There are two categories of muscle fibre: red and white. These exhibit different characteristics on stimulation.

1. When red fibres are stimulated, the resulting force twitch is slow rising and longer lasting, and is called a slow twitch.
2. When white fibres are stimulated, the resulting force twitch is fast rising and short lived, and is called a fast twitch.

| Red fibre | – | Slow rising and long lasting | = | Slow twitch |
| White fibre | – | Fast rising and short lived | = | Fast twitch |

Biochemistry

A further classification has been proposed, designating two types of fibre[3,4].

| Type I | – | Acid stable and alkaline labile |
| Type II | – | Acid labile and alkaline stable |

The myosin ATPase affinity (ATPA) is an indicator of the fibre's contractile speed[5]. Therefore fibres can be subdivided according to the different sensitivities of the myosin ATPAs[6].

The fibre's capacity to perform work is related to the presence or absence of oxygen.

Anaerobic fibre –   Pallid appearance   – More readily fatigued

Aerobic fibre   –   Reddish appearance   – Resistant to fatigue

Another classification of muscle fibres is based on the mechanical response of all muscle fibres of a motor unit when their motor neurone is stimulated by a single electrical impulse, (contractile response) or by a sustained train of stimuli (contractile fatigue response)[7] (Table 4.1).

Table 4.1 Classification of muscle fibres based on contractile response and contractile fatigue response

Class	Single impulse	Sustained train
FF	Fast	Easy fatigue
FI	Fast	Slow fatigue
FR	Fast	Very slow fatigue
S	Slow	No fatigue (resistant)

Definitions
Recruitment: The point at which a motor unit is brought into play, as detected by EMG.
Firing rate: The rate at which a motor unit fires is measured in pulses per second (pps).
Control properties of motor units:
1. The recruitment and firing behaviour of motor units during the process of force generation.
2. It is through these modes that the central and peripheral nervous systems affect the performance of muscles.

The motor neurone pool

The concept of the motor neurone pool (MNP) is that it is an aggregate of interacting neurones, located in the anterior horn of the spinal cord, whose collective behaviour is associated with the control of function in either one muscle or a number of muscles (at any given time.)

The input to the MNP consists of:
1. Afferent information from the peripheral receptors and the Renshaw system, and
2. The drive from higher centres.

The output of the MNP consists of efferent information transmitted down the α and γ motor neurones, and possibly also the β motor neurones.

The muscle spindle

This is a fusiform capsule, attached at both ends to parallel muscle fibres. Its twofold function is to monitor length and changes in length of the muscle. The intrafusal muscle fibres number 5 to 25. Wrapped around each of the intrafusal fibres are endings of two groups of afferent nerve fibres.

Group 1: (a) These go to the MNP, where they have monosynaptic terminations and play an excitatory role in the same muscle. (b) These have disynaptic terminations and play an inhibitory role in the antagonistic muscle, thus causing reciprocal inhibition. (c) There are also longer pathways of reciprocal excitation relayed by oligosynaptic routes[8,9].

Group 2: (a) These are disynaptic and excitatory in the same muscle. (b) It is not known whether these have any antagonistic connections.

Both Group 1a and Group 2 fibres alter their firing rate on change in length of their mechanoreceptor endings (on spindle elongation or contraction.)

Elongation   –   Increased firing rate

Shortening   –   Decreased firing rate

The rate of change in length of the spindle also modifies the firing rate. Group 1a respond both to length and velocity of change; their response is both static and dynamic. Group 2 respond to changes in length only; their response is static only.

Both α and γ systems are coactivated during contraction. This means that, when the MNP of any muscle is excited, both the extrafusal and the intrafusal fibres are involved.

The Golgi organs
These are found in the aponeuroses, and they respond to changes in tension, rather than to changes in length. They are innervated by 1b disynaptic fibres:
1. Inhibitory, (negative) to the homonymous MNP.
2. Excitatory, (positive) to the antagonist MNP[10].
They are sensitive to individual motor unit activity and have a wide range of sensitivity, responding also to stimulation from the muscle as a whole[11].

Behaviour of muscle spindles and Golgi organs in stretch and contraction
Slow stretch

Spindles   – positive to homonymous MNP; negative to antagonist MNP

Golgi organs – negative to homonymous MNP; positive to antagonist MNP

It is seen that the actions of these two structures are opposed in slow stretch.

Brisk stretch
Counteracting reflex response takes place, 1a fibres dominating. This is the stretch reflex. Thus is it seen that the musculoskeletal system provides a mechanism whereby it compensates for changes in muscle length and in the load put upon a muscle.

Contraction

Spindles   – negative to homonymous MNP; positive to antagonist MNP

Golgi organs – negative to homonymous MNP; positive to antagonist MNP

Here it is seen that their actions are complementary.

Renshaw cells
It has been found in motor neurone axons that antidromic impulses moving towards the cell body inhibit neighbouring motor neurones, and that such impulses cause discharges of certain interneurones in the ventral horn, called Renshaw cells. This forms a feedback (reflex) circuit with recurrent inhibition, whose significance is not yet understood.

Other muscle receptors
In addition to the above, muscles contain a variety of other sensory fibres, whose function is not clear.

Control properties of motor units

Firing rate

This is muscle dependent. In small muscles firing rates reach higher levels than in large muscles.

DeLuca[12] compared deltoid and first dorsal interosseous muscles in secretaries, long distance swimmers, weight lifters and pianists. He found:
In the deltoid
1. Rapid increase in firing rate
2. A plateau in all four groups
3. Relatively slow decline in firing rate.
In the first dorsal interosseous
1. Linear relationship between firing rate and force
2. No plateau in all four groups
3. Relatively rapid decline in FR.

Firing rate at recruitment and derecruitment

Both recruitment and derecruitment firing rates are higher in the deltoid than in the first dorsal interosseous muscle. However, the derecruitment firing rate is lower than the recruitment firing rate in the deltoid, whereas this is not the case in the first dorsal interosseous.

The important conclusion to be drawn is that large and small muscles behave differently in these respects. The dynamics of the firing rates also differ between the two types of muscle.

Firing rates during strenuous contraction

The firing rates of high-threshold units sometimes double from 30 pps to 60 pps. This is found in the first dorsal interosseous muscle. It is associated with a sense of fatigue, and it is not found in the deltoid.

Firing rate as a function of time and adaptation

The firing rate declines independently of the force output of the muscle, and is apparently a reflection of motoneuronal adaptation and/or a decrease in the excitation of the muscle. This has been observed in isometric and force-varying contractions. Therefore firing rate adaptation is at least in part a motoneurone product[12].

Under constant current stimulation of motoneurones:
1. Fast twitch, fast fatiguing firing rates decrease.
2. Slow twitch, fatigue resistant firing rates do not alter.

The concept of the common drive

Is there a strategy (or are there strategies) in the generation or modulation of muscle force? Can this be revealed in firing rate and recruitment? There is much evidence that firing rates of active motor units increase proportionately to increased force output[13-19]. This implies that increased excitation to the motor neurone pool increases the firing rates of all the active motor units; that is there is a unison behaviour of the firing rates of motor units as a function of both time and force.

DeLuca (1982) has shown that the nervous system:

1. Does not control the firing rates of motor units individually,
2. Acts to modify excitation or inhibition of the motor neurone pools uniformly[20].

The modulations in firing rates occur simultaneously and in similar amounts in motor units. Fluctuations in force output are causally related to variations in firing rate. Therefore, if an increase in force output of a muscle is required, all the active motor units increase their firing rates proportionately.

The common drive in relation to antagonistic muscles
During voluntary stiffening of the first interphalangeal joint, the firing rates of inputs in the two muscles concerned (extensor and flexor) are highly correlated.

During random flexion/extension isometric, (resisted) contractions of these muscles, the firing rates of the antagonist muscle were highly negatively correlated.

This implies the existence of an ordered modulation of the firing rates of the motor units in the two muscles. The nervous system regards them as one unit and controls them in like fashion. In this case, when the two antagonistic muscles are activated simultaneously to stiffen the joint, the homonymous MNP consists of the MNPs of both muscles[20].

Firing rates at force reversal
It has been shown that disfacilitation begins **before** force reversal, which achieves a smooth and accurate change from one to the other direction[18].

Recruitment/derecruitment within a MNP
Recruitment
This progresses from the smallest to the largest motor neurone[21]. The most convenient in situ measure of the motor neurone size in a contracting muscle has been found to be the conduction velocity of the axon. Axons with lower conduction velocities are consistently more excitable than are those with higher conduction velocities. The lower conduction velocities are, of course, found in the smaller axons.

Derecruitment

When the force output of a muscle is voluntarily decreased, motor units are derecruited in reverse order of recruitment[20]. This observation implies that disfacilitation of the MNP also obeys the principle of ordered behaviour. There are reports suggesting that recruitment order may be altered but, in the opinion of Basmajian and DeLuca[77], there are possible technical shortcomings, (for example electrode migration) which mean that this question is still open.

Recruitment as a function of muscle

Small muscles recruit all motor units below 50% maximum voluntary contraction (MVC). Larger muscles recruit motor units up to 80% of the full range of voluntary force, and possibly further.

Recruitment as a function of time

The faster twitch muscle fibres comprising the motor units which are recruited at higher force thresholds decrease their mechanical output at a faster rate than do the earlier recruitment, slower twitch muscle fibres. Therefore, are motor units recruited during a sustained contraction? As yet it is not possible to issue a clear satatement on this matter.

Firing rate and recruitment interaction
Within a muscle

Referring to the peripheral control system, it will be seen that considerable anatomical and functional coupling exists among the motor units within a muscle[22]. When a muscle is recruited during slow force increasing 1–2% of maximum voluntary contraction (isometric), it has often been observed that previously activated motor units are disfacilitated.

This is noted as a decrease in firing rates of previously activated motor units as the firing rate of the newly activated motor unit increases and the force output of the muscle increases. The interaction between recruitment and firing rate provides an apparently simple strategy for ensuring smooth force output.

In different muscles

It is apparent that small muscles are controlled by different firing rate/recruitment schemes from larger muscles. Smaller muscles recruit their motor units within the range 0–50% of maximum voluntary contraction and rely exclusively on firing rate increase to augment their force output between 50–100% MVC. The firing rates of these muscles continually increase with increase in force output, reaching values as high as 60 pps.

Larger muscles recruit motor units at least up to 90% MVC, and possibly higher. Their firing rates have a relatively smaller dynamic swing, peak at 35–40 pps and tend to demonstrate a plateau effect. Smaller muscles rely primarily upon firing rate, whereas larger muscles rely primarily upon recruitment to modulate their force output.

This work reveals two features:

1. There is a common drive.
2. There is a significant difference in the control mechanisms between small and large muscles in both firing rate and recruitment.

Studies on the EMG signal amplitude and force reveal similar differences between large and small muscles, although "this distinction in their behaviour may possibly reflect the differences in the firing rate and recruitment properties of small and large muscles, as well as other anatomical and electrical considerations"[77].

This last quotation typifies the stringency of the standards which have been deployed throughout the text by Basmajian and DeLuca. This difference in behaviour between different muscle sizes to our knowledge has never been predicted, and should warn all to be cautious when considering the many, at times elaborate, hypotheses to be found in this field.

Muscle interaction

The control strategies discussed so far can now be considered in relation to muscle interaction. Before control is further discussed, a number of reflex phenomena should be noted.

It has been shown that, when subjects fall to the ground onto the outstretched hand, all the muscles which surround the elbow are strongly activated some tenths of a second before the hand touches the surface. Consequently, the musculature is prepared to protect the joint. This is partly a conditioned reflex and partly a non-conditioned reflex, arising from tonic neck and labyrinthine reactions. Similar results have been shown in the lower limb. Myotatic relfexes were found to play no significant role in the decelleration, as they came much too late[23].

It has also been shown by EMG that the human gastrocnemius has a stretch reflex, called the functional stretch reflex, elicited by a sharply applied and maintained dorsiflexion of the ankle. It occurs after a delay of 120 milliseconds[24].

Gravitational forces elicit a body jerk in muscles of the trunk and lower limbs whenever an external force is removed suddenly[25]. O'Connell demonstrated the effect of sensory deprivation on the ability of the human being to achieve the erect posture when he is dropped vertically some moderate, but to him unknown, distance[26].

No hypothesis concerning muscle interaction can afford to ignore reflex factors.

Synergistic muscles

These are defined as those muscles actively providing an associated contribution to a particular muscular function.

It is self-evident that contraction of any one muscle may be accompanied by the synergistic activity of a companion muscle acting on the same joint.

Such activity is particularly evident in the mechanically complicated joints surrounded by small muscles. An example of this type of synergistic behaviour is to be found in the work of Weathersby, who reported considerable activity in certain forearm flexors during ordinary movements of the thumb[27].

What is less apparent, but nonetheless instinctively obvious, is the often noted synergistic activities of other muscles to stabilize joints. Gelhorn, demonstrated the role of far-removed synergists in movements of the wrist[28]. While flexor carpi radialis was activated in very slight flexion of the wrist, triceps brachii became active with increasing effort in the prime movers, the extensors of the wrist remaining relaxed meanwhile. Only with very strong static flexion of the wrist would activity appear in the antagonists, and that only occasionally.

Using as a model the act of prehension of the hand, the plasticity of synergists during voluntary movements has been demonstrated. Thus the interplay of the flexors of the fingers and of the thumb with those of the forearm was shown during normal activity to vary very significantly and to depend upon information of peripheral origin: the position of joints, the angle at which the synergists act, the nature of the objects grasped, etc.[29].

The complexity and variability of control factors in these movements could scarcely be greater.

"It has been found that anticipatory movements are present in the lower limbs, hips and trunk before the onset of voluntary movements in the arms."[30]

Muscle role

A muscle is a contractile organ. Mechanically it can only generate tension and hence can only pull. Thus at least two opposing muscles are required to control the simplest possible joint function.

The agonist muscle is that which initiates a desired contraction, thus it is the prime mover muscle.

The antagonist muscle is any muscle which actively provides a negative contribution to a particular function during a contraction.

A synergist muscle actively provides an additive contribution – positive or negative – to a particular function during a contraction.

Thus the classification of any given muscle in these categories is entirely dependent upon the intended movement or task.

Coactivation and reciprocal inhibition

Four separate mechanisms have been found to govern the contractions of an agonist/antagonist muscle set.
1. Centrally mediated reciprocal inhibition.
2. Centrally mediated coactivation.
3. Peripherally mediated reciprocal inhibition.
4. Peripherally mediated coactivation.

Sherrington demonstrated the existence of a centrally mediated reciprocal inhibition, when he applied electrical stimuli to various areas of the motor cortex of a cat and noted that some muscles contracted, while their antagonists relaxed[31,32]. He also observed that, in decerebrate cats, one stimulus applied peripherally elicited opposite reactions in an agonist/antagonist muscle set. This led him to postulate the concept of peripherally mediated reciprocal inhibition.

Although Sherrington elaborated on the concepts of reciprocal inhibition he did recognize that agonist/antagonist muscle sets could be voluntarily excited to contract at the same time. This centrally mediated coactivation is a realizable and at times used control strategy.

A relatively recent finding in this area has been the existence of peripherally mediated coactivation. This mechanism was first reported by Fenyes et al.[33] and it is important to note that the current understanding of this phenomenon is very limited and somewhat insecure.

Sherrington's dual observations have led to an active debate concerning central versus peripheral influences in agonist/antagonist muscle controls. Lashley, pointed out that there are examples of motor tasks involving movements that are too rapid to be controlled by proprioceptive afferent cues from the moving limb[34]. In such cases a central programme would be required to generate the pattern of excitation and inhibition needed to produce these movements.

The involvement of higher centres in reciprocal inhibition has been reasserted. Cheney et al. concluded that the synaptic terminations of some motor cortex cells with the flexor and extensor spinal motor neurones are reciprocally organized[35]. Along the same line of investigation, Terzuolo et al. demonstrated that, in ballistically initiated movements performed by monkeys, the agonist/antagonist reciprocity is eliminated after cerebellar ablation[36]. Ballistic contraction is defined as one that is executed with the greatest speed physiologically possible.

These studies suggest that separate systems control co-contraction and reciprocal inhibition in antagonistic muscles. They also support the idea, originally put forward by Tilney and Pike in 1925, that the cerebellum plays an important role in switching from reciprocal inhibition to co-contraction[37].

It has been shown that, during rapid movements, the activity of both

agonist and antagonist muscles display a triphasic pattern[36,38-52].
1. An initial burst of agonist activity, with the antagonist silent.
2. Limb accelleration, followed by a reduction of agonist activity, with a burst of activity in the antagonist.
3. Limb decelleration, with a subsequent resumption of agonist and antagonist activity.

The generally accepted explanation for this triphasic sequence is that the nervous system avoids damage that might result from the explosive force being generated by the agonist muscle during ballistic contraction.

Most of these studies on ballistic movements indicate that, if the subject is instructed to precontract the antagonist muscle against a fixed load and to activate the agonist as quickly as possible, the earliest sign of rapid voluntary movement is not the activation of the agonist with a rapid burst, rather inhibition of the antagonist muscle. This has been referred to as the silent period.

Hallet et al. suggested that, in ballistic movements, the triphasic pattern is originated by purely preprogrammed signals with little influence from the periphery[46]. Conversely, Angel did not support the notion of complete preprogramming of the agonist/antagonist triphasic pattern of activation, arguing that the contraction is affected by feedback signals from the periphery[53].

Jacobs et al. concluded that both spinal and supraspinal control mechanisms are necessary in regulating agonist/antagonist function[52,54]. They studied the EMG activity associated with rapid limb movements in the cat and concluded that, in the triphasic activity pattern, the antagonist burst and the sudden agonist burst represent reponses to muscle stretch whose amplitude is modulated by descending commands.

Waters and Strick studied the EMG activity in human subjects required to track a visual object with ballistic movements by pointing at it[55]. They concluded that antagonist muscle activity during ballistic movements may be influenced by the subject's movement strategy.

Basmajian and DeLuca[77] have noted that during an isometric constant force contraction in which the antagonist muscles are not active, the strategy used to stop the contraction differs depending on the requirements of the individual. If the contraction may be terminated with no time constraints, the agonist simply relaxes and the contraction ends. If the contraction is to be terminated faster than the agonist can relax, then the antagonist becomes active to achieve the task.

Lagasse suggested that separate motor systems control speed and force and that, while the interaction between agonist and antagonist muscles is fundamental for maximum speed of joint movement, it is relatively unimportant in static force generation[56].

Others found a pattern of responses in which low unsustained activity occurs in an antagonist at low speeds of voluntary flexion and extension at the elbow[57-62]. At middle speeds there were successive activities in the agonist/antagonist muscles, including common electrical silence. At high speeds of flexion and extension there was powerful overlapping of phasic activities in agonist and antagonist. They focussed their attention not on the speed per se but on the tension in the agonist.

It is generally accepted that slow movements are under peripheral influence, at least in the process of learning new skills[63]. However, Polit and Bizzi showed that trained deafferented dorsal root severed monkeys can peform arm target aquisition movements in the presence of external mechanical disturbances and in the absence of afferent feedback[64]. This was thought to be possible because a given coactivation of agonist and antagonist muscles defines an equilibrium position for the joint. Modification in this level of activation will change the equilibrium position.

The work of Day et al. conflicted with this interpretation; their results show the target aquisition with the thumb distal phalanx in a deafferented patient could not be properly achieved in the presence of external mechanical disturbances[65].

In a later study, Bizzi et al. argued that posture control could indeed be achieved by presetting the level of coactivation of antagonistic muscles[66]. However, during movements there is also active control of the trajectory, in addition to control of the final position. Thus some control algorithm other than simply presetting agonist/antagonist coactivation is used during movement.

Practical clinical consequences

For several decades, ideas concerning abnormal patterns of motor activity have existed.

The material presented above is, by comparison, relatively recent and, while it does not provide direct refutation of such ideas, its complexity and unpredictability surely reflect a need for reassessment and caution with regard to any hypothesis in this field.

Once again, this shows the importance of the laboratory to any clinician. In the absence of relevant evidence, hypothesis may be almost unlimited. On the other hand, hypothesis must be constrained by such relevant evidence as does exist. As expressed elsewhere in this book, we feel that validated material, much of it recent, should be borne in mind by the clinician.

Spinal muscle function
General

Spinal muscle function is a basic consideration on clinical grounds, because exercises, whatever their intended or believed purpose, can only be effective if the muscles under consideration are in fact being exercised.

Any opinion concerning 'patterns of motor activity' should relate to what muscles have been shown to do.

What spinal muscles do is important to the clinician, because this seldom correlates fully with the functions ascribed to them, world wide, in anatomical and other texts, which, as will be shown, are commonly both inadequate and inaccurate.

Specific
We consider here three groups of muscles related to spinal movement.
1. The erector spinae.
2. The deep muscles of the back.
3. The muscles of the abdominal wall.

Erector spinae
With regard to these muscles, electromyography shows that:
1. One main function is to control 'paying out', which, indeed, is as important as the function of extension[67].
2. In very rapid flexion, little or no activity is required or in fact appears. On the other hand, as the slowly flexing trunk is lowered, the activity in erector spinae increases apace and then decreases to quiescence when full flexion is reached[67].
3. If an attempt is made then to force flexion further, silence continues to prevail in the erectors[67].
4. In full flexion, then, the weight of the torso is borne by the posterior ligaments and fasciae[67].
5. The erector spinae again comes into action when the trunk is raised once more to the erect position[67].
6. In the initial stages of flexion of the trunk in bending forward, the movement is controlled by the intrinsic muscles of the back[68].
7. In full flexion while seated (usually considered by school teachers as a 'bad' posture) if the position is maintained comfortably for long periods the erector spinae remain relaxed[68].
8. Most subjects standing in a relaxed erect posture show a low level of discharge in the erector spinae[68].
9. Small adjustments of the position of the head, shoulders or hands can be made which abolish the activity of the muscle, i.e. an equilibrium or balance can be achieved[68].
10. Extension of the trunk is initiated, as a rule, by a short burst of activity[68].
11. While standing upright, flexion of the trunk to one side is accompanied by activity of the erector spinae of the opposite side, i.e. the muscle is not a

72

prime mover, but an antagonist[68].

12. However, if the back is already arched in extension, not even this sort of activity occurs[68].

13. The erector spinae contract (apparently vigorously) during coughing and straining. This occurs even in the midst of their normal silence, whether the subject is erect or full-flexed[68].

14. With the subject standing, the activity in erector spinae ceases earlier during forward bending than it does when seated[68].

15. In some patients complete relaxation is found in the sitting posture, but not in standing[68].

16. The erector spinae remain relaxed during the initial movement of lifting weights of up to 56 lb[68].

17. It is movement at the hip joints that accounts for the earliest phase of apparent extension of the trunk[68].

18. However, it is the ligaments of the back that are required to carry the added weight, without help from the muscles[68].

19. The recording of activity from both right and left erectors during bending to either side shows that there seems to be a pattern of co-operative activity and not a simple simultaneous antagonism[69].

20. During the performance of various trunk movements, muscles show patterns of activity that clearly show two functions – sometimes they initiate movements and at other times they stabilize the trunk[70].

21. Almost all the movements recruit all the muscles of the back in a variety of patterns, although the predominance of certain muscles is obvious[70].

22. Morris *et al.* found that muscles that might be expected to return the spine to the vertical position often remained quiet; they suggest that factors such as ligaments and passive muscle elasticity play an important role[70].

23. During easy standing, longissimus is slightly to moderately active; it can be relaxed by gentle ('relaxed') extension of the spine[70].

24. During forced full extension, flexion, lateral flexion and rotation in different positions of the trunk, it is almost always prominently active[70].

25. A position of complete silence is easily found for iliocostalis in the erect position, but with slight forward swaying activity is instantly recruited[70].

26. Forward flexion and rotation in the flexed position bring out its strongest contractions, but it is also fairly active in most movements of the spine[70].

27. In almost all vigorous exercises performed from the orthograde position, the most active muscle is spinalis; next in order is longissimus, and least active is iliocostalis lumborum[71].

28. Nevertheless, all three muscles and the main mass of erector spinae act powerfully during strong arching of the back in the prone posture[71].

29. During push-ups there is considerable individual variation but, typically, the lower back muscles remain relaxed[71].
30. Simple side-bending exercises of the trunk do not recruit erector spinae as long as there is no concomitant backward or forward bending. This refutes earlier opinions, whose authors had ignored movements in the ventrodorsal plane that do involve erector spinae[71].

Comment
Gray's *Anatomy*[78] defines the function of erector spinae thus:
"Bilateral contraction results in extension of the column, and unilateral contraction results in lateral bending of the vertebral column to the side of the contracted muscle."
It will be seen that there exists a marked discrepancy between this definition and the realities revealed by scientific investigation, the results of some of which were first published nearly forty years ago.

The deep muscles
1. The same muscle group displays different patterns of activity in the thoracic as compared with the lumbar level[72].
2. Variations in the pattern of activity during forward flexion, extension and axial rotation suggest that the transversospinal muscles adjust the motion between individual vertebrae[72].
3. The experimental evidence confirms the anatomical hypothesis that the multifidi are stabilizers rather than prime movers of the whole vertebral column[72].

Changes in the lumbar curvature during sitting and standing
4. The lumbar muscles are inactive during relaxed sitting but show some activity in straight sitting and in the standing posture[72].
5. When the back of a seated subject is supported, levels of both intradiscal pressure and EMG signal fall[73].

Forward flexion in sitting and standing positions
6. As noted before, Floyd and Silver first showed that the back muscles became electromyographically inactive at a critical point during extreme flexion[68].
7. Donisch and Basmajian found spontaneous electrical silence of the lumbar muscles in extreme flexion in most subjects, but only half of them showed spontaneous inactivity of their thoracic muscles in both seated and standing positions[72].
8. During the Valsalva manoeuvre, with increased intrathoracic and intra-abdominal pressure while holding a sandbag of 11.25 kg, all thoracic and a number of lumbar muscles showed activity instead of electrical silence[72].
9. In extension from the flexed to the upright posture, back muscles do not

always become active immediately extension is begun. Instead there are frequently short bursts of activity that occur (especially in the lumbar region) when the movement of extension is half completed[72].

10. With regard to axial trunk rotation, less than half of the examined subjects showed expected activity of the transverse and paraspinal muscles of the thoracic region; whereas more than half of the subjects showed the expected activity in the lumbar region. This finding is somewhat surprising, considering that most of the actual rotatory movement occurs in the thoracic region[72].

11. Paradoxical activity in the deep muscles of the spine was found in 5 subjects at the thoracic and in 3 subjects at the lumbar levels[72].

12. Activity in the rotatores multifidi during ipsilateral rotation has also been occasionally found[72].

13. All subjects showed bilateral activity at the thoracic level. In more than half of these this activity did not appear to be related to the direction of the rotatory movements[72].

Comment

Again the complexity and unpredictability of muscle function in the back will surprise many clinicians, particularly those who, unaquainted with this material, may hold convictions which might bear reconsideration. Possibly the most apt comment is that of Basmajian and DeLuca, "Perhaps the designation of specific function is almost impossible in the back, where we have a complex arrangement of muscle bundles acting on a multitude of equally complex joints. Those who insist on finding prime movers, antagonists and synergists in the genuine musculature of the back will always be disappointed."[77]

Musculature of the anterior abdominal wall

These muscles are of importance in this context for two reasons: first in that they assist in spinal movements, and second in that they prestress the spine and are thereby relevant to the rational prescription of exercises aimed at the prevention of back pain.

1. Floyd and Silver frequently found some difference between the right and the left sides of the abdominal musculature, even when electrodes were carefully matched[68]. They ascribed this to a basic asymmetry in function and found individual variations in the amount of difference.

2. With the head raising movement used commonly as an exercise for strengthening abdominal muscles, the recti were powerfully active, while the external oblique and the part of the internal oblique that was studied were only active at first[68]. Even with increased effort they became only moderately active.

3. One might conclude from their finding that only the rectus is benefitted maximally by the head raising exercise, in spite of the exercise being advocated to increase the general 'tone' of the abdominal wall[68].

4. In contrast to the head raising exercise, the bilateral leg raising exercise brought all the abdominal musculature into activity to stabilize the pelvis[68].

5. One-sided leg raising was less effective, calling upon activity predominantly on the same side of the abdomen[68].

6. In the relaxed standing position, all the electrodes except those over the lower part of the internal oblique picked up no activity. Internal oblique apparently is on constant guard over the inguinal region[68].

7. When the subjects (whether recumbent or erect) were made to strain or to 'bear down' with the breath held, the external obliques and the internal obliques (lower parts) contracted to a degree that was directly related to the effort, but rectus abdominis, in contrast, was very quiet. This was later confirmed by Ono[79]. Surely it is surprising that physical therapists have not seized upon these findings for application in the strengthening of weak or stretched obliques. Perhaps they are not dramatic enough[68]!

8. With forced expiration, with coughing, and with singing, the pattern was similar to that in straining; i.e. marked activity in the obliques and none in the rectus[68].

9. Floyd and Siler[68] have proved conclusively that the apparent hardening of the recti on straining is usually only a passive bulging of the muscles and their sheaths. "One can only hope that this knowledge, available now for several decades, will soon reach the practicing surgeon."[77]

10. However, there is exuberant activity in the recti bilaterally during a cough. So there is a difference between the reactions of the recti to the increase of intra-abdominal pressure from bearing down and the sharp short increase of coughing[74].

11. In movements of the trunk, performed without resistance in either the sitting or standing posture, the obliques and recti remain quiescent. However, lateral bending of the trunk does produce activity in the more posterolateral fibres of external oblique[75].

12. Inclining the trunk backwards gives activity in all the muscles, but forward bending is unaccompanied by activity[75].

13. "Rotation of the pelvis on the thorax (hip roll) and the reverse curl are excellent activators of the internal oblique in this (supine) position."[75]

14. Less effective are 'chin up', 'pull up' and 'pelvic tilt' in the supine position, isometric contraction of the abdominal wall, 'low bicycle with tilt', vertical jumping and straight leg raising in the supine position[76].

15. The upper and lower parts of the rectus abdominis vary in response to different movements[76].

16. Most of the activity in the recti during trunk flexion from the the supine position occurs during the first part of the movement[76].
17. Trunk raising elicits more activity than trunk lowering[76].
18. Maximal abdominal muscle activity occurs during hook-lying (knees bent) unsupported slow and fast sit-ups[76].

Comment

Gray's *Anatomy*[78] defines the activities of the rectus abdominis and internal and external obliques as follows:
1. "With the pelvis fixed they flex the lumbar spine."
2. "With the thorax fixed they:
   a. have the same function
   b. draw the front of the pelvis upwards."
3. "Working unilaterally they bend the spine to the ipsilateral side."
4. "The external oblique tends to rotate the trunk to the opposite side, the internal oblique to the same side."

In the light of the material presented, these classic definitions are simplistic and misleading, with regrettable consequences for case analysis and management.

Comment on muscular function

This chapter reveals the extreme complexity of muscular function, and it will be particularly noted that this does not correspond with the relatively elementary definitions given in so many texts, world wide, up to the present time. We re-emphasize that some of this work is of very long standing.

Ideas relating to assessment and management that have been shown to be mistaken or inadequate are likely to prove unhelpful to both clinician and patient.

The most surprising feature to us is how unexpected and unpredicted the emerging realities are. Despite the myriad hypotheses that have been postulated over the past hundred years or more with regard to muscular function, no-one, to our knowledge, predicted that:
1. The control strategies for large and small muscles would differ significantly,
2. The erector spinae would show most activity in flexion,
3. In the Donisch Basmajian experiment[72] less than half of the examined subjects showed this expected activity of the transversospinal muscles of the thoracic region, whereas more than half of our subjects showed the expected activity in the lumbar region. This finding is somewhat surprising, considering that most of the actual rotatory movement takes place in the thoracic region.

4. The ligaments would play the part they do:
   a. In full flexion there is no muscular activity, and the weight of the torso is borne by the ligaments and fasciae.
   b. A further example, not directly related to spinal activity, concerns the shoulder joint. "Hardly any informed person would doubt that, when gravity acts on the upper limb, and certainly when the limb carries a heavy load, muscles are the chief agents in preventing the distraction of the joints. Yet, as a result of many studies, we have concluded that this is a false belief."[77] Thus, common sense may be demonstrable non-sense!
   c. "Contrary to expectation, the vertically running muscles that cross the shoulder joint and the elbow joint are not active to prevent distraction of these joints by gravity. Much more surprising is the the fact that they do not spring into action when light, moderate or even heavy loads are added, unless the subject voluntarily decides to flex his shoulder or his elbow and thus to support the weight in bent positions of these joints."[77]
5. Muscle activity in axial rotation of the trunk would prove paradoxical.

The current prescription of exercises and the formulation of hypotheses regarding muscle function that do not relate to this material must inevitably be diminished to the point of naivety.

References

1. Ekstedt (1964). Human single muscle fibre action potentials. *Acta Physiol. Scand.*, **61** (Supp.), 226
2. Buchthal *et al.* (1957). Multi electro study of the territory of a motor unit. *Acta Physiol. Scand.*, **39**, 83–103
3. Engel (1962). The essentiality of histo and cyto chemical studies of skeletal muscle in the investigation of neuro muscular disease. *Neurology*, **12**, 778–794
4. Engel (1974). Fibre type nomenclature of human skeletal muscle for histo chemical purposes. *Neurology*, **24**, 344–348
5. Barany (1967). ATPase activity of myosin correlated with speed of muscle shortening. *J Gen. Physiol.*, **50**, 197
6. Brooke and Kaiser (1976). Three myosin adenosin triphosphatase systems. The nature of their pability and sulfhydryl depend? *J. Histochem. Cytochem.*, **18**, 670–672
7. Burke *et al.* (1971). Mammalian motor units. Physiological histochemical correlation in three types in cat gastrocnemius. *Science*, **174**, 709
8. Jankowska *et al.* (1981). Pattern of 'non reciprocal' inhibition of motor neurones by impulses in group la muscle spindle afferents in the cat. *J. Physiol.*, **316**, 393–409
9. Jankowska *et al.* (1981). Oligo-synaptic excitation of motor neurones by impulses in group la muscle spindle afferents in the cat. *J. Physiol.*, **316**, 441–425
10. Watt (1976). Analysis of muscle receptor connections with spike triggered averaging. 1. Spindle primary and tendon organ afferents. *J. Neurophysiol.*, **39**, 1375–1392
11. Binder *et al.* (1977). The response of golgi tendon organs to single motor neurone contractions. *J. Physiol.*, **271**, 337–349

12. DeLuca *et al.* (1982). Behaviour of human motor units in different muscles during linearly varying contractions. *J. Physiol.*, **329**, 113–128
13. Leifer (1969). Characterisation of single muscle fibre discharge during voluntary isometric contraction of the biceps brachii muscle in man. *PhD thesis*, Stanford University, Stanford, Ca
14. Person and Kudina (1972). Discharge frequency and discharge pattern in human motor units during voluntary contractions of muscle. *Electroencephalogr. Clin. Neurophysiol.*, **32**, 471–483
15. Milner-Brown *et al.* (1973). Changes in firing rate of human motor units in linearly changing voluntary contractions. *J. Physiol.*, **230**, 371–390
16. Tanji and Kato (1973). Recruitment of motor units in voluntary contraction of a finger muscle in man. *Exp. Neurol.*, **40**, 759–770
17. Monster and Chan (1977). Isometric force production by motor units of extensor digitorum communis muscle in man. *J. Neurophysiol.*, **40**, 1432–1443
18. Monster (1979). Firing rate behaviour of human motor units during isometric voluntary contraction. Relation to unit size. *Brain Res.*, **171**, 349–354
19. Kanosue *et al.* (1979). The number of active motor units and their firing rates in voluntary contraction in the human brachialis muscle. *Jpn. J. Physiol.*, **29**, 427–443
20. DeLuca *et al.* (1982). Controls scheme governing concurrently active human motor units during voluntary contractions. *J. Physiol.*, **329**, 129–142
21. Henneman *et al.* (1965). Excitability and inhibitability of motor neurones of different sizes. *J. Neurol. Physiol.*, **28**, 599–620
22. Broman *et al.* (1985). Motor unit recruitment and firing rates interaction in the control of human muscles. *Brain Res.*, **337**(2), 311–319
23. Carlsön and Johansson (1962). Stabilization of/and load on the elbow joint in some protective movements. An experimental study. *Acta Anat.*, **48**, 224–231
24. Watt and Jones (1966). On the functional role of the myotatic reflex in man. *Proc. Can. Fed. Biol. Soc.*, **9**, 13
25. Denslow and Gutensohn (1967). Neuromuscular reflexes in response to gravity. *J. Appl. Physiol.*, **61**, 311–334
26. O'Connell (1971). Effect of sensory deprivation on postural reflexes. *Electromyography*, **11**, 519–527
27. Weathersby (1966). The forearm stabilizers of the thumb. An electromyographic study. *Anat. Rec.*, **154**, 439
28. Gellhorn (1947). Patterns of muscular activity in man. *Arch. Phys. Med.*, **28**, 568–574
29. Livingstone *et al.* (1951). Plasticité d'une synergie musculaire dans l'exécution d'un mouvement voluntaire chez l'homme. *J. Physiol. Paris*, **43**, 605–619
30. Bouisset and Zattara (1981). A sequence of postural movements preceeding voluntary movements. *Neurosci. Lett.*, **22**, 263–270
31. Sherrington (1906). *The Integrative Action of the Nervous System.* 2nd Edn. (New Haven, Conn.: Yale University Press)
32. Sherrington (1909). Reciprocal innervation of antagonist muscles. On double reciprocal innovations. *Proc. R. Soc. London. Ser. B.*, **91**, 249–268
33. Fenyes *et al.* (1964). Clinical and EMG studies of 'spinal reflexes' in premature and full-term infants. *J. Neurol. Neurosurg. Psychiatr.*, **23**, 63–68
34. Lashley (1951). The problem of serial order in behaviour. In Jefferies (ed.) *Cerebral Mechanisms in Behaviour.* Hixon Symposium. (New York: Wiley)
35. Cheney *et al.* (1982). Reciprocal effect of single cortico-moto neuronal cells on wrist extensor and flexor muscle activity in primate. *Brain Res.*, **247**, 164–168
36. Terzuolo *et al.* (1973). Studies on the control of some simple motor tasks. 2. On the cerebellar control of movements in relation to the formulation of intentional commands. *Brain Res.*, **58**, 217–222
37. Tilney and Pike (1925). Muscular co-ordination experimentally studied in its relation to the cerebellum. *Arch. Neurol. Psychiatr.*, **1**, 289–334
38. Hufshmidt and Hufshmidt (1954). Antagonist inhibition as a sign of a sensory motor reaction. *Nature* (London), **174**, 607

39. Barnett and Harding (1955). The activity of antagonist muscles during voluntary movement. *Ann. Phys. Med.*, 2, 290–293
40. Basmajian (1957). New views on muscular tone and relaxation. *Can. Med. Soc. J.*, 77, 203–205
41. Bierman and Ralston (1965). Electromyographic study during passive and active flexion and extension of the knee in the normal human subject. *Arch. Phys. Med.*, 46, 71–75
42. Gottlieb *et al.* (1976). Interactions between voluntary and postural mechanism of the human motor system. *J. Neurol. Physiol.*, 33, 365–381
43. Patton and Mortenson (1970). A study of some mechanical factors affecting reciprocal activity in one joint muscle. *Anat. Res. Rec.*, 166, 360
44. Terzuolo and Viviani (1974). Parameters of motion and EMG activities during some simple motor tasks in normal subjects and in cerebellar patients. In Cooper, Riklam and Schneider (eds.) *The Cerebellum, Epilepsy and Behaviour*, pp. 173–215. (New York: Plenum Press)
45. Simoyama and Tanaka (1974). Reciprocal 1A inhibition at the onset of voluntary movements in man. *Brain Res.*, 82, 334–337
46. Hallet *et al.* (1975). EMG analysis of stereotyped voluntary movements in man 1. *J. Neurol. Neurosurg. Psychiatr.*, 38, 1154–1162
47. De Sousa *et al.* (1975). Atividade de musculos antagonistas. Estudio electromiografico. *Rev. Hosp. Clin. Fac. Med. S. Paulo*, 30, 471–473
48. Morin *et al.* (1976). Role of muscular afferents in the inhibition of the antagonist motor nucleus during a voluntary contraction in man. *Brain Res.*, 103, 373–376
49. Jacobs (1976). Antagonist EMG temporal patterns during rapid voluntary movement. *PhD dissertation*, University of Toledo, Ohio.
50. Hallett and Marsden (1979). Ballistic flexion movements of the human thumb. *J. Physiol.*, 294, 33–50
51. Brown and Cooke (1981). Responses to force perturbations preceding volutary arm movements. *Brain Res.*, 220, 350–355
52. Ghez and Martin (1982). The control of rapid limb movement of the cat. *Exp. Brain Res.*, 45, 115–125
53. Angel (1977). Antagonist muscle activity during rapid arm movements. Central versus proprioceptive influences. *J. Neurol. Neuropsychiatr.*, 40, 683–686
54. Jacobs *et al.* (1980). Antagonist EMG temporal patterns during rapid voluntary movements. *Neurology*, 30, 36–41
55. Waters and Strick (1981). Influence of 'strategy' on muscle activity during ballistic movements. *Brain Res.*, 207, 189–194
56. Lagasse (1979). Prediction of maximum speed of human movements by two selective muscular co-ordination mechanisms and by maximum static strength. *Percept. Motor Skills*, 49, 151–161
57. Goubel and Bouisset (1967). Relation entre l'activite electromyographique integrée et la travail méchanique effectué au cours d'un mouvement monoarticulaire simple. *J. Physiol.*, 59, 241
58. Lestienne and Bouisset (1968). Pattern temporel de la mise enjeu d'un agoniste et d'un antagoniste en fonction de la tension de l'agoniste. *Rev. Neurol. Paris*, 118, 550–554
59. Goubel *et al.* (1968). Determination dynamique de la compliance musculaire in situe. *J. Physiol.*, 60, 255
60. Pertuzon and Lestienne (1966). Charactère electromyographique d'un mouvement monoarticulaire executé a vitesse maximale. *J. Physiol.*, 60, 513
61. Lestienne and Goubel (1969). Contribution relatif de deux agonistes un travail avec et sans raccourcissement. *J. Physiol.*, 61, 342–343
62. Bertoz and Metral (1976). Behaviour of a muscular group subjected to a sinusoidal and trapezoidal variation of force. *J. Acta Physiol.*, 29, 378–384
63. Desmedt *et al.* (1978). Ballistic skilled movements. Load compensation and patterning of motor commands. *Prog. Clin. Neurophysiol.*, 4, 21–55
64. Polit and Bizzi (1979). Characteristics of motor programmes underlying arm movements in monkeys. *J. Neurol. Physiol.*, 41, 542–556

65. Day *et al.* (1981). Manual motor function in a deafferented man. *J. Physiol.*, **320**, 23–24
66. Bizzi *et al.* (1982). Mechanical properties of muscles. Implications for motor control. *Trends Neurol. Sci.*, **5** (11), 395–398
67. Allen (1948). Muscle action potential used in the study of dynamic anatomies. *Br. J. Phys. Med.*, **11**, 66–73
68. Floyd and Silver (1951). Function of erector spinae in flexion of the trunk. *Lancet*, **20**, 133–138
69. Friedebold (1958). Die Aktivitit Normaler Ruckenstreckmuskulatur. Elektro-Myogramm unter vershierschiedenen haltungsbedingungen. Eine Studie zur Skelettmuskelmeckanik. *Z. Orthop.*, **90**, 118
70. Morris *et al.* (1962). An electromyographic study of the intrinsic muscles of the back in man. *J. Anat.*, **96**, 509–520
71. Pauly (1966). Electromyographic analysis of certain movements and exercises. Part 1. Some deep muscles of the back. *Anat. Rec.*, **155**, 223–234
72. Donisch and Basmajian (1972). Electromyography of deep muscles in man. *Am. J. Anat.*, **133**, 25–26
73. Andersson *et al.* (1975). The sitting posture. An electromyographic and discometric study. *Orthop. Clin. N. Am.*, **6**, 105–120
74. De Sousa and Furlani (1974). Electromyographic study of the M. rectus abdominus. *Acta Anat.*, **86**, 281–298
75. Partridge and Walters (1959). Participation of the abdominal muscles in various movements of the trunk in man. Electromyographic study. *Phys. Ther. Rev.*, **39**, 791–800
76. Flint and Gudgell (1965). Electromyographic study of abdominal musculature activity during exercises. *Res. Quart.*, **36**, 29–37
77. Basmajian and DeLuca (1985). *Muscles Alive*. (Baltimore: Williams and Wilkins)
78. Gray (1973). *Anatomy*, 35th Edn. (London: Churchill Livingstone)
79. Ono (1958). Electromyographic studies of the abdominal wall muscles in visceroptosis. I. Analysis of patterns of activity of the abdominal wall muscles in normal adults. *Tohoku J. Exp. Med.*, **68**, 347–354

5
CONTROL OF THE MUSCULOSKELETAL SYSTEM

Reflex and perceptual considerations
In this chapter we draw heavily on the presentations made by Professor B. Wyke at the FIMM congress in 1983 in Zürich[1].

Perception
Postural sensation: This is defined as the perceptual awareness of the static spatial relationships of one part of the body to another, or more colloquially as 'knowing where the various bits of your body are, without looking at them'.
Kinaesthesis: This is defined as perceptual awareness of the amplitude, velocity and direction of joint movement, active or passive.

Reflexogenic
Arthrostatic: This is defined as the reflex activity of immobile joints.

Arthrokinetic: This is defined as the reflex activity of joint movement, active or passive.
   It will be noted that in postural sensation the only mechanoreceptors to be involved will be Type I. With regard to kinaesthesis and arthrokinetic reflexes, mechanoreceptors I, II and possibly III may be involved.

   The effects of removal of mechanoreceptors in trauma or degeneration lead to disturbances of perception, postural and kinaesthetic, and of reflexes, arthrokinetic and arthrostatic, which in practice are really quite devastating. For example, in severe injuries of the capsule of the ankle joint, this can be shown by standing the patient with such an injury in front of a screen, with eyes closed, first on one foot and then on the other. When standing on the sound foot, he will have the normal amplitude of postural sway of about 1.5° to either side, and normal spatial relationships to the other leg, arms, shoulders and hands. When standing on the injured side, all this is distorted. There is a postural sway of approximately 8° to either side, and all other postural relationships are distorted. In other words, there is a widespread disruption of postural reflexes if input from an ankle is lost. The same can be demonstrated with the hip.

This again is an example of the integral part that the peripheral joints play in the whole activity of the musculoskeletal system.

It can be seen that the system is subject to constant perceptual and reflex activity, and that there are widespread and unforeseeable consequences if the input is distorted from any source.

This illustrates the point, perhaps at times insufficiently appreciated, that the musculoskeletal system is at all times subject to complex and unpredictable changes.

Further, this means that in musculoskeletal practice it is unrealistic to consider any one part in isolation. "No man is an island". It is therefore unsound to make assumptions based on previous observations. The only relevant data are those currently exhibited.

The cervical reflexes

These are discussed for two reasons. First because of their extraordinary power. This arises because the population density (defined as the number of receptors per unit tissue volume) is far higher in the upper cervical spine than it is at progressively lower levels. It follows that the central effects of discharge from the mechanoreceptors in the neck are very powerful, while the lumbar contribution is relatively feeble. This was shown by Coutts et al. as long ago as 1948, when the rotation of the head of an experimental animal was shown to produce reflex adjustments of the entire body[2]. This phenomenon is currently used in rehabilitation units in teaching hemiplegic patients to walk with the help of neck movements.

They have also been the subject of relatively recent experimental work which provides valuable insight into their activity and function in normal, pain-free situations, and also in painful situations.

Cervical articular nerve stimulation

A single articular nerve contributing to the supply of the receptors in a single cervical apophyseal joint capsule is dissected out at various levels. This articular nerve, containing the afferent fibres innervating the mechanoreceptors and nociceptors in the fibrous joint capsule, is then placed on stimulating electrodes, so that the afferent fibres of different diameters in the nerve may be stimulated at varying stimulus parameters. Simultaneous, multichannel electromyography enables one to examine the reflexogenic consequences of this cervical articular mechanoreceptive afferent activity. These reflexogenic effects operate plurisynaptically and plurisegmentally and in this respect they are identical to the systems operating in peripheral joints.

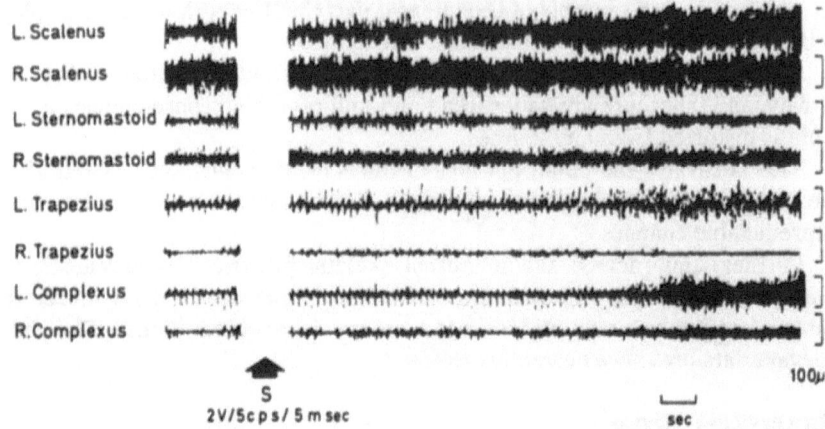

Figure 5.1 Cervical articular mechanoreceptive reflex effects on neck muscles. At the arrow (S), a single cervical articular nerve supplying the left C3–C4 cervical apophyseal joint (isolated by microdissection in an anaesthetized cat) was repetitively stimulated electrically for 3 s with stimulus parameters (indicated below signal) that selectively excite the mechanoreceptive afferent fibres in the nerve. The tracings are simultaneous electromyograms from homologous pairs of neck muscles, displaying the co-ordinated long-duration reflexogenic effects of articular mechanoreceptive afferent activation. (From Paterson and Burn (1986) *Examination of the Back*, Lancaster, MTP Press)

Figure 5.1 demonstrates the changes in motor unit activity in homologous pairs of neck muscles on introducing a low-intensity stimulus.

Since the excitability of nerve fibres is proportional to their diameter, (which is to say that the larger fibres have the lower threshold) it follows that, when one applies suitably selected low-intensity stimuli to the articular nerve, one may stimulate the mechanoreceptive fibres without activating the much finer nociceptive afferents contained in the same nerve. This mimics experimentally what occurs in normal head and neck movements.

When one increases the stimulus to the nerve trunk to a sufficient degree, one can activate the nociceptive afferents at the same time as one activates the mechanoreceptive afferents. When this additional nociceptive input is introduced, one reproduces in the laboratory what occurs in a patient who has a painful disorder involving one of of his cervical apophyseal joints.

The effect of mechanoreceptive input is to alter motor unit activity, some muscles showing facilitation, others inhibition, either to varying and unpredictable degrees.

Figure 5.2 shows what happens if one adds nociceptive input by increasing the stimulus to a sufficient degree: the former picture is wholly distorted.

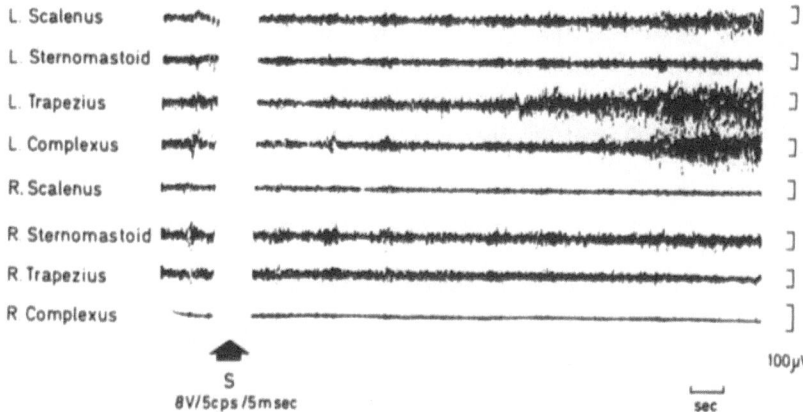

Figure 5.2 Cervical articular nociceptive reflex effects on neck muscles. At the arrow (S), the same cervical articular nerve as in Figure 5.1 was repetitively stimulated electrically for 3 s with stimulus parameters (indicated below signal) that excite the nociceptive (as well as the mechanoreceptive) afferent fibres in the nerve. The simultaneous electromyograms (from the same neck muscles as Figure 5.1) display the altered patterns of reflex activity evoked by the additional activitity of nociceptive afferents coming from the C3–C4 joint. (From Paterson and Burn (1986) *Examination of the Back*, Lancaster, MTP Press)

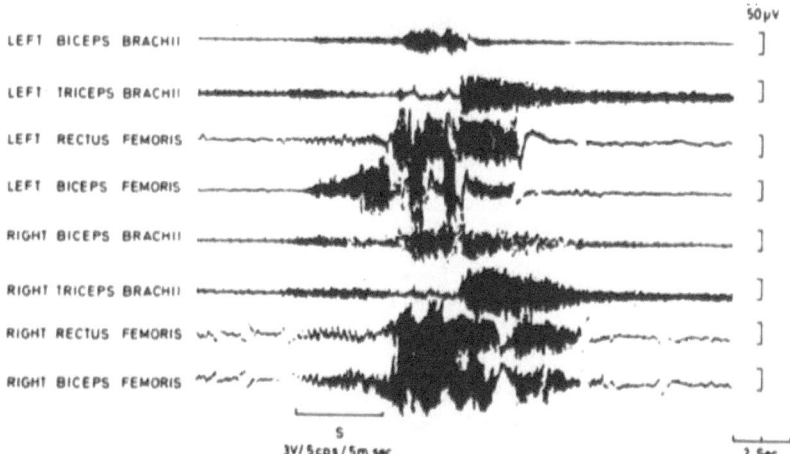

Figure 5.3 Cervical articular mechanoreceptive reflex effects on limb muscles. At the signal (S), a single cervical articular nerve supplying the left C3–C4 cervical apophyseal joint (isolated by microdissection in an anaesthetized cat) was repetitively stimulated for 3 s with stimulus parameters (indicated below signal) that selectively excite the mechanoreceptive afferent fibres in the nerve. The tracings are simultaneous electromyograms from homologous pairs of upper and lower limb muscles, displaying the co-ordinated reflexogenic effects (of varying duration) of articular mechanoreceptive afferent activation, and indicate that such inputs affect limb as well as neck (see Figure 5.2) muscles. Repetition of the experiment with additional nociceptive afferent excitation (as in Figure 5.2) produced a different pattern of reflex effects on the limb muscles (not illustrated here). (From Paterson and Burn (1986) *Examination of the Back*, Lancaster, MTP Press)

85

Figure 5.3 shows that the effects of stimulating cervical apophyseal joint capsular nerves are seen not only in the cervical musculature, but also powerfully and reciprocally co-ordinated in the musculature of all four limbs, showing facilitation and inhibition in alternating patterns.

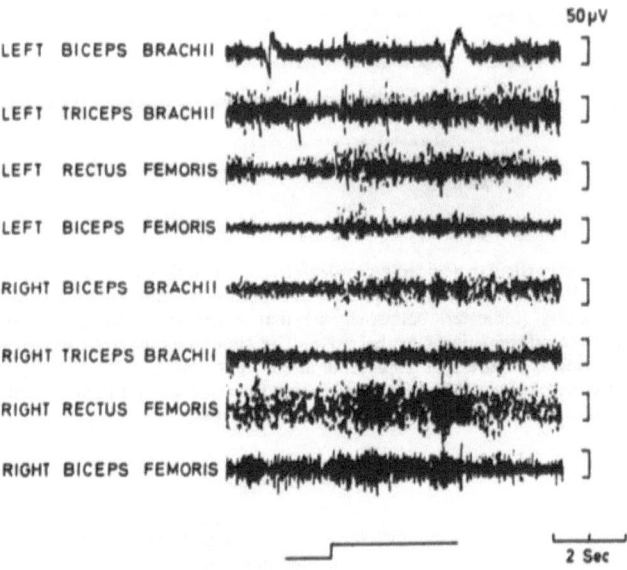

Figure 5.4 Reflex effects of cervical articular manipulation. At the event signal, vertical traction was applied rapidly across the apophyseal joints between the C3 and C4 vertebrae (isolated by surgical microdissection from all tissues other than their nerve and blood supply in an anaesthetized cat). The simultaneous electromyograms from homologous pairs of upper and lower limb muscles display the articular mechanoreceptive reflex effects of such cervical manipulation (the accompanying reflex effects on the neck muscles are not illustrated here). (From Paterson and Burn (1986) *Examination of the Back*, Lancaster, MTP Press)

Figure 5.4 shows that cervical nociceptive input, as previously described in relation to the cervical musculature, again completely distorts the previous pattern in all four limbs.

Practical clinical consequences
1. Cervical pain inevitably causes distortion of the normal reflexogenic control in the musculature of all four limbs.
2. These reflexes show quite clearly not only the complex and unpredictable way in which the musculoskeletal system functions in normal, pain-free circumstances, but that the addition of pain distorts this in a widespread and unforeseeable manner.

3. These findings are crucial to case analysis, in that there is intricate and constantly changing activity, which demands repeated reassessment.
4. This material is relevant to all treatments involving mechanoreceptor stimulation (such as massage, TNS and manipulation). Clearly the application of any of these treatments to the neck must of necessity have consequences far more widespread than many clinicians using them currently appreciate.

References

1. Wyke (1983). *Articular Neurology*. Presented at the FIMM Congress, Sept. 1983, Zurich
2. McCouch, Deering and Ling (1951). *J. Neurophysiol.*, **14**, 191

6
RELEVANT PSYCHOLOGY

In this section we lean heavily on the chapters in Wall and Melzack's *Textbook of Pain* by Craig, Weisenberg, Sternbach, Reading, Merskey and Pilowsky.

Introduction
A basic psychological approach to pain may be summarized as follows:
1. Using the gate control theory as a conceptual basis, pain is viewed as consisting of several components.
   a. Pain has a sensory component, similar to other sensory processes.
   b. Pain also has essential aversive, cognitive, motivational and emotional components that lead to behaviour designed, for example, to escape or avoid the stimulus.
2. Great importance is attached to central nervous system processes.
   a. Higher cortical areas are involved in both discriminative and motivational systems that influence reactions on the basis of cognitive evaluation and past experience.
   b. The gate control theory emphasizes the significant role of psychological variables, and how they affect the reaction of pain.
   c. Especially with chronic pain, successful pain control often involves changing the cognitive motivational components, while the sensory components remain intact.
   d. Hypnosis, anxiety reduction, desensitization, attention distraction, as well as other behavioural approaches, can be effective alternatives and supplements to pharmacology and surgery in the control of pain. (Fields and Basbaum). For this reason, psychological factors are inevitably involved in management.

Cognitive aspects of pain
Cognition has been defined as, "a generic term, embracing the quality of knowing, which involves perceiving, recognising, conceiving, judging, sensing, reasoning and imagining". This lengthy definition illustrates the complexity of cognitive considerations[1].

Can cognition be shown to be an effective form of treatment?
It has been shown that instructions can affect pain reactions. When patients were asked to imagine they would receive one thousand dollars if they delayed shouting "stop" while receiving electrical pain stimulation, they increased pain tolerance and pain sensitivity range compared with a group not so instructed[2]. A number of other 'instructional' series have shown this to be an effective strategy[3,4].

The results of another series, involving a variety of different techniques, indicated that relaxation training produced an increased pain tolerance, while distraction and image retaining resulted in a higher pain threshold score[5]. Self-statements did not result in any significant main effects or interactions, and in fact reduced the effectiveness of distraction and imagery used. It appears that, while effective, what has been replicated in other studies is that not all reinterpretive or imagery strategies necessarily lead to reduced pain reaction. For example, in 1972 it was found that hypnotic analgesia plus pleasant imagery conditioning was not as effective as an analgesia suggestion alone in modifying tolerance[6].

When using any strategy, it must fit the context and be accepted by the person involved. "What is acceptable and relaxing to one person may produce tension and aversion in another."[78, p.164] This illustrates that, while cognitive treatments can be effective, like so many other treatments, they are unpredictably so[7,8].

Psychological theory – control
Dissonance and attribution theory have been considered in the past, but of particular interest over recent years has been 'control' as a concept[9,10]. Despite much work, the issue of control and predictability, as for many other areas of pain perception, is not entirely clear[11–14].

Turk defined six major categories of cognitive strategy[15].
1. Imaginative inattention.
2. Imaginative transformation of pain.
3. Imaginative transformation of context.
4. Attention diversion, external.
5. Attention diversion, internal.
6. Sensitization.

Turk's survey revealed that there were 15 studies showing more effective pain tolerance for cognitive strategy, while 12 studies showed that these strategies were not superior to control groups, and later studies reviewed by Tann support these conclusions[16].

Comment
The variety of these results again demonstrates unpredictability.

Problems of clinical studies

The problems of pain assessment in the laboratory and clinical context are reviewed elsewhere (see p. 251). It is important to note the type of study control groups used to follow up results. Of the 13 studies reviewed by Turner and Chapman, only 5 were controlled, and 8 had follow-up reports varying from 5 weeks to 12 months[17].

The number of patients studied in these series varied from 1 to 11[18-22]. This shows that, not only are the numbers small, but they vary widely, with inevitable consequences for predictability.

In a study on tension headache patients in four groups, a cognitive self-control group focussed upon maladaptive cognitive responses that mediated tension headache[23]. Patients were taught to find the cues that triggered tension and anxiety, and were taught cognitive strategy to interrupt them. The second group was provided with cognitive self-control plus progressive relaxation. The third group used discussion techniques to focus on symptoms, without being provided with any coping skills. The fourth group was a monitoring no-treatment control. The treatment groups showed significant reduction in headache activity compared with the control group, but no differences between groups. This study raises significant questions regarding just what are the important ingredients in treatment.

"These studies, as well as others not mentioned, support the effectiveness of cognitive strategies in clinical settings. What remains clear, or remains unclear, however, is what the critical ingredients should be, as many of the studies used combined procedures or did not have control groups. Dependent measures also are not used consistently across studies, leaving doubt as to what outcomes can be expected."[78, p.168]

Practical clinical consequences

In view of this material, cognition is clearly relevant, but its practical use remains empirical, as with so many treatments (see p. 270).

Behavioural aspects of pain

Behaviourism

As a concept, this is derived from experimental physiological psychology, including Pavlovian conditioning, and it is an endeavour to present psychology as far as possible as a natural science.

It is a reaction against the 'mentalism' of both philosophical psychology and psychoanalysis.

It focuses on acts that can be observed, and avoids speculation on motivation and affect, save as hypotheses to be tested experimentally.

Analysis of pain behaviour
Pain behaviour is usually classified in two groups.
1a. Respondent pain behaviour is that which is elicited by antecedent noxious stimuli or injury signals.
1b. Respondent behaviour may include reflex autonomic responses, such as cardiovascular changes, pupillary dilatation, sweating, etc. It may also include muscle spasm, gasping and similar automatic or reflex-like responses. These behaviours can be conditioned: for example, the mere sight of a nurse with a syringe may evoke acute pain behaviours.
2a. Operant pain behaviour is that which is reinforced by subsequent environmental effects.
2b. Operant behaviours are, for example, inactivity, medication use and complaints of pain.

Pain behaviours
These are:
1. The result of pain.
2. Determined by environmental consequences, such as taking to bed, taking analgesics, etc.
3. They will disappear or persist depending upon the reinforcement, whether this be positive of negative, or whether a positive reinforcement is absent.

Features of reinforcement
They are initially temporary. Once behaviour has started to come under control of environmental factors, reinforcements may vary it.
   If behaviour is to become persistent, reinforcement has to be initially consistent, but thereafter its rate may become intermittent[24]. Positive reinforcements include sympathetic attention, bed-rest and the use of analgesics.
   Avoidant behaviour acts as an indirect positive reinforcement by avoiding situations or circumstances likely to give rise to pain. This is a frequently encountered problem, and the generation of avoidant behaviour is rapid and its maintenance all to easy with only sporadic reinforcement.

Comparison between behaviour and cognition
Those who 'believe in' cognition assert that, "If one alters the experience then behavioural changes will follow. Specifically, if one can abolish or significantly reduce the pain as experienced, then invalidism, hypochondriacy, drug taking and all the rest of the chronic pain behaviours will disappear or diminish significantly. First change the experience [they would say] and the rest will follow."

The behaviourists believe the reverse. Change the behaviour and changes in subjective experience will follow. If pain behaviour is eliminated patients will feel little or no pain. 'Feelings' are a matter for speculation and behaviour alone is real and verifiable.

These differences in principle are fundamental, but in fact have been amalgamated in cognitive behavioural therapy.

Practical clinical consequences

The importance we place on behavioural considerations in case analysis is stressed elsewhere (see Case Analysis, p. 160).

Pure behavioural treatment has produced impressive results in the treatment of chronic pain. In practice, however, such treatment is extremely rare, as most clinicians acknowledge the significance of cognitive and affective factors and regard all three as being inextricably intertwined.

Emotional aspects of pain

Clinical relevance

Several analytical studies have indicated that emotional factors commonly account for the greatest variance in meaningful components extracted from patients' descriptions of both back pain and experimental electric shock stimulation[25,26].

Analyses of a number of major pain syndromes have led to interesting conclusions regarding the role of emotion in pain. It has been observed that pain severity is worse in some syndromes than in others, but that this variation is small[27].

It has been observed that high-intensity chronic back pain and cancer pain are associated with particularly high emotional loadings[28].

It is also shown that migraine and tension headaches can be distinguished on a variety of sensory and emotional scales on the McGill Pain Questionnaire[29]. However, given the great difficulties of taxonomy with regard to these two conditions, this finding has to be viewed with some caution (see Clinical Presentations, p.167).

Pain anticipation and emotion

The anticipation of pain and a reaction to it are not unique to human beings. However, foresight contributes to greater rumination over diminished capacities and thwarted goals, as well as anxious anticipation of prolonged distress, physical disabilities, disfigurement and death[30].

Added to the various morbid psychological states already described is the psychological impact of non-painful symptoms and the consequences of injuries and diseases, such as immobilization, nausea, vomiting and diarrhoea.

In addition, the emotional and behavioural damage can be further compounded by reactions to painful treatment. People with severe intractable pain appear particularly susceptible to these added components of mental anguish[31].

Emotional processes are most conspicuous when renewed or more severe pain is anticipated. Impending threats can precipitate dispassionate preparation or serious distress in the form of disorganized hysterical behaviour, inappropriate avoidance strategies or substantial physiological arousal.

In these circumstances, an observer can know that adequate nociceptive input for intense emotional expression does not exist, yet observe a vigorous display of distress that seems the same as that from a response to severe noxious input. This behaviour can be put to use, for example in preparation for painful medical or dental procedures[32].

In contrast, apprehension of severe pain can have serious debilitating effects, including substantial fear, behavioural disorganization, denial of somatic problems and a refusal to seek care. For this reason, explanation is of great importance in management. Distress in these circumstances is a matter demanding recognition and therapeutic attention.

Distress as an enhancer of pain
There is some evidence in support of this idea.

Chronically anxious and depressed people appear particularly vulnerable to pain. Indeed, pharmacological and behavioural procedures which decrease anxiety and depression often substantially reduce clinical pain.

It has been observed that low back pain patients who were psychologically disturbed had a higher incidence of recent distressful life events than had patients who were not disturbed[33].

It has also been observed that unhappy childhoods, premarital personality problems and current marital problems were more characteristic in chronic pain patients without demonstrable organic pathology than in those with organic lesions accounting for their pain[34].

It is also noteworthy that stress reduction or avoidance (e.g. from vocational or domestic duties) as a consequence of pain complaints may promote or reinforce the pain behaviour[35].

Distress as a precipitator of pain
Distress may also precipitate pain complaints because they provide a legitimate access to sources of care[36]. Pain patients frequently deny personal and interpersonal distress, despite substantial manifest evidence, and emphasize their somatic problems. This pattern has been identified as prognostic of poor success with conventional medical care[37].

Thus, psychological processes cannot be ignored, even if there is an organic basis for pain disorders.

Pain behaviour and emotional components

The extraordinary efforts to protect oneself which are associated with the anticipation of pain are matched by increasing demands for care, as the distress occasioned by pain increases.

The emotional component of pain appears to be intimately related to motivational properties, appearing to activate efforts to take care of oneself[38].

Among headache patients, it has been noted that, the stronger the distress, the more the complaints and pill taking[39].

Cognitive appraisal and emotional aspects of pain

The emotional intensity and quality of pain experiences have come to be recognized as interacting within the individual's interpretation and appraisal of events that precipitate pain, the nature of the disorder and its impact on their lives[40,41].

For example, it has been observed that severe wounds suffered by soldiers in battle and civilians in accidents led to striking differences in pain behaviour. The soldiers complained and demanded care far less than the civilians, apparently because the injury signalled escape from the life threatening demands of battle and the return home. However, injury and hospitalization were construed by the civilians as representing a severe threat to comfortable established lives. This study provided dramatic evidence that cognitive appraisal affected both emotional responses during pain and the manner in which the individual responded to the demands of injury and disease[42]. The significance of affect in pain has been well known for a very long time. In 1580, Montaigne, wrote, "Nous sentons plus un coup de razoir du Chirurgien que dix coups d'Épée en la chaleur du combat". We feel the cut of the barber's razor more keenly than ten sword wounds received in the heat of battle.

Evidence now indicates that people in pain eagerly, and sometimes desperately, search for information that would give meaning to the experience, provide relief and enhance recovery[43]. Since erroneous expectations about pain tend to precipitate emotional distress, techniques to provide accurate information about the impact of physical trauma have proved to be effective in avoiding and reducing stress for children and adults about to undergo noxious diagnostic or therapeutic procedures[44].

Idiosyncratic styles of interpreting the meaning of painful experiences influence the emotional immpact. Thus low back pain patients who are also depressed have been found to systematically misinterpret or distort the

94

nature and significance of their dilemma, and to interpret it in a negative way[45]. In this investigation, cognitive errors were:

1. Catastrophizing – anticipating or misinterpreting events as being disproportionately severe.
2. Over-generalizing – assuming the outcome of different experiences will be the same.
3. Selective abstracting – selectively attending to negative aspects of experience.

These are particularly prominent when the depressed low back pain patients are focussing on their disorder. It emphasizes the relevance of psychological factors to the musculoskeletal clinician – they cannot be ignored. The consequence of this with regard to chronic pain is that much clinical time has to be spent in finding out how accurate is the patient's appraisal of his condition and in correcting the inaccuracies.

The effect of various therapies on the emotional component of pain

Psychological and physical intervention strategies may influence one component and not another[46]. For example, various analgesic interventions appear to moderate the severity of distress, leaving sensory qualities relatively unaffected[44].

Frequent reports of the potent impact of prefrontal leucotomy, hypo-analgesia and opiate analgesics on the emotional rather than the sensory qualities of pain led Barber to conclude, "apparently the sensation of pain in itself is not necessarily 'painful'".[46] Thus analgesic procedures may yield effects by reducing or eliminating emotional discomfort, rather than by changing somatosomatic experience.

Again, Gracely's series comparing the action of diazepam with fentanyl showed, "This finding contradicts the prevalent assumption that narcotics produce analgesia primarily by influencing emotional discomforts"[47].

Practical clinical consequences

A multidimensional approach will reveal a complex organization of sensory, emotional, motivational and cognitive systems that dynamically interact in any pain experience.

The relevant emotional processes are themselves complex. The evidence is clear that therapeutic interventions designed to reduce or eliminate pain in fact influence a number of the components of the response. The distinction between sensory and emotional qualities is most pertinent here. It would seem (perhaps more frequently than has been acknowledged) that the impact of analgesic agents has been to change emotional qualities of fear, anxiety and depression, rather than to achieve sensory attenuation.

Psychotherapy may work by the provision of support and reassurance.

Many psychoactive drugs serve to reduce anxiety, while antidepressant drugs reduce emotional distress, rather than affecting sensory components.

Relaxation training, distraction strategies and biofeedback may disrupt the pain/anxiety/tension cycle. Placebos may reduce anxiety. Surgical strategies, including prefrontal lobotomies, appear to interrupt destructive moods and emotional distress.

Psychological aspects of acute and chronic pain

The distinction between these two states is important. They present different features and radically different problems for clinical management. An analogy may be drawn here with the physiology of pain (see The Dorsal Horn, p.45).

The functions of pain

In the acute phase, pain is usually thought of as a warning signal of potential injury. It also may be an accompaniment to recovery from abrupt injury, and may serve to enforce rest or still behaviour. From the medical point of view, acute pain may be thought of both as a sensation of actual or impending injury and as a need state for rest. Thus pain for stillness may also be basic for survival[48].

With regard to chronic pain, the situation is quite different. It was described by Leriche in 1939, ". . . reaction or defence? Fortunate warning? But as a matter of fact, the majority of diseases, even the most serious, attack us without warning . . . when pain develops . . . it is too late . . . the pain has only made more distressing and sad a situation already long lost . . . In fact pain is always a baneful gift, which reduces the subject of it, and makes him more ill than he would be without it"[49]. "Chronic pain is usually destructive physically, psychologically and socially."[50]

This has been best and most classically described by Weir Mitchell, describing a wounded soldier in the American Civil War.

"He begged at times to be killed, at others to go home . . . sometimes he would lie open-eyed, regarding furiously the passers-by who shook his bed as they walked, every movement seeming to add to his torment . . . Under active treatment the pain lessened but, . . . from being a man of gay and lively temper, known in his company as a good natured jester, he became morose and melancholy and complained that reading gave him vertigo, and that his memory of recent events was bad."[51]

The psychological consequences of pain

One classification of pain is temporal, dividing it into three forms, each of which appears to have different psychological features.

Phasic pain
This is of short duration and ordinarily occurs at the onset of injury. It is primarily characterized by withdrawal from the source of injury and patterns of verbal and non-verbal expressive behaviour recognizable as pain to observers[52]. (See the quotation from Montaigne given in the last chapter.) This reaction is not inevitable.

Acute pain
Nowhere is the relationship of injury to pain more variable than in the period immediately after acute injury[53].
Acute pain brought about by tissue damage comprises both phasic pain and a tonic stage which persists for variable periods of time until healing takes place. Acute tissue damage tends to provoke fear and anxious concern for oneself. If the damage or the source of distress persists, the pain can come to be perceived as unbearable and uncontrollable, and very high levels of anxiety can be precipitated.

Chronic pain
This persists beyond the period of time required for healing, and it is most destructive because of its potential for substantial impact on the psychological and social well-being of the patient.
The longer the pain persists, the greater the probability that the patient will become fearful, irritable, somatically preoccupied, erratic in the search for relief and, above all, depressed[36,54].
These changes affect not only the patient but others concerned with him or her, including the family, friends, employer and health care professionals[55].
While depression may be severe, in chronic pain it has been observed that only 10% of a continuous series of chronic pain patients presenting to a pain clinic displayed depressive symptoms, and the sample's mean depression score was low, as compared with a psychiatric patient sample[56].
In another series, 83 pain clinic patients, (all with demonstrable physical lesions) had a mean score on the questionnaire of 7.13, which placed them in the non-depressed group. Even 12 patients who were receiving tricyclic anti-depressants were also in this category. Thus, although occasional cases of depression are recognized in pain clinic patients, they are generally identified more often with pain in psychiatric populations, and even then are present in only a minority of the psychiatric patients with pain[57].

Practical clinical consequences
While acute pain is clearly accompanied by psychological changes, these resolve on resolution of the pain. In contrast, the psychological consequence

of chronic pain is that its very chronicity determines the degree of neuroticism, rather than the source or nature of the pain. The fact that 10% of pain clinic patients have treatable depression shows that, while a relatively minor factor, it should not be ignored.

Miscellaneous psychological features of musculoskeletal interest
Is there a correlation between personality and pain?

Many authors (over 30 were listed in a study in 1967) have commented on these[58]. They are said to include particularly guilt, resentment, hostility, multiple somatic complaints, excessive consultations and numerous operations.

Many such reports are anecdotal, but there has been demonstrated an increased frequency of surgery in psychiatric patients with pain, and increased frequency of resentment in the same group, compared with those without pain[59,60]. The marital relationships of such people have been noted to be disturbed[60].

Among other theories advanced, it has been maintained that many patients can only adapt themselves to life by reason of having a traumatic social or personal relationship, such as a bad marriage in which they played a masochistic role or by suffering from pain[61,62].

Such views tend to be speculative and are not supported by controlled evidence.

Cultural influences on pain behaviour
These have been much discussed and are significant. However, they seem capable of manipulation. For example, "especially impressive was the marked change in behaviour in Italian parturients in a large obstetric centre in Turin, noted between two visits made five years apart. During the first visit, in 1954, the labour ward was a sea of cacophony, caused by the screaming, pleading and praying of nearly 50 labouring women. In contrast, five years later, one heard only an occasional moan from a similar number of parturients who had had an intensive course of psychoprophylaxis. Most went through the entire labour and delivery with minimal pain and pain behaviour, but later stated that they had had moderate to severe pain"[63].

While cultural differences may exist, this shows quite clearly that they may be modified.

Psychological mechanisms of pain
Psychological problems as a cause of pain have been mentioned elsewhere (see p.93). Mechanisms that have been proposed are perhaps somewhat tenuous, but they should be considered.

The first occurs where anxiety concerning a physical lesion actually increases the pain. The mechanism of this effect is unknown, but it has frequently been observed. It would conform with the gate theory, in that effects transmitted down through descending pathways might increase the pain. It is certainly a fact that pain in clinical practice is frequently much relieved by measures which relieve the patient's anxiety about the provocative lesion. All this, however, is speculation.

Pain may also at times, though very rarely, be due to psychotic hallucination. The most clear cut and the most rare example of this is schizophrenia. Schizophrenic hallucinations are almost never concerned with pain. Schizophrenics frequently have body experiences of other people doing things to them, such as hypnotizing them, influencing them with rays, and so on, but it is astonishing how rarely they indicate that these bodily changes are painful. In a series of 78 patients with schizophrenia, only one was found whose pain might be attributed to her delusion, and, as it happens, this patient was suffering from an atypical form of the disease[64].

This is of particular interest to musculoskeletal practitioners because some clinicians, using mobility testing, have found 'abnormalities in 9 out of 25 cases of schizophrenia. This seems to be a striking discrepancy, and it must be noted that the diagnostic procedures used in mobility testing are wholly subjective. This reinforces our reservations, expressed elsewhere, with regard to the validity of such tests.

It further demonstrates the extreme importance of taking a multidisciplinary approach to musculoskeletal problems, because relevant clinical information may be found, and therefore should be sought, in all associated disciplines.

Discrimination between organic and non-organic pain
Such studies, using, for example, the Minnesota Multiphasic Personality Inventory (MMPI) scores, are rather few or slight. However, these have been successfully used to predict which patients would respond to somatic treatment, e.g. chemonucleolysis or surgery, or to conservative therapies[65-69]. However, there are those who do not accept the validity of these studies.

It has been shown that there are occasions when such distinctions can be made on the basis of the patient's response to the adjectival checklists of the McGill Pain Questionnaire (MPQ)[70].

It has been shown that patients who do not have a detectable lesion, but who do not have psychiatric illness either, use language that suggests that they fall into the group of patients with organic lesions not yet discovered[70].

The diagnostic value of such findings seems currently rather limited (see Discriminant Validity, p.100).

In the past numerous patients have been dismissed as not exhibiting abnormal physical signs as a direct result of those signs having not been sought by reason of their being unknown. In manipulative practice, for example, it is common to see patients with headache of vertebral origin who have been labelled neurotic, who do in fact exhibit the local signs described in basic case analysis (see p.151 *et seq.*).

Pain patterns which may be recognized in patients whose pain is primarily of psychological origin
Such pain is more common in women than in men.

In men it will often be associated with a disability that has occurred at work, and where there is an element of compensation. In chronic pain of psychological origin, the pain is usually severe. The pain is frequently felt in more than one part of the body, and this feature, in the absence of a well-recognized organic diagnosis, is significant.

The pain is bilateral or symmetrical in half the patients, and there is a tendency revealed in some studies for it to be commoner on the left side[71].

Psychological pain is usually continuously present, rather than having irregular fluctuations. It hardly ever keeps the patient awake at night and rarely, if ever, awakens him from sleep. If this occurs, it is a strong pointer to there being an organic component.

Physical factors sometimes relieve pain, even if it is of psychological origin. Mild analgesics, heat or cold may help. The response never appears to be great, or at least not for long. Nevertheless, this is yet another indication of the complexity of this problem, both diagnostic and in management.

It will be seen that this is of little practical help to the musculoskeletal clinician, because, as these points show, such a distinction is difficult to establish with any certainty. Nonetheless, he should be aware of the problems and complexities.

Pain and illness behaviour
Introduction
Illness behaviour has been defined as the way in which individuals think, feel and act in relation to their health status. Thus, clinically, pain and illness behaviours are inseparable, and self-report can present only a part of the whole picture[72].

Illness behaviours may be divided into adaptive and pathological. The latter is termed abnormal illness behaviour (AIB) and becomes clinically significant when there appears to be a marked discrepancy between the patient's behaviour and identified pathology[73,74].

The determinants of illness behaviour
These are cognitive, emotional and behavioural.

100

Abnormal illness behaviour

This has been defined as the persistence of an inappropriate or maladaptive mode of perceiving, evaluating and acting in relation to one's own state of health, despite the fact that a doctor (or other appropriate social agent) has offered a reasonably lucid explanation of the nature of the illness, and the appropriate course to be followed, based on a thorough examination and assessment of all parameters of functioning (including the use of special investigations) and taking into account the individual's age, educational and sociocultural background.

This is best appreciated placed in the context of the concept of the 'sick role'. This is conditionally granted to individuals who show evidence of a state or disease over which they have no control, and which brings them little benefit compared with the suffering and loss of pleasures they are experiencing. Those accorded the 'sick role' are exempted from the discharge of their usual duties to an extent appropriate to the nature of their disease. For a period, therefore, the individual is granted special privileges, but these are graded and withdrawn by degrees, as the disease is resolved.

This brings up a distinction between illness and disease. Illness has been defined as, "an organismic state which fulfills the requirements of a relevant reference group for admission to the sick role"[74]. Abnormal illness behaviour is considered an illness when the motivation seems predominantly unconscious. When conscious, it is labelled malingering.

AIB classification
Psychotic AIB
1. Depressive psychosis. This can involve hypochondriacal illusions, for example in the unshakeable belief the patient has cancer.
2. Schizophrenia with pain. This may also involve hypochondriacal and somatic illusions, but, as has been observed above, it is extremely rare.

Neurotic AIB
1. Hypochondriacal reactions. These are characterized by an over concern with health, out of proportion to the degree of objective pathology identified.
2. A phobic attitude towards illness. This is a situation in which a patient focusses on the symptoms and, for example, is convinced that chest pains and palpitations are indicative of heart disease, or that headaches mean a brain tumour.
3. A conviction as to the presence of disease associated with a non-response to reassurance.
4. A preoccupation with bodily symptoms.

5. Conversion reactions. Here the patient denies preoccupation or fears about illness, but rather complains of pain and the consequences of the symptom.

Illness behaviour assessment

Many patients show a mixture of features. To facilitate evaluation, an illness behaviour assessment schedule (IBAS) has been evolved. This is a method of assessing both the patient's and the doctor's views of the patient's health status. It can also serve as a check list to ensure that areas relevant to the diagnosis have been covered, whilst providing information concerning cognition and emotion.

The IBAS format is:

Items 1 to 6. The patient's perception of the information he has received, and his acceptance of it.

Items 7 to 8. His ideas of the type of illness he has.

Items 9 to 11. His awareness of symptoms and associated preoccupations or phobic attitudes.

Item 12. His idea about aetiology.

Items 13 to 19. His emotional state and the extent to which somatic illness is being used defensively.

This offers a basis on which to establish whether a patient is showing clear-cut abnormal illness behaviour. It also allows (items 14 and 15) a means of evaluation between anxiety and depression.

Illness behaviour questionnaire

Another approach to assessment is the illness behaviour questionnaire (IBQ). This consists of seven scales.

1. General hypochondriasis (GH). High scorers on this scale have fearful or phobic attitudes to illness, with some insight into the inappropriateness of these attitudes and a higher level of arousal or anxiety.
2. Disease conviction (DC). High scores indicate a strong affirmation as to the presence of physical illness and resistance to reassurance by doctors.
3. Psychological versus somatic perception of illness (P/S). High scorers exhibit a tendency to blame themselves for the illness, and to be accepting of the need for psychiatric help. A low score indicates the rejection of the possibility that psychological factors are important and a tendency to focus on somatic problems.
4. Affective (emotional) inhibition (AI). High scores indicate a difficulty in expressing personal feelings to others.
5. Affective (emotional) disturbance (AD). A high score indicates the presence of feelings of anxiety and depression.

6. Denial (D). High scores on this scale indicate that the subject denies current life problems and, in addition, attributes his situation entirely to physical illness.
7. Irritability (I). High scores on this scale indicate feelings of anger and an awareness of interpersonal friction.

This is currently used in the study of chronic pain syndromes and other conditions.

Practical clinical consequences

Abnormal illness behaviour, defined as a marked discrepancy between physical findings identified and pain behaviour, does exist, and musculo-skeletal clinicians should therefore be aware of this. If suspected, the patient should be referred appropriately.

Pain assessment

Objectives

1. Case analysis, with a view to selecting the most appropriate treatment.
2. a. Monitoring pain fluctuation during treatment, and so not having to depend upon retrospection, so often fraught with bias.
   b. Reliable monitoring of the pain, which permits controlling features to be identified. Because pain relief is seldom total (particularly in chronic pain patients) measurement may identify the degree and nature of the change that is brought about by treatment.
3. Evaluation of treatment efficacy, so that treatment and its specific effects can be distinguished from the non-specific placebo effects well documented in pain[75].

Features of pain relating to clinical assessment

Suffice it to say here that it is now recognized that pain is a complex experience, with evidence confirming that it involves variation in several dimensions, depending on ever-changing states, continuously influenced by a multitude of extrinsic and intrinsic stimuli[76].

Four main components have been described: nociception, sensation, suffering and behaviour[77].

This model discards the notion of a linear relationship between the amount of noxious input and the intensity of the pain experienced.

Comparison between laboratory and clinical conditions

There is a lack of emotional and cognitive connotation surrounding experimentally induced pain.

In the laboratory it is possible to measure the pain stimulus and thereby relate subjective report to the amount of stimulation in a way that is not generally possible in the clinic.

While placebos are effective in approximately 35% of cases in a clinic, this is reduced to 3.2% in the laboratory. The missing ingredient in the laboratory is the anxiety associated with the disease process; reduced pain reactions in the clinic often result from reducing anxiety[78].

The laboratory presents a different context within which the complexity of the pain response is partially ignored. In the laboratory the pain is of short duration, with no concern for effectiveness following the termination of the experimental session. In the clinic, treatment often involves chronic pain, so that long-term follow-up studies are of great importance. Simply reducing pain during treatment is far from adequate.

With regard to treatment, the laboratory setting permits readier separation of treatment and no-treatment control groups. The clinical setting, in which there is a live suffering patient, demands that practitioners do not withhold treatment.

Multiple input strategies are common in the clinical setting, so that it is not always possible to know exactly what has been manipulated, or what is the ingredient that seems to be crucial.

No-treatment control patients, aside from the ethical issues of non-treatment, will not be content to sit by idly, simply asking questions. They will seek help elsewhere.

Placebo control groups cannot be seen as non-intervention controls, since placebo intervention can of itself produce powerful effects and even long-term therapeutic success[41]. For example, it has been demonstrated that two mock equilibrations for myofascial pain dysfunction syndrome were effective in producing total or near total remission of symptoms in 16 out of 25 patients. 13 of the patients for whom follow-up proved possible remained symptom free 6 to 29 months later[79].

But, "Laboratory pain in induction methods have helped to increase our understanding and knowledge of pain mechanisms in man . . . Laboratory induced pain response parameters are useful for human analgesic assays of drugs and other pain relieving treatment modalities, such as acupuncture, transcutaneous electrical nerve stimulation, hypnosis, relaxation and cognitive strategies. In short, laboratory pain induction methods in normal man have become important tools in furthering our knowledge and understanding of pain mechanisms."[80]

Pain parameters

There are three main parameters to be considered here; subject report, behavioural assessment and physiological assessment.

Subject report

This is unique. "Accurate appraisal of the biochemical, neuronal and psychological mechanisms of pain and analgesia depends heavily on the assessment of pain in human subjects. Man's unique verbal abilities open the window to private experience, and only through such an experience is pain defined."[81]

Abandoning the idea of a one-to-one relationship between sensory input and the amount of pain expressed subjectively or behaviourally evades the question as to whether the pain," is real or is all in the mind".

Such an outmoded view can create problems.

1. The patient's complaints may be taken at face value and aggressive therapy instituted.
2. Alternatively, such a presentation may be taken as indicative of a psychological 'overlay', and the patient referred for psychotherapy[76].

A multidisciplinary approach has much to commend it. "Various analgesic interventions appear to moderate the severity of affective distress, leaving sensory qualities relatively unaffected. . . . Thus analgesic procedures may yield effects by reducing or eliminating affective discomfort, rather than by changing aesthetic experience."[46]

It can be seen that, not only is assessment multidisciplinary, but many of the treatments involved in the management of pain themselves intrude into several clinical fields, other than those to which they were initially or primarily directed.

Thus there is no justification for the fact that traditionally, "doctors and patients become extremely angry with each other when there is a mismatch between disease and the amount of pain which the doctor expects, especially if the patient has the impertinence to fail to respond to his expected therapy. At this point the doctor begins to question if the pain is real or in the mind. What is this curious question asked by the observer, but never by the person in pain?"[82]

Subject report procedures

It is clearly impossible to take a clinical history without resort to verbal report. The patient's statements are used to gauge both the severity of the pain and its qualitative nature, since the language used may convey to the clinician an indication of the kind of injury or damage. For example, the use of 'burning' may be related to nerve injury, while 'aching' may refer to a more visceral complaint[83]. But, "to describe pain solely in terms of intensity is like specifying the visual world in terms of light flux, without regard to pattern, colour, texture and the many other dimensions of the visual experience"[27].

The limitation of self-report extends to the diagnostic problem of coming to know and understand another person's pain experience. Communications of pain appeal to the observer's ability to match the message with memories of his own experiences and contacts with other people expressing similar distress[84]. Those in a position to act upon the reports of another's distress are obliged to presume at least strong similarities between their own and the suffering person's experiences. This assumes experiences that can overlap only partially[85].

The difficulties of subjective report have been aptly put by a worker from another field. "The problem, however, starts earlier. The communication between a patient and his physicians. This is where it starts and where information has to be obtained. Its limits are best illustrated with lesions of the afferent system, such as for instance in regenerating nerves. Many prominent investigators, dissatisfied with the unintelligible verbalisations of the sensory experiences of their patients, were sufficiently fascinated by the problem to submit to having their own nerves crushed or cut and resutured, in order to observe and describe the sensory experiences during the subsequent stages of re-innervation. Starting in 1905, these experiments were repeated by many in the subsequent 60 years. None of these investigators ever agreed with each other, thereby demonstrating that it is impossible to convey the contents of a distorted message to an outside observer .... the textbooks, however, ignore this whole episode."[86]

The assessment of verbal reporting

In this a number of difficulties are encountered. The report may be subject to response bias or falsification. The report of pain may not be proportional to the severity of the noxious stimulus. Verbal report may be discordant with other indices. Assessment itself may have a reactive effect in terms of sensitizing the patient to the pain and so affecting the rating given[87].

These problems have seemed to some to be insurmountable. For example, some have drawn attention to the similar anatomical pathways of pain thought to give rise to distinctive experiences. Others, behaviourists, have concluded that pain language was confounded by too many unidentified variables to be of diagnostic use. "Such extreme positions ignore the possibility of concommitant monitoring across response channels and the fact that the clinical utility of each measure or response channel investigated will need to be established empirically rather than assumed, since it will vary according to the circumstances of the investigation."[87]

Many somatically orientated physicians are alert to the difficulties of using the site of vertebral pain for diagnostic purposes; for them the fact that some authorities regard pain language as being useless from a diagnostic point of view will come as an unpleasant surprise. This is discussed in greater detail in Case Analysis, p.151.

Rating scales
These are the most commonly reported measures in clinical pain research. Examples are verbal rating scales (VRS) and visual analogue scales (VAS). Their use presents certain problems.

They are linear, and therefore only one aspect of pain is consistently recorded.

With regard to time variations, memory capacity is an individual function, and anyway pain often fluctuates.

Low reliability may reflect poor sensitivity of a single rating scale. However, reliability is likely to be increased if a number of judgements is used for each dimension under study.

The more complex the task, the more likely is distortion. One study comparing the VRS and VAS scales assumed that the tendency for visual analogue scales to yield more uniform distribution was a reflection of their superior sensitivity[88]. However, this has been criticized, since the psychophysical literature suggests a tendency for responses to be spread over a constrained response range, regardless of intensity, spacing or frequency of the underlying stimulus continuum[89].

Studies have been undertaken on the degre to which various rating scales (visual, verbal or numerical) influence the responses obtained. Results vary. In one study, comparing VRS with VAS, the authors concluded that the VAS "reflected more precisely what a patient actually feels than the VRS."[90] A second study on the two scales revealed few differences[91], while a third study, comparing visual, adjectival and numerical scales, found a consistent preference for the adjectival scale[92]. Thus results are, indeed, far from uniform; consensus remains beyond our reach.

Correlation between scales has been studied, since scales tapping the same dimensions would be expected to be highly correlated. Such high correlations have been generally reported[93-95], but one problem is that these have been due to the operation of a 'halo effect', whereby the rating on the first scale dominated those provided on subsequent ones.

The principal objection to all these endeavours is that they are unidimensional and therefore fail to reflect the complexity of the pain experience, with its sensory, emotional and evaluative components[83].

Cross modality matching
Tursky devised scales reflecting sensory, emotional and reaction verbal descriptors, and these were subsequently extended using scales of sensory intensity, unpleasantness and painfulness[83]. This method reflects only the intensity of the sensations recorded, but it does offer a means, despite ignoring qualitative differences, of comparing measures in clinical and experimental pain.

One study using these techniques has demonstrated that values asssigned to the words within each scale are consistent, both within and between individual subjects[96].

Gracely *et al.* generated independent ratio scales of sensory and emotional pain descriptors that are differentially sensitive to placebo, tranquillizer and narcotic intervention. A minor tranquillizer (diazepam) aimed specifically at emotional distress generated by experimentally induced pain, resulted in changes in the use of emotional but not sensory pain descriptors. In contrast, the narcotic (fentanyl) was found substantially to reduce the sensory intensity, but not the unpleasantness of experimentally induced pain[47].

Other work in the assessment of chronic or facial pain patients, requiring them to match electrical stimulation of the tooth pulp to their clinical pain with various psychophysical methods, have shown that these methods are valid. "In practical terms, this work has demonstrated the utility of verbal scales which reflect different dimensions of the pain experience."[89]

It will be seen that this work would surprise clinicians who are not psychologically orientated, who may prescribe both narcotic and non-narcotic analgesics.

The McGill pain questionnaire (MPQ)

This consists of 78 adjectives, arranged in 20 groups, reflecting similar pain qualities within each group[97].

Using emotional, sensory and evaluatve descriptors, it is multidimensional and thereby is a departure from unidimensional rating scales[27].

Previous attempts have been made to systematize pain language in relation to the seriousness of the condition, the location of pain, and whether the pain is of psychiatric origin[98,99].

The MPQ, however, by imposing an organization of pain adjectives, achieves the objective of quantifying the language.

It has been frequently used in clinical evaluations[29,100–102] and in the laboratory[25,103]. It reflects three dimensions.

Sensory groups – 1 to 10
Emotional groups – 11 to 15 and 20
Evaluative groups – 16
The three remaining groups, 17 to 19, constitute a sensory miscellany.

The questionnaire uses a number of indices:
1. A pain rating index, based on the scale values of words checked, which can be computed for the total questionnaire and for each of the three subscales.

2. A rank score, reflecting the rank values in each subgroup of the words checked, can also be computed for the total and for each of the subscales.
3. The number of words checked.

Validity
Does the MPQ support the hypothesis of sensory, emotional and evaluative differences? Much work has been done in an effort to elucidate this.

One series produced results that were interpreted as suggesting that acute pain may involve less differentiation of the sensory, emotional and evaluative reaction to components than does chronic pain[94].

All studies confirm the distinction between sensory and emotional subgroups and lend support to the practice of deriving representative scale scores[104,105].

An evaluative or reactive component has also been distinguished, but less consistently.

The MPQ has been further investigated in relation to psychological state. The suggestion is made that patients with demonstrable depression or other indices of psychopathology should show distinctive profiles on the MPQ, and in particular on the emotional subscale. Work done led the authors of one study to conclude that the emotional scale of the MPQ showed satisfactory validity, since patients who had low scores on the emotional dimension of pain recorded significantly greater scores on depression, anxiety and somatization scales[106].

A similar series on cancer patients found differing results; but, on further work, it was found that those patients with pain resulting from cancer reported a reliably greater emotional component of their pain than did patients complaining of the same intensity of pain, whose pain was of benign origin[28].

Comment
Therefore the MPQ has validity.

Comparison with other methods
A number of series involving clinical and experimental work have shown that the magnitude of correlations obtained compares favourably with that obtained from comparisons on linear rating scales[29,94,103,104,107,108].

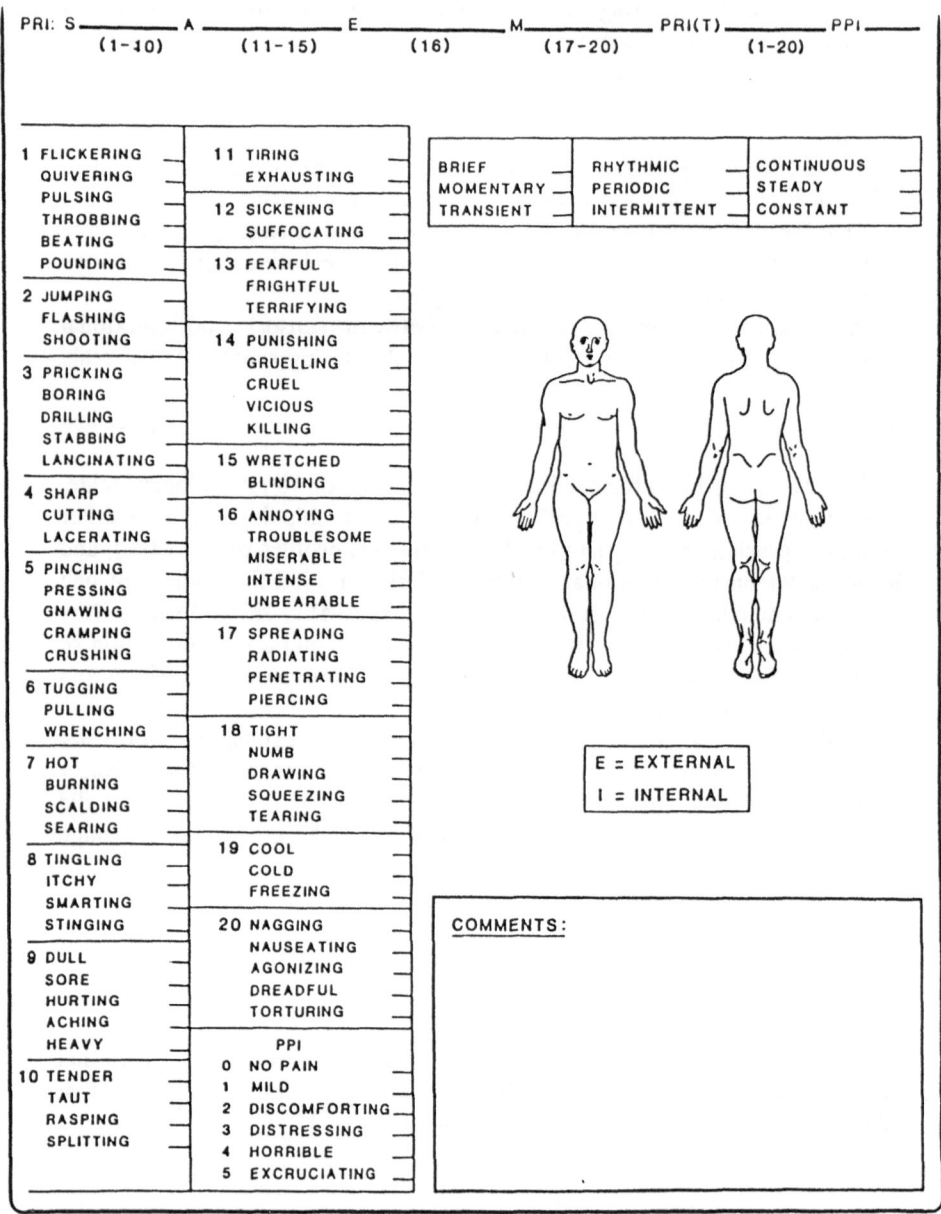

Figure 6.1 The McGill pain questionnaire

The diagnostic potential of the MPQ
A comparison of MPQ profiles of women experiencing chronic pelvic pain and postepisiotomy pain showed that acute pain patients displayed a greater use of sensory word groups testifying to sensory input for the damaged perineum. Chronic pain patients used emotional and reactive subgroups with greater frequency[94].

A further study, in a survey of 95 patients covering 8 clinical pain syndromes, generated functions yielding a direct classification of 77% on the basis of MPQ scores, although this figure may be overoptimistic in the absence of a validation sample[85].

In another series, results showed that the MPQ scores yielded higher direct classification rates than a checklist format, although the functions derived did not offer clinical utility[109].

A further series reviewed patients displaying greater psychological disturbance and showed higher numbers of words attracting higher rank scores[110]. It was concluded that the MPQ might be a useful means of measuring emotional disturbances secondary to pain, in chronic pain patients where the incidence of psychological difficulties is likely to be high[36].

Therefore, although the MPQ indeed offers discriminant validity, it does not provide the means for arriving at a valid diagnosis.

Behavioural assessments
Behaviour can be observed and thereby objectively measured or assessed. There are three main categories of behaviour assessment[111].

Somatic interventions, such as taking medication, seeking surgery or nerve blocks.

Impaired functioning, in terms of reduced mobility or range of movement, avoidance of occupational commitments, or impaired interpersonal relationships.

Pain complaints, in the form of moaning, contortions or facial expressions.

Behaviour assessment is particularly important because of the complexity of the pain experience, and subjective report (as has been shown) has limitations in case analysis. Subjective report and behavioural indices are not perfectly correlated.

In a study on the relationship between complaint behaviour and exercise in chronic pain patients, in order to test the assumption of the correlation between these two indices, consistently negative correlations between exercise rates and pain complaints emerged. Thus, for the chronic pain patients studied, the more exercises performed, the fewer the pain complaints and/or visible/audible expressions of pain[112].

A further series on self-reported behaviour, consisting of self-reporting avoidance and complaints by migraine and tension headache patients, related these indices to subjective pain reports. Correlations between behaviour and diary records of intensity, frequency and duration were low. The exception was medication rate, since this correlated with more frequent headaches. MPQ scores were correlated with behaviour, in particular avoidance correlated with the emotional dimension, medication rate with sensory pain, and complaint behaviour with both sensory and emotional scores. Personality and mood indices also related to behavioural parameters. The author suggested that concordance may become attenuated as chronicity increases, once again demonstrating that more intense pain does not necessarily imply more pain behaviour[29].

Discussing results obtained by using psychosocial pain inventory (PSPI) Sternbach writes, "this suggests that the extent to which pain behaviour comes under environmental influence may have little to do either with personality variables or with pain description, but rather with the laws of learning, according to which behaviour is governed by its consequence."[113]

Medication requirements can also be considered as a category of behavioural measurement, as these have been shown to be influenced by many factors other than the level of pain experienced. For example, it has been shown that the administration of analgesics by hospital staff is influenced by staff attitudes and the sex of the patient, in addition to the level of pain reported by the patient. This resulted in drugs being withheld from male patients on occasions when female patients tended to receive more powerful analgesics than were necessary. A study of the influence of personality on pain behaviour showed that patients who scored highly on extroversion scales were more likely to complain and receive more medication even though self-reported linear analogue scales suggested no greater subjective experience than for introverted patients[114].

A further interesting piece of work compared drug intake before and during hospital admission. In only 22% of the sample were the hospitalized patients taking less medication than previously reported. The trend as a whole was for patients to report less narcotic intake prior to admission than was actually requested during hospitalization[115].

This material demonstrates clearly the important fact that behavioural features are not only a reality, but are independent of subject report.

Physiological parameters of pain
"In general there would seem to be little basis for discrete physiological changes related to the pain experience."[87]

Conclusions

A distinction may be drawn between the three main response channels, subjective, physiological and behavioural, with each lending itself to further subdivisions.

Assumptions should not be made about the degree of concordance between these response channels, since varying levels of agreement will emerge, with relative importance attached to the verbal report or the behavioural indices, depending upon the setting.

Behavioural indices may assume greater importance as chronicity increases, and failure to monitor this may lead to errors.

Subjective report may be given greater credence in the initial evaluation. In chronic pain, the confining influence of response sets, reinforcing contingencies and emotional disturbance on pain reports are well known.

"In conclusion, the range of measures reviewed illustrates the absence of an ideal method to monitor and investigate pain mechanisms . . . Having accepted a complex dynamic model of pain, it follows that there is no ideal assessment method. A selection of dependent measures will be determined by the context in which the evaluation takes place and the clinical objectives. In general independent and parallel monitoring across the three main response channels will improve the information yield."[87]

Clinical conclusions to relevant psychology

It is apparent that the problems confronting the pain clinician, both diagnostic and therapeutic, are indeed complex. To clinicians from other disciplines the practical importance of psychological factors may come as something of a surprise. For example, "Even those patients with an objective basis for their chronic pain disability respond well to an operant pain management programme. Clearly psychological processes cannot be ignored, even if there is an organic basis for pain disorders".[55, p.158]

If the psychological features of low back pain are as marked as those of cancer pain, their relevance to the musculoskeletal clinician is inescapable.

Not to be aware of the limitations of subject report and the relevance of the behavioural aspects of pain assessment is bound to impair the value of history taking in case analysis.

References

1. Stedman (1976). *Medical Dictionary*. 23rd Edn. (Baltimore: Williams and Wilkins)
2. Wolff *et al.* (1965). Effect of suggestion upon experimental pain response parameters. *Perception Motor Skills*, 21, 675–683
3. Wolff and Horland (1967). Effect of suggestion upon experimental pain. A validation study. *J. Abnorm. Psychol.*, 72, 402–407
4. Blitz and Dinnerstein (1968). Effects of different types of instructions on pain parameters. *J. Abnorm. Psychol.*, 73, 276–280

5. Meichenbaum (1977). *Cognitive Behaviour Modification*. (New York: Plenum Press)
6. Greene and Reyher (1972). Pain tolerance in hypnotic analgesic and imagination states. *J. Abnorm. Psychol.*, **79**, 29–38
7. Worthington (1978). The effects of imagery content, choice of imagery content, and self verbalisation on the self control of pain. *Cognitive Ther. Res.*, **2**, 225–240
8. Scott (1978). Experimenter-suggested cognitions and pain control. *Psychol. Rep.*, **43**, 156–158
9. Zimbardo *et al.* (1966). Control of pain motivation by cognitive dissonants. *Science*, **151**, 217–219
10. Zimbardo *et al.* (1969). The control of experimental pain. In Zimbardo (ed.) *The Cognitive Control of Motivation*, p. 100. (Glenview. Ill.: Scott, Foreman)
11. Corah (1973). Effect of perceived control on stress reduction in paedodontic patients. *J. Dent. Res.*, **52**, 1261–1264
12. Geer *et al.* (1970). Reduction of stress in humans through non-veridical perceived control of aversive stimulation. *J. Pers. Soc. Psychol.*, **16**, 734–738
13. Glass *et al.* (1973). Perceived control of aversive stimulation. *J. Pers.*, **41**, 577–595
14. Melzack and Perry (1975). Self regulation of pain. The use of alpha feedback and hypnotic training for the control of chronic pain. *Exp. Neurol.*, **46**, 452–469
15. Turk (1978). Cognitive behavioural techniques in the management of pain. In Foreyt and Rathjen (eds.) *Cognitive Behaviour Therapy. Research and Application*, p. 199. (New York: Plenum Press)
16. Tan (1982). Cognitive and cognitive behavioural methods for pain control. A selective preview. *Pain*, **12**, 210–228
17. Turner and Chapman (1982). Psychological interventions for chronic pain. A critical review. 2. Operant conditioning, hypnosis and cognitive behavioural therapy. *Pain*, **12**, 23–46
18. Cantela (1977). The use of covert conditioning in modifying pain behaviour. *J Behav. Ther. Exp. Psychiatry*, **8**, 45–52
19. Rybstein-Blinchik and Grzesiak (1979). Reinterpretive cognitive strategies in chronic pain management. *Arch. Physical Med. Rehabil.*, **60**, 609–612
20. Stenn *et al.* (1979). Biofeedback and a cognitive behavioural approach to treatment of myofascial pain dysfunction syndrome. *Behav. Ther.*, **10**, 29–36
21. Hartman and Ainsworth (1980). Self regulation of chronic pain. *Can. J. Psychiatry*, **25**, 38–43
22. Wernick *et al.* (1981). Pain management in severely burnt adults. A test of stress innoculation. *J. Behav. Med.*, **4**, 103–109
23. Holroyd and Andrasik (1978). Coping and the self control of chronic tension headaches. *J. Consulting Clin. Psychol.*, **46**, 1036–1045
24. Ferster and Skinner (1957). *Schedules of Reinforcement*. (New York: Appleton-Century-Crofts).
25. Crockett *et al.* (1977). Factors of the language of pain in patient and volunteer groups. *Pain*, **4**, 175–182
26. Leavitt *et al.* (1978). Affective and sensory dimensions of back pain. *Pain*, **4**, 273–281
27. Melzack (1975). The McGill Pain Questionnaire. Major properties and scoring methods. *Pain*, **1**, 275–279
28. Kremer *et al.* (1982). Pain measurement. The affective and dimensional measure of the McGill Pain Questionnaire with a cancer population. *Pain*, **12**, 153–163
29. Hunter and Philips (1981). The experience of headache. An assessment of the qualities of tension headache pain. *Pain*, **10**, 209–219
30. Melzack and Dennis (1980). Phylogenetic evolution of pain expression in animals. In Kosterlitz and Terenius (eds.). *Pain and Society*, p. 13. (Weinheim: Verlag Chemie)
31. Bond (1980). The suffering of severe intractable pain. In ibid., p. 53
32. Melamed and Siegel (1980). *Behavioural Medicine. Practical Applications in Health Care*. (New York: Springer Verlag)
33. Leavitt *et al.* (1980). Psychological disturbance and life event differences among patients with low back pain. *J. Consulting Clin. Psychol.*, **48**, 115–116

34. Merskey and Boyd (1978). Emotional adjustment and chronic pain. *Pain*, **5**, 173–178
35. Fordyce (1976). *Behavioural Methods in Chronic Pain and Illness*. (St Louis, Mo.: C.V. Mosby)
36. Sternbach (1974). *Pain Patients. Traits and Treatments*. (New York: Academic Press)
37. Wilfling *et al.* (1973). Psychological demographic and orthopaedic factors associated with the prediction and outcome of spinal fusion. *Clin. Orthopaed.*, **90**, 153–160
38. Blendis *et al.* (1978). Abdominal pain and the emotions. *Pain*, **5**, 179–191
39. Philips (1982). The nature and treatment of chronic tension headache. In Craig and McMahon (eds.) *Advances in Clinical Behaviour Therapy*. (New York: Brunner, Mazel)
40. Turk *et al.* (1983). *Pain and Behavioural Medicine. Theory, Research and a Clinical Guide.* (New York: Guilford)
41. Weisenberg (1977). Pain and pain control. *Psychol. Bull.*, **84**, 1008–1044
42. Beecher (1959). *Measurement of Subjective Response. Quantitative Effects of Drugs*. (New York: Oxford University Press)
43. Craig (1978). Social modelling influences on pain. In Sternbach (ed.) *Psychology of Pain*, p.73. (New York: Raven Press)
44. Johnson and Rice (1974). Sensory and distress components of pain. *Nurs. Res.*, **23**, 203–209
45. Le Fevre (1981). Cognitive distortion and cognitive factors in depressed psychiatric and low back pain patients. *J. Consulting Clin. Psychol.*, **49**, 517–525
46. Barber (1959). Towards a theory of pain. Relief of chronic pain by pre-frontal leucotomy, opiates, placebos and hypnosis. *Psychol. Bull.*, **56**, 430–460
47. Graceley *et al.* (1978). Narcotic analgesia. Fentanyl reduces the intensity but not the unpleasantness of painful tooth-pull sensations. *Science*, **203**, 1261–1263
48. Wall (1979). On the relation of injury to pain. *Pain*, **6**, 253–264
49. Leriche (1939). *The Surgery of Pain*. pp. 23–24. (Baltimore: Williams and Wilkins)
50. Bonica (1953). *The Management of Pain*. pp. 154–156. (Philadelphia: Lea Febiger)
51. Mitchell (1965). *Injuries of Nerves and the Consequences*. pp. 65–66. (New York: Dover)
52. Craig and Prkachin (1982). Non verbal measures of pain. In Melzack (ed.) *Pain Management and Assessment*. (New York: Raven Press)
53. Melzack, Ty and Wall (1982). Acute pain in an emergency clinic. Latency of onset and descriptor patterns related to different injuries. *Pain*, **14**, 33–43
54. Bonica (1979). Important clinical aspects of acute and chronic pain. In Beers and Bassett (eds.) *Mechanisms of Pain and Analgesic Compounds*, p. 183. (New York: Raven Press)
55. Craig (1983). Emotional aspects of pain. In Wall and Melzack (eds.) *Textbook of Pain*, p.156. (London: Churchill Livingstone)
56. Pilowsky *et al.* (1977). Pain, depression and illness behaviour in a pain clinic population. *Pain*, **4**, 183–192
57. Pelz and Merskey (1982). A description of psychological effects of chronic painful lesions. *Pain*, **14**, 293–301
58. Merskey and Spear (1967). *Pain. Psychological and Psychiatric Aspects*. (London: Baulliere, Tindall and Cox)
59. Spear (1967). Pain in psychiatric patients. *J. Psychosom. Res.*, **11**, 187–193
60. Merskey (1965). Psychiatric patients with persistent pain. *J. Psychosom. Res.*, **9**, 299–309
61. Engel (1959). 'Psychogenic' pain, and the pain prone patient. *Am. J. Med.*, **26**, 899–918
62. Blumer (1975). Psychiatric considerations in pain. In Rothman and Simeone (eds.) *The Spine*. (Philadelphia: W.B. Saunders)
63. Bonica (1983). Local anaesthesia and regional blocks. In Wall and Melzack (eds.) *Textbook of Pain*, p. 382 (London: Churchill Livingstone)
64. Watson *et al.* (1981). Relationships between pain and schizophrenia. *Br. J. Psychiatry*, **128**, 33–36
65. Wiltse and Rocchio (1975). Preoperative psychological tests as predictors of success of chemonucleolysis in the treatment of low back syndrome. *J. Bone Joint Surg.*, **57A1**, 478–483
66. Smith and Duerksen (1980). Personality in the relief of chronic pain. Predicting surgical outcome. In Smith, Merskey and Gross (eds.) *Pain Meaning and Management*, p. 22. (New York: Spectrum)

67. Ootsdam *et al.* (1981). Predictive value of some psychological tests on the outcome of surgical intervention in low back pain patients. *J. Psychosom. Res.*, **3**, 227–235
68. McCreary *et al.* (1979). The MMPI as predictor of response to conservative treatment of low back pain. *J. Clin. Psychol.*, **35**, 278–284
69. Waring *et al.* (1976). Predictive factors in the treatment of low back pain by surgical intervention. In Bonica and Albe-Fessard (eds.) *Advances in Pain Research Therapy*, pp. 939–942. (New York: Raven Press)
70. Leavitt and Garron (1979). Validity of a back pain classification scale among patients with low back pain not associated with demonstrable organic disease. *J. Psychosom. Res.*, **23**, 301–306
71. Merskey and Watson (1979). The lateralisation of pain. *Pain*, **7**, 271–280
72. Mechanic (1962). The concept of illness behaviour. *J. Chronic Dis.*, **15**, 189–194
73. Pilowsky (1969). Abnormal illness behaviour. *Br. J. Med. Psychol.*, **42**, 347–351
74. Pilowsky (1978). A general classification of abnormal illness behaviour. *Br. J. Med. Psychol.*, **51**, 131–137
75. Beecher (1972). The placebo effect as a non-specific force surrounding disease and the treatment of disease. In Jongen *et al.* (eds.) *Pain. Basic Principles, Pharmacology and Therapy.* (Stuttgart: Georg Thieme)
76. Sternbach (1978). Clinical aspects of pain. In Sternbach (ed.) *Psychology of Pain*, p. 241. (New York: Raven Press)
77. Fordyce (1978). Learning processes in pain. In ibid., p. 200
78. Weisenberg (1983). Cognitive aspects of pain. In Wall and Melzack (eds.) *Textbook of Pain*, p. 167. (London: Churchill Livingstone)
79. Goodman *et al.* (1976). Response of patients with myofascial pain dysfunction syndrome to mock equilibration. *J. Am. Dent. Assoc.*, **92**, 755–758
80. Wolff (1983). Methods of testing pain mechanisms in normal man. In Wall and Melzack (eds.) *Textbook of Pain*, p. 192. (London: Churchill Livingstone)
81. Graceley (1980). Pain measurement in man. In Bonica (ed.) *Pain, Common Discomfort and Humanitarian Care*, p. 111. (London: Elsevier; Amsterdam: North Holland)
82. Wall (1978). The gate control theory of pain mechanisms. A re-examination and re-statement. *Brain*, **101**, 118
83. Tursky (1976). Development of a pain perception profile. A psycho-physical approach. In Weisenberg and Tursky (eds.) *Pain. New Perspectives in Therapy and Research*, p. 171. (New York: Plenum Press)
84. Craig (1982). Modelling and social learning factors in chronic pain. In Bonica (ed.) *Advances in Pain Research and Therapy.* (New York: Raven Press)
85. Dubuisson and Melzack (1976). Classification of clinical pain descriptors by multiple group discriminant analysis. *Exp. Neurol.*, **51**, 480–487
86. Noordenbos (1983). Prologue. In Wall and Melzack (eds.) *Textbook of Pain*, (London: Churchill Livingstone)
87. Reading (1983). Testing pain mechanisms in persons in pain. In Wall and Melzack (eds.) *Textbook of Pain*, p. 196 (London: Churchill Livingstone)
88. Scott and Huskisson (1976). Graphic representation of pain. *Pain*, **2**, 175–184
89. Graceley (1980). Psycho-physical assessment of human pain. In Bonica and Albe-Fessard (eds.) *Advances in Pain Research and Therapy*, **3**, p. 805. (New York: Raven Press)
90. Ohnhaus and Adler (1975). Methodological problems in the measurement of pain. A comparison between the verbal rating scale and the visual analogue scale. *Pain*, **1**, 379–384
91. Joyce *et al.* (1975). Comparison of fixed interval and visual analogue scales for rating chronic pain. *Eur. J. Clin. Pharmacol.*, **8**, 415–420
92. Kremer *et al.* (1981). Measurement of pain. Patient preference does not confirm pain measurement. *Pain*, **10**, 241–248
93. Woodforde and Merskey (1972). Some relationships between subjective measures of pain. *J. Psychosom. Res.*, **16**, 173–178
94. Reading (1982). An analysis of the language in pain in chronic and acute patient groups. *Pain.* (In press)
95. Downie *et al.* (1978). Studies with pain rating scales. *Ann. Rheum. Dis.*, 378–381

96. Graceley *et al.* (1978). Validity and sensitivity of ratio scales of sensory and affective verbal pain descriptors. Manipulation of affect by diazepam. *Pain*, 5, 19–29
97. Melzack and Torgerson (1971). On the language of pain. *Anaesthesiology*, 34, 5059
98. Agnew and Merskey (1978). Words of chronic pain. *Pain*, 3, 73–81
99. Devine and Merskey (1965). The description of pain in psychiatric and general medical patients. *J. Psychosom. Res.*, 9, 311–316
100. Reading and Newton (1977). On a comparison of dysmenorrhea and intrauterine device related pain. *Pain*, 3, 265–276
101. Fox and Melzack (1976). Transcutaneous electrical stimulation and acupuncture. Comparison of treatment for low back pain. *Pain*, 2, 141–148
102. Rybstein-Blinchik (1979). Effects of different cognitive strategies on chronic pain experience. *J. Behav. Med.*, 2, 93–101
103. Klepac *et al.* (1981). Sensitivity of the McGill Pain Questionnaire to intensity and quantity of laboratory pain. *Pain*, 10, 199–207
104. Reading (1979). The internal structure of the McGill Pain Questionnaire in dysmenorrhea patients. *Pain*, 7, 353–358
105. McCreary *et al.* (1981). Principal dimensions of the pain experience and psychological disturbance in chronic low back pain patients. *Pain*, 11, 85–92
106. Kremer and Atkinson (1981). Pain measurements. Constructive validity of the affective dimension of the McGill Pain Questionnaire with chronic benign pain patients. *Pain*, 11, 93–100
107. Buren and Kleinknecht (1979). An evaluation of the McGill Pain Questionnaire for use in dental pain assessment. *Pain*, 6, 23–33
108. Reading (1980). A comparison of pain rating scales. *J. Psychosom. Res.*, 24, 119–126
109. Reading (1982). A comparison of response profiles obtainable on the McGill Pain Questionnaire and an adjective check-list. *Pain*. (In press)
110. Atkinson *et al.* (1982). Diffusion of pain language with affective disturbance confounds differential diagnosis. *Pain*, 12, 375–384
111. Fredericksen *et al.* (1978). Methodology in the measurement of pain. *Behav. Ther.*, 9, 486–488
112. Fordyce *et al.* (1981). Pain complaint exercise performance in chronic pain. *Pain*, 10, 313–322
114. Bond and Pilowsky (1966). Subjective assessment of pain and its relationship to the administration of analgesics in patients with advanced cancer. *J. Psychosom. Res.*, 10, 203–208
115. Ready *et al.* (1982). Self reported versus actual use of medications in chronic pain patients. *Pain*, 12, 285–294

7
RELEVANT PATHOLOGY –
GENERAL CONSIDERATIONS

Rheumatological considerations
Inflammatory conditions are encountered surprisingly rarely, and they are mentioned here merely as a reminder, fuller accounts being found in the appropriate texts.

Rheumatoid arthritis
The commonest inflammatory condition presents typically with positive Rose–Waaler and latex tests, a raised erythrocyte sedimentation test and erosive X-ray changes. Manipulation has no place in the treatment of this disease. In the active phase it would be pointless and painful, while in the quiescent phase manipulation of the neck (for example) with the possibility of jamming the odontoid process into the spinal cord, is potentially fatal and absolutely contraindicated.

The seronegative arthritides
Reiter's disease, psoriatic and colitic arthritides present little diagnostic difficulty. Ankylosing spondylitis does, as its onset is frequently insidious and, in 75% of cases, presents with low back pain. Careful examination of the spine is essential – restriction of movement, particularly of rotation of the thoracic spine, and a diminished respiratory excursion in the young male being significant. These findings may be associated with iritis, aortic incompetence or colitic symptoms. The essential imvestigative finding is radiological evidence of sacroiliitis. Diagnosis is important, as a policy of maximum mobility and full activity seems to affect the prognosis and ultimate restriction of movement markedly for the better. Manipulation in the active phase has no place, and the clinician may miss the diagnosis, if this procedure affords transient relief. In the quiescent phase, manipulation is indicated where it is thought appropriate, and in the absence of contraindication.

Scheuermann's disease
This is equally common in the two sexes. It usually presents between the ages of 13 and 17, with poor posture and aching in the region of the kyphosis,

accentuated by standing and relieved by lying down. The kyphosis is thoracic in 75% of cases and thoracolumbar in 24%, rarely purely lumbar. The thoracic cases present with accentuated dorsal kyphosis and increased lumbar lordosis. The thoracolumbar cases present with a long kypohosis and a short lumbar lordosis. Initially the defect can be cured, but after 6–9 months the deformity becomes fixed. There may be local tenderness, but there are no other marked clinical signs.

In the active phase in severe cases, results using a Milwaukee splint for a year are excellent, so that early diagnosis of this not uncommon condition is important. Whereas manipulation in the acute phase is useless and may delay diagnosis, it can be of service in the quiescent phase, given appropriate indications. Mild cases frequently elude diagnosis entirely, and it is common to find radiological evidence of Scheuermann's disease in adults who give no history of symptoms in adolescence.

Polymyalgia rheumatica
This is a rare condition that can readily mislead the medical manipulator; more so the lay manipulator. Presenting in the elderly, with a history of marked early-morning stiffness and 'girdle' pain, it may be seen by the clinician when symptoms have diminished. Signs are rare, and the pain and stiffness may lead him to feel that manipulation may be of help. This is a potentially disastrous error. Thrombosis of the retinal artery is a feature of the condition, which may, of course, cause blindness. The action to be taken is blood estimation of the ESR and start treatment with steroids without waiting for the result.

Benign and malignant neoplasms
Neoplasms of any sort are of rare occurrence in musculoskeletal medical practice, but they are, of course, of prime importance. Among those which should be borne in mind are the following.

Benign
  Bony
    Chondroma
    Osteochondroma
    Benign osteoblastoma
    Aneurysmal bone cysts

  Non-bony
    Osteoclastoma   Neurofibroma
    Haemangioma   Cystic lesions of nerve roots
    Meningioma

Malignant
  Primary
    Bony   *Non-bony*
    Cordoma   Hodgkin's disease
    Myeloma   Reticular cell sarcoma
    Sarcoma

  Secondary
    Bony
    Most often from primaries of: Breast
                                  Lung
                                  Kidney
                                  Prostate
                                  Thyroid

Root pain
Aetiology

"Possibly the great majority of root compression is due to disc protrusion and is asymptomatic."[1] "It is quite amazing to what extent a nerve root can become squeezed and deformed by a slowly growing osteophytic protrusion without any clinical evidence of irritation or dysfunction. Reactive fibrosis may also involve a root sheath and periarticular tissues, obliterating the root pouches, and yet the root may remain functionally intact. Such changes, however, always make the root extremely vulnerable to all kinds of stress and strain."[2]

In a series of myelographic investigations of 300 people with neither symptoms nor signs, 37% were found to have evidence of trespass into the neural canal, multiple defects were shown in 18 %, and in 9% the changes were marked[3]. The causes of root compression are those of a space-occupying lesion; these are many, and disc protrusion is only one.

Physiology

In this respect, matters are far from clear. Mild pressure on roots is not necessarily painful[4]. Some of the pain associated with root problems is referred from neighbouring structures, such as muscle insertions, joint capsules or ligaments[5,6]. In these problems there may be deafferentation (partial or complete interruption of input) of transmission neurones in the cord, which may then develop spontaneous activities[7,8].

Dermatomal overlap is a marked and unpredictable feature[9] and A-δ and C primary afferents have never been mapped specifically in any species[10].

It has been shown in Relevant Physiology (p. 38) that the spread of primary afferent fibres is wide; they may travel for up to 12 segments in the spinal cord before contacting spinal cord neurones[11-14].

Receptive fields in the dorsal horn show marked plasticity[15] and "individual receptive fields of substantia gelatinosa neurones on which the afferents terminate may be variable and subject to descending control."[16,17]

Local anaesthetic blocks can abolish pain when given distal to the site of root damage, so some normal afferent impulses may play a facilitating role[18].

Mechanoreceptive afferent fibres may well play a part in pain states[19-22]. The extent of lesions in these situations is often difficult to assess. Minor interference with pial vessels can cause a massive decrease in the perfusion of the entire dorsal horn[23]. The ventral roots contain some afferent fibres, which may contribute to pain[24,25].

Diagnosis

The aetiology of root pain is not understood in the majority of cases. Methods of examination and special investigations also present difficulties of interpretation which make accurate diagnosis impossible in many cases. Therefore the use of the term root pain, so widely employed over recent years, will often give the clinician a false sense of certainty, which is clearly of potential disadvantage to the patient.

This emphasizes, once again, that accurate diagnosis in musculoskeletal medicine is seldom attainable.

Pain associated with nerve damage

Introduction

"The mid-nerve part of the normal mammalian axon is specialised for impulse propagation and is very poorly suited to impulse generation. Axon membrane accommodation is brisk. For example, when a prolonged, supra-threshold depolarising current pulse is injected into normal myelinated fibres, they fire only once, at the outset of the stimulus, and do not produce a repetitive impulse train. Similarly, gentle external pressure on a nerve does not generate impulses or evoke a sensation of pain. Even when axons are severely stretched or cut across they usually produce at most a brief injury discharge, and then fall silent."[26]

However, recently "it has been conclusively demonstrated that compression of a nerve, even for as short a time as 20 minutes, can produce ectopic foci of discharges along the nerve at a site remote from that of the pressure. It is not difficult to imagine ectopic foci occurring along the whole stretch of the ulnar nerve after chronic compression in patients following trauma, and this explains why repeated attempts to relieve the pain of ulnar neuritis by transposition of the nerve may only worsen the pain."[27]

Therefore damaged peripheral nerve can assume properties other than those of undamaged nerve.

Nerve changes following injury
Immediate
Following external injury and an immediate discharge, sprouting takes place. In a few weeks many sprouts are formed and may spread into surrounding tissues. In a simple crush injury all fibres may sprout into a Schwann cell tube, but in other injuries this will not be wholly successful, and a partial neuroma will form.

The consequences of this are several: the generation of spontaneous nerve impulses which decreases over a month, with some sprouts continuing to produce nerve impulses indefinitely. These sprouts are also extremely sensitive to mechanical distortion, however slight. They are also very sensitive to adrenalin, and this may well provide an explanation of the various sympathetic discharges.

Longer term changes
Longer term effects include sprouts establishing contact with one another. This allows ephaptic transmission to take place and for there to be the possibility of direct afferent transfer of impulses. This means that damaged nerves may themselves contribute to pain states.

"Normal nerves are capable of generating rhythmic discharge only at specialised terminal endings. Damaged nerves can acquire this capability at ectopic sites. Once a rhythmic impulse generator has been established, spontaneous discharge may occur. Correspondingly, the nerve may become sensitive to a broad range of depolarising stimuli including changes in mechanical, chemical, ionic and metabolic conditions."[26]

Moreover, not only may injured nerves generate impulses, but they can also amplify normal impulse discharges. "The most striking of these processes depends on the fact that rhythmic impulse generators have threshold properties. In fibres and dorsal root ganglion cells that are silent but are near the threshold of the rhythmic impulse generators, small stimuli that bring the rhythmic generator to threshold have disproportionately large and prolonged effects."[26]

The import of this is that damaged nerve acquires abnormal properties of its own, which may generate, maintain or enhance pain in an unpredictable manner.

Central consequences following nerve injury

Short term

With regard to dorsal root ganglia, nerve impulse generation increases rapidly, rising to a maximum in about 3 weeks and declining over months, but never ceasing so long as the neuroma exists. There is increased sensitivity to mechanical distortion and to adrenalin. There are chemical changes in that there is a loss of substance P and other peptides in the spinal cord afferent terminals. There is also a decrease of conduction velocity which reverses only after many months.

The functional consequences of these changes are not clear, but there is marked evidence that there are central consequences of peripheral lesions.

Longer term

There is some dispute as to whether there is atrophy of the central terminals of sensory afferents, but there is no doubt that some dorsal root ganglia cells die, and that in consequence some deafferentation (partial or complete interruption of input) takes place.

Therefore any peripheral nerve injury has central consequences which are unpredictable and which may in themselves be a cause of pain[28].

Summary

A review of these various factors has led an author concerned, inter alia, with the running of a problem back service to write, "this, together with the reduced number of fibres and spontaneous discharges, produces a totally altered profile to the central nervous system, and this in turn may give rise to abnormal firing centrally, and the production of pain". "Indeed, now that so many of these mechanisms have become apparent, one wonders why pain is not a commoner accompaniment of nerve injury."[29]

The significance of peripheral nerve injury is currently insufficiently appreciated by physicians interested in musculoskeletal medicine. Recent work has shown how complex these injuries are and how intractable they can be.

The fact that peripheral nerves are accessible to study has permitted the observation that damaged nerve can behave independently. The factors involved in this are complex and difficult to elucidate and to quantify. As this is the case for peripheral nerves, the physiology within the CNS is hardly likely to prove less complicated, with the further consequences that this must have for diagnosis. The same considerations apply to therapy, and the implication of this is to emphasize empiricism at the periphery and therefore, surely, centrally.

The prolapsed intervertebral disc (PID)
Historical considerations
At one time made to the exclusion of almost all others by clinicians dealing with low back pain, this diagnosis has an interesting history. "Sciatica was first described by the early Greek and Roman physicians. However, it was not related to the dysfunction of the sciatic nerve until 1764, when Domenico Cotugno of Naples published his 'De Ischiade Nervosa Commentarius'."[30] Irritation of the sciatic nerve and its component nerve roots was subsequently found to result from underlying conditions such as spinal arthritis, intraspinal and extraspinal neoplasms and spondylolisthesis. More recently it became apparent that sciatica may be at times caused by nerve root compression from a herniated nucleus pulposus of a lumbar intervertebral disc.

"We have our heritage from Dr. Barr of Boston who, one Sunday morning in 1932 in the Pathology Laboratory of Massachusetts General Hospital, was the first person to understand that the material recently removed from one of his patients as a chondroma was in reality a disc hernia. He solved one important part of the low back pain problem, but as we all know by now, it was only a minor part."[31]

Although as a diagnosis it is nowadays far less frequently made, it is nevertheless a matter to be discussed, because in the English speaking world the ideas of Dr Cyriax are still a subject of controversy and debate. It is therefore pertinent to review these ideas in the light of current evidence.

Incidence
According to Dr Cyriax:
1. "The great majority of soft tissue symptoms in the neck originate from various different stages of the same disorder (the PID) and respond to the same treatment of manipulative reduction of disc displacement . . . "[32]
2. "In the thoracic spine disc lesions account for a higher proportion of thoracic pain than is often realised . . ."[32]
3. "In the lumbar spine medical examination shows a great preponderance of lumbar disorders are attributable to disc lesions[32]".

Others regard this diagnosis as an infrequent cause of back pain. Amongst them are Bradford and Spurling (1945)[33], Barr (1951)[34], Friberg (1954)[35], Rabinovitch (1961)[36], Hirsch (1965)[37], De Palma and Rothman (1970)[38], Scott-Charleton and Roebuck (1972)[39], Arnoldi (1972)[40], Mooney and Robertson (1976)[41], Nachemson (1976)[31], Weinstein, Ehni and Wilson (1977)[42], Sunderland (1978)[43], Andersson (1982)[44], O'Brien (1983)[45], Spangfort (1983)[46], DuBuisson (1983)[1] and Lewit (1985)[47].

We have found no opinion to the contrary in the literature, save that of Dr Cyriax himself.

The Cyriax diagnosis
In view of the foregoing, how was Dr Cyriax's conclusion as to the frequency of this diagnosis arrived at?

History
First by taking a history "based on information he (the clinician) will decide whether it is a disc lesion or one of the uncommon causes of backache".
The word 'uncommon' here seems to prejudge the issue to some extent.

Examination
Movements: These consist of what are known as joint signs, that is to say gross global movements which may be painful, restricted, or both. However, it must be observed that there are many potential causes of such findings, other than the PID.

Straight leg raising: This is regarded as a means of stretching the dura mater (i.e. it is a dural sign) and "limitation indicates that the dural sleeve at the levels of the L4 to S2 roots cannot move properly".
Here it must be remembered that the straight leg raising test is complex (see Case Analysis, p.151).
Moreover, "one of the interesting features of deep pain is the segmental muscle spasm which accompanies all deep pain of more than momentary duration."[48] Pederson et al. (1956)[49] have quite clearly demonstrated the limitation of straight leg raising due to painful lesions in a number of different tissues, as have King (1977)[50], Mooney and Robertson (1976)[41] and Kirkaldy-Willis and Hill(1979)[51].

Root signs: These comprise weakness, reflex changes and alterations in sensation.

Weakness: The very real difficulties of clinical assessment of weakness are discussed at p.154.

Reflex alterations: It has been shown by Mooney and Robertson (1976)[41] that these can be caused by injecting zygoapophyseal joints with hypertonic saline; this being reversed by the subsequent injection of local anaesthetic. Their studies confirm that, lacking definitive neurological signs, it is impossible by pain complaints alone to specify precise sites of abnormality or the exact nature of pathology. "There is some question as to what constitutes a true neurologic sign; we no longer consider diminished straight leg raising or reflex changes to necessarily implicate nerve root pressure by disc protrusion."[41]

The disc and nerve root compression: It is stated that, "a lateral disc displacement may interfere only with the dural sleeve of the nerve root or with the parenchyma as well". However, as has been shown:
1. The aetiology of root pain is far from clear.
2. In many cases marked root involvement can take place without symptoms.
3. The disc is but one of many structures which can impinge upon the nerve root.

Protruded material: It is stated that symptoms can be caused by protrusion of a disc which may be composed of cartilage (annular) or part of the nucleus pulposus (nuclear). In fact, Mcnab (1977)[52] observed that it is unusual at operation to find disc herniation consisting solely of material extruding through a defect in the annulus, the displaced material almost invariably consisting of differing amounts of nucleus, annulus and cartilage plates.

Sylvest, Hentzer and Cobayasi (1977)[53] studied the material found at operation on 5 patients with a protruded disc, and 1 with a ruptured disc. "Division of material into annulus fibrosus and nucleus pulposus proved inaccurate. Chondrocytes were always the predominant cell type and could be divided into three categories:
1. healthy cells,
2. a chondrocyte arrangement showing cloning cells and evidence of increased secretion,
3. a type characterising a stage of cell death."

The caudal epidural
With regard to special investigations, the caudal epidural is used not only therapeutically but also as a means of confirming the diagnosis of a PID. "The only structures rendered anaesthetic are the exterior surface of the dura mater and the nerve roots. Presumably the posterior surface of the posterior longitudinal ligament and the anterior surface of the ligamentum flavum are numbed too, but the effect of 0.5% procaine does not penetrate to the substance of those tissues, . . . cessation of symptoms after injection shows the solution has been able to pass between two surfaces, and there is only one tissue apt to protrude posteriorly without invasion, a disc lesion."[32]

However, "it used to be thought that the dura mater was impermeable to local anaesthetics and that epidural anaesthetic blockade occurred at the mixed nerve and dorsal root ganglia beyond the dural sleeves surrounding each pair of anterior and posterior spinal roots. Radioactive tracer studies have shown that the dura mater is not impermeable, and that subarachnoid and epidural local anaesthetics act at precisely the same sites, namely the spinal roots, mixed spinal nerves and the surface of the spinal cord to the depth of a millimetre or more, depending on the lipid solubility of the anaesthetic."[54,55].

" . . . myelographic studies show that contrast agents such as metrizamide can travel from the lumbar region to the basal cisterns in a matter of aminutes, and to the lateral ventricles within an hour . . ."[56].

Thus the use of the caudal epidural in this way as a means of diagnostic validation is shown to be unsound.

The diagnostic realities
In fact, the diagnosis of disc protrusion is far from easy. "Studies to identify the causes of surgical failures reveal that inaccuracy of diagnosis and poor selection of patients were more important factors than technical errors during the operation itself."[31,57-59]. To quote Spangfort (1983) "the point is to establish the presence and location of the offending disc herniation, and unfortunately surgical exposure is still the only way to do so with absolute certainty."[46]

Conclusion
To quote Dr Cyriax yet again, "a lumbar disc lesion may be characterised by:
1. A history consistent with a displacement.
2. Pain and limitation of lumbar movements in the non-capsular pattern, consistent with displacement.
3. Dural symptoms and signs.
4. Nerve root symptoms and signs (impaired mobility)
5. Nerve root symptoms and signs (impaired conduction)

Often items 3, 4 and 5 will be absent, leaving the diagnosis to be founded on history and movements alone, reinforced by attendant congruous negative findings."[32]

In view of the material presented here and elsewhere in this book, we feel that this last assertion may most aptly be described as being rather sanguine. In fact, it may be asked, in the light of what is now massive evidence, why these ideas should still be a matter for discussion and controversy. The root cause must undoubtedly lie with Dr Cyriax's remarkable gifts as a writer and teacher, with his clarity and conviction.

Osteoarthrosis/osteoarthritis
Inflammatory considerations
1. As this heading suggests, there is still controversy as to whether there is an inflammatory element in this heterogeneous disease complex.
   a. There is, however, considerable clinical and pathological evidence of an inflammatory component in this disease, and many authors continue to call it osteoarthritis[60].

b. Supportive evidence for the presence of an inflammatory component in osteoarthritis is provided from both clinical and pathological observation. Patients with osteoarthritis in whom clinical features of inflammation predominate, i.e. pain, heat, redness, swelling and loss of function and morning stiffness, have been described by several authors[61-64].

c. In a review of random synovial specimens from 15 consecutive patients with osteoarthritis who underwent hip or knee arthroplasty, Goldenberg et al.[65] found synovial lining cell hyperplasia in 8, vascular changes in 10 and leukocyte infiltration in 9. Only 2 of these synovia were normal, whereas 6 showed mild synovitis, 3 moderate synovitis and 4 demonstrated markedly inflamed synovium indistinguishable histopathologically from rheumatoid arthritis.

d. Cooper et al. found inflammatory cells around blood vessels or in focal aggregates and lining cell hyperplasia as commonly in synovial tissue from patients with osteoarthritis as in samples from patients with rheumatoid arthritis[66].

e. Schumacher et al. examined the knees of 150 consecutive autopsies which included 30 patients with severe osteoarthritis and 78 with minimal or no osteoarthritis[67]. Of the latter group only 12 synovial membranes showed either lining cell proliferation or lymphocyte infiltration compared with 36 from 78 knees with moderate or severe osteoarthritis.

f. Bullough examined femoral heads from patients with rheumatoid and osteoarthritis, and also found extensive pathological evidence of inflammation[68].

g. It is perhaps useful, therefore, to adopt the view expressed by Hart that only if these changes cause symptoms should we diagnose osteoarthritis.[69]

2. The evidence that there is an inflammatory element to osteoarthritis reinforces the clinical impression that this condition is episodic.

Degenerative considerations

Degenerative changes in the spine are common, and indeed Vernon-Roberts has shown that by the age of 40 all discs show degenerative changes to a greater or lesser degree[70]. As we show, X-ray changes are not correlated with symptoms, and moreover we know that the incidence of back pain diminishes after the age of 55[71,72].

Every general practitioner will be familiar with the patient who has been told by another clinician that, because of degenerative changes in his spine shown radiologically, his back pain is fixed, and there is little or nothing anyone can do for him.

In view of the above material, this is simply not the case. The solutions to the problems which still dominate the field of musculoskeletal medicine must ultimately come from the stables of orthodox academic neurology, orthopaedics and rheumatology. Indeed, it is interesting to observe how much clinically relevant material has come from these sources over the past few years.

What is disturbing, however, is that this material has often not reached people engaged in clinical practice, especially in general practice. The use made of the X-ray of the degenerative spine is perhaps the most striking example of this phenomenon.

Referred pain, tenderness and associated reflex phenomena
The localization of pain
Skin pain: Localization of skin pain in normal circumstances is accurate to within about 1 cm of the point stimulated. Discrimination is also accurate. This latter is the capacity to distinguish two spatially separate stimuli.

Deep or referred pain: Deep pain, unlike skin pain, is usually diffuse, poorly localized and often felt at some distance from the point stimulated, when it may be described as being referred.

Over the years, many deep structures have been systematically investigated by passing needles into them, scratching or pricking, or by the injection of irritant solutions. Ligaments, muscles and joints have all been studied in this manner and present broadly similar results.

Patterns of distribution have been plotted, but "there are individual variations, determined by variation in the segmental innervation of the joints concerned, as well as the individual's past experience".[73]

The complexity of the innervation of the spine "accounts for the accepted difficulty of determining the anatomical source of low back pain in patients."[73]

The mechanisms of referred pain are not fully understood, but it has been shown that:
1. Nociceptive afferents from visceral tissues project onto the same cells in lamina 5 of the basal spinal nucleus as do the afferents from segmentally related areas of skin.
2. Because of this convergence of visceral and cutaneous nociceptive inputs on the relaying cells in lamina 5, their excitation is the essential prerequisite for centripetal transmission of nociceptive activity into the brain, and thus the evocation of the experience of pain.
3. It will be apparent that normally trivial stimuli applied to related areas of skin may induce these relay cells to fire, should their excitability be sufficiently increased by pre-existing afferent activity emanating from

visceral nociceptive nerve endings[74].

As long ago as 1939, Kellgren demonstrated the existence of referred pain following the injection of hypertonic saline solutions into the vertebral connective tissues[75].

Clinical research

In 1951, Frykholm, in his operations on cervical spines under local anaesthesia, found that, on stimulating the dorsal root, the patient experienced pain in the distribution of the dermatome[76]. If the anterior root was stimulated, the patient felt pain situated in muscles which had been painful and tender before operation.

In 1959, Cloward described referral of pain to periscapular areas on injecting for discography under local anaesthesia into the anterior parts of various cervical discs, C3/C4, C4/C5, C5/C6 and C6/C7. He identified the painful areas as being C3/C4 for the upper fibres of the trapezius, C4/C5 for the upper scapular medial border, C5/C6 for the middle of the medial border of the scapula and C6/C7 medial at the inferior angle[77].

This author not only demonstrated the existence of referred pain, but fell into the error of assuming that the site of the referred pain gave a clear indication of its site of origin[77]. This has been shown not to be the case, not only by Holt in 1964[78], but also by Klafta and Collis in 1969[79], who performed 549 cervical disc injections over a 10-year period, in an endeavour to evaluate the diagnostic usefulness of pain associated with discography. Pain similar to the presenting pain was produced in 22% of cases, dissimilar pain in 67% and no pain at all in 11%[79].

The dermatome

Kirk and Denny-Brown in 1970[80], and subsequently Denny-Brown *et al.* in 1973[80a], have shown experimentally that an isolated dermatome can vary enormously in extent and, indeed, that the dermatomes should be considered as a neurophysiological entity which can vary almost from moment to moment.

In 1978, Last wrote, "the dermatome charts of the limb are are probably as accurate today as maps of the world were in the 16th. century"[81].

With regard to cells of lamina 1 of the dorsal horn, "the area of the receptive fields of the majority of cells is restricted to some fraction of their dermatome, but some extend to include as much as a whole leg."[82]

To quote Mooney and Robertson (1976), "It is apparent to us that the localisation of pain in the low back, buttock and leg is a non-specific finding"[41]. Discussing the apophyseal joint syndrome, they say, "on the other hand, the very same referral pattern can no doubt be caused by irritation within the spinal canal".

In 1983 Bourdillon wrote, "a remarkable property of referred pain is that it can appear to be exactly the same when produced by either of two (or more) separate sources"[83].

If it has been shown that the same cells in lamina 1 of the dorsal horn have a multiplicity of functions, and that they subserve different functions at different times, and that their receptive fields can extend from a fraction of a dermatome to a whole leg, then to use the dermatome as a diagnostic tool is unphysiological[84].

Tenderness

Tenderness may be defined as pain provoked by an innocuous stimulus.

As with referred pain, tenderness is not fully understood. "Tenderness is partly explained by a sensitisation of nociceptors, but in some pathological states, such as referred pain, innocuous stimuli to normal tissue may produce pain. There are reasons to believe that impulses from low threshold afferents may summate with those from nociceptors."[84, p.9]

As Wall says, "the central nervous system in tenderness and referred pain can change the way in which it handles an input from another source."[85]

Referred pain may or may not be accompanied by secondary hyperaesthesiae. In 1977, McNab found that injection of hypertonic saline into the lumbosacral supraspinous ligament could not only radiate pain down the leg but could also be associated with tender points in varying sites, commonly situated over the sacroiliac joint and in the upper and outer quadrant of the buttock[52].

O'Brien, in 1979, on palpating the lumbosacral promontory via the abdominal wall, found tenderness in more than three quarters of patients with low back pain[86]. In a control group of 50 asymptomatic individuals only two exhibited tenderness, and both of them had experienced back pain in the preceding three months.

Frykholm[76] and Cloward[77] both demonstrated referred tenderness. Unfortunately the diagnostic use of this phenomenon remains as restricted as that of referred pain.

Reflex skin tenderness

When skin is injured it becomes quite tender, as does, to a lesser extent, a variable area of surrounding skin. However, areas of sore skin can also appear on the face after stimulating the mucosa of the paranasal sinuses, and can appear in association with visceral disease when their distribution follows a segmental pattern[73]. This is assumed to be a reflex phenomenon, but it is not fully understood. Nevertheless, it has practical implications, in that it forms the basis of the skin pinching test. (See Case Analysis, p.154).

Palpable peripheral changes – trigger points
Introduction
"A very tender type of tissue in the human body, so frequently a cause of pain in all sorts of conditions; traumatic, rheumatic, postural, occupational etc.; is the tissue of junction between muscle, tendon, intermuscular septum or similar structure with periosteum or bone. This of course includes joint capsules, ligaments, tendon insertions and structures of that kind."[39] These points, called 'trigger points' by Travell were described by her as having the following characteristics.
1. A circumscribed deep tenderness.
2. A localized twitch or fasciculation when pressing or pinching the muscular location of the trigger area.
3. Pain referred elsewhere when the trigger point was pressed upon[87].

History
These points have a long history, being first mentioned in a publication in Germany in 1843[88] and consistently reported on since then in many countries. They have acquired many titles, "fibrositis, interstitial myofibrositis, muscle callus, muscle gelling or myogelloses, muscle hardening, muscular rheumatism, soft part rheumatism, myofascial pain syndrome, myofasciitis, trigger points, myalgia, myalgic spots"[89]. In the United Kingdom, they were described in a classic paper, published in 1947, as being herniations of lobulated fat and labelled fibrositis[90].

Clinical features
It has always been observed that they are lumps, or thickenings or hardenings, although not always tender. Further that massage and other local treatments to these painful thickenings bring relief (at least temporarily and sometimes permanently) to many patients. As to their nature, "many patients with a painfully pressure sensitive spot in their muscles also have a palpable hardening associated with it. Other patients have the pain but not the hardening. Most German authors, and the originators of the fibrositis concept, concentrated on the nature of the hardening as a means of understanding the cause of the pain. Taking this approach, one can consider seven possible causes for the palpable hardness. Increased fibrous connective tissue, oedema, altered viscosity of muscle, ground substance infiltrate, contracture of muscle fibres, vascular engorgement, fatty infiltration."[91]

In fact, no-one so far has been able to identify these problems histologically. It is therefore reasonable to suggest that the term fibrositis should not be used, since its existence has never been proved[74]. The association between trigger points and acupuncture points for pain are discussed in Management: Acupuncture, p.228[92]. Trigger points are further discussed in Clinical Presentations, pp. 172, 176.

Muscle spasm

This has been defined as "excessive motor unit activity."[74]

"One of the interesting features of deep pain is the segmental muscle spasm which accompanies all severe and deep pain of more than momentary duration."[48] This has been demonstrated in the trunk, where injecting deep structures either at the front or the back of the body produces segmental pain and striking rigidity of the appropriate segment of the abdominal or chest wall. This also takes place in the limbs but, because the segmental musculature is more widely distributed, this may be less obvious. Nevertheless, it is of clinical importance[73]. (See Clinical Presentations, pp. 173, 175).

"Experimental injury of anaesthetised animals provides clear evidence that hypertonus per se will follow damage of acute onset to musculoskeletal tissues."[49]

Wyke shows that, "type 4 joint receptors in joint capsules, fat pads and ligaments, when subject to sufficient irritation, will provoke intense, non-adaptive motor unit responses simultaneously in all muscles related to the joint as well as in more remote muscles elsewhere in the body."[93]

Mooney and Robertson report patients with straight leg raising reduced to about 45–60° and positive EMG readings at the point of limitation[41]. Injection of a single facet joint is followed by the return of normal range of straight leg raising and myoelectrical silence.

Muscle spasm may or may not be painful, but if maintained for a prolonged period in any muscle a dull aching pain develops in that muscle, which also becomes tender[74].

Summary

Referred pain

The vagaries of referred pain are important.

1. "In the first place it is clear that widespread pain in the limbs or trunk may result from circumscribed lesions, particularly if the source of pain is situated deeply in the trunk of limb girdles."[73]
2. "Secondly, the site in which the pain is felt is only an indirect guide as to its source of origin, so that in every case it is well to preserve an open mind at the outset, and examine carefully all structures which by virtue of their segmental innervation could give rise to the pain under consideration."[73]

Trigger points

1. Trigger points are therefore of great importance to the clinician interested in musculoskeletal medicine. If found in isolation, without obvious spinal or visceral causes, they can be treated effectively in the great majority of cases.

2. No spinal examination is complete without a thorough examination of the musculoskeletal system including a search for trigger points, since their site is unpredictable.

Muscle spasm
This may be defined as excessive motor unit activity.
1. When one considers the nociceptive innervation of lumbosacral tissues, it is quite clear that any posture, maintained over a long period of time, can affect muscles, fasciae, ligaments and articular capsules. All these nociceptor systems, severally or together, are capable of stimulating painful paravertebral muscle spasm.
2. This accounts for the exceptional difficulty of determining the anatomical source of low back pain in patients.

Practical clinical consequences
The syndrome: In the light of this material and of similar problems encountered in the dorsal horn, it can be seen that to use the site of pain or tenderness as a means of arriving at a specific diagnosis, indicating a specific tissue, is unrealistic in the majority of cases of back pain that we meet. Over the years, many syndromes, i.e. collections of symptoms and signs, have been presented as being reliable diagnostic tools. Examples are sudden onset backache, impacted synovial meniscoid villus, the cocktail party syndrome, the locking of an arthrotic facet joint, the adolescent acute back and slow onset backache and sciatica, or the equinox syndrome. In view of the material presented, such syndromes must be regarded with very considerable doubt. Indeed, in this area it is doctors themselves who have, sadly, greatly contributed to the confusion which is so marked a feature of this field.

"The range of labels used in connection with back pain is a fair reflection of medical ignorance and factional interests."[99] Further, this has had the added disadvantage of persuading the clinician that he has the correct diagnosis of the patient's problems and, thereby, in his persisting with a particular line of treatment which, in view of the evidence, is not reasonable.

Local examination: It is surely reasonable to utilize the phenomena associated with pain as the basis of local examination, always bearing in mind that, as epiphenomena, these will be present in an unpredictable proportion of cases to an unpredictable degree. After all, this forms an important part of a diagnosis of acute appendicitis. Indeed, many clinicians, in many countries, have made use of these over the years, attaching to them a great variety of different hypotheses and labels. This variety of terminology is one of the key reasons for the confusion currently existing in this field, but it in no way detracts from the usefulness of local examination.

The autonomic system and musculoskeletal medicine

Although the subject of much controversy, there are certain realities with regard to autonomic function and its association with musculoskeletal pain which are quite clear. It has been shown that the irritation of spinal joint nociceptors simultaneously evokes a large number of reflex alterations, including:

1. Paravertebral muscle spasm,
2. Alterations in cardiovascular, respiratory and endocrine function[94]. On injection of 6% saline into thoracic paravertebral muscle tissue, not only is referred pain induced, but also pallor, sweating, fall in blood pressure, subjective faintness and nausea.

"As the discharges from certain of the nuclear subgroups within the hypothalamus continuously controls the global afferent activity in the sympathetic and parasympathetic outflows from the neuraxis, and as neurones within these same hypothalamic nuclei are also the source of the hypophyseoportal hormones that regulate the secretary activity of the adenohypophysis as well as the antidiuretic and oxitocic hormones, it will be apparent that the above mentioned thalamohyopthalamic projection system provides the means whereby nociceptive afferent activity entering the brain evokes the complex of visceral reflex effects such as those involving the cardiovascular and gastrointestinal systems and the hormonal changes that are inevitably associated with the experience of pain."[74]

Therefore autonomic activity is an integral part of the physiology of pain,

Practical clinical consequences

Autonomic pain

For many years it has been held that autonomic pain could be identified as a separate and isolated phenomenon, in some way quite different from somatic pain. In view of the evidence, it is clear that this notion has to be discarded.

Pain from muscles and joints can produce visceral symptoms; for example, referral of pain to the chest can cause a feeling of intense constriction and to the abdomen a sensation of nausea and fullness. Therefore the separation of visceral and somatic problems is not always easy and requires careful consideration. (See Clinical Presentations, p.174).

The important point with regard to this group of pains is that the quality of deep pain, whether visceral or somatic in origin, is identical; being that of deep pain as a whole. Visceral pain, like deep somatic pain, is diffuse, and its distribution follows the same segmental origin and pattern, and may exhibit the same reflex phenomena. Again, the difficulty of correctly evaluating the somatic and visceral problems can be considerable[73].

Pain measurement

For many years autonomic activities have been used as a means of measuring pain intensity objectively. However, this is not possible, because, "in short, the visceral hormonal changes in the experience of pain are epiphenomena that are evoked in parallel by the arrival of nociceptive afferent activity in the thalamus and are not directly related quantitatively"[74]. Hence clinical attempts to use measurement of changes in heart rate, in arterial blood pressure, in electrical skin resistance or temperature, or in plasma catecholamine concentration as indices of the intensity of the painful experiences are entirely fallacious, as they are based on the false assumption of an equation between the hypothalamic reflex effect of the peripheral nociceptive stimulation and the affective response thereto[74].

Therefore, sadly, all such endeavours are futile. "In general, there would seem to be little basis for discrete physiological changes related to the pain experience."[95] Thus, in pain assessment the clinician is compelled to fall back on the psychological parameters of the McGill questionnaire which, whatever its admitted shortcomings, gives a more objective evaluation of these matters than does any other.

The facilitated cord segment

In osteopathic theory, the autonomic nervous system has been used in a concept known as the 'facilitated cord segment' as a means whereby spinal problems can be involved with and cause organic disease. "The increased, summated state creates what is called a facilitated cord segment, because the threshold for the efferent discharges is lowered and the transmission of impulses is therefore facilitated. These discharges lead to abnormal function, in the first place to hyperfunction, and then to hypofunction, and then if the abnormal stimuli persist for long enough, pathological changes can then ensue. The irritated spinal segment is vulnerable to other noxious influences, and even if a mechanical cause in itself is not sufficient to evoke abnormal responses, the combination of it with other factors is sufficient to introduce abnormal symptoms. Mechanical lesions are aetiological in many diseases, because adhesions weaken those viscera which are reflexively and segmentally associated with them. They cannot and should not be discounted in any disease."[96]

"So we can contend that by restoring normal mechanics we are achieving in a natural way the restoration of autonomic balance by calming the stimulated and over-excited segment."[96]

This concept has an interesting history. It was based on a paper published by Denslow, Korr and Krems in 1947, in which they studied EMG response to various pressures applied to musculature[97]. "It is concluded that low threshold segments are those in which a relatively large portion of the motor neurones are contained in a state of facilitation due to chronic presumptive bombardment by impulses from some unknown source. Presumptive evidence indicates that the facilitating impulses arise from segmentally related structures." This is the only evidence produced for this idea, and subsequent work by the same authors and others was unable to substantiate it because, since the changes they monitored were reflex, they were found at the end of the day to be unpredictably variable. No other evidence has ever been produced to support what at the time appeared a perfectly legitimate hypothesis.

On the other hand, the body of evidence now in favour of the complexity, plasticity and co-activity of neurology is vast. (See The Dorsal Horn, p.47). "Upper cervical roots spread six segments, and lower ones fourteen, six above and seven below the segment of entry in the cat, and L3 to S2 roots all show some projection in all of these segments, the most dense being in their own segment."[98] The immensely widespread activity shown by the cervical reflexes is such that 'localized' concepts of organic disease must be looked at somewhat askance.

This does not condemn osteopathy, as to do so on these grounds would be as unreasonable as to reject orthodox medicine on the grounds of the prevalence of the diagnosis of the disc lesion that was so dominant a generation ago.

Visceral and somatic pain
Perhaps most important for the current situation in this field is the fact that too few doctors appreciate that, as Kellgren has shown in Copeman's *Textbook of the Rheumatic Diseases*, "there are no simple criteria by which we can distinguish between pain of visceral and somatic origin."[73] Therefore, its assessment should be an integral part of the evaluation of conditions presenting as being ostensibly visceral in origin. By the same token, of course, visceral problems can present as being overtly spinal in origin.

The scale of this close association is so great and the current situation so unsatisfactory, that it highlights the fact that musculoskeletal considerations are a part, and an important part, of orthodox medicine.

References

1. Dubuisson (1983). Nerve root damage and arachnoiditis. In Wall and Melzack (eds.) *Textbook of Pain*, p. 442. (London: Churchill Livingstone)
2. Frykholm (1971). The clinical picture. In Hirsch and Zotterman (eds.) *Cervical Pain*, p. 5. (Oxford: Pergamon Press)
3. Hitzelberger and Witton (1968). Abnormal myelograins in asymptomatic patients. *J. Neurosurg.*, **28**, 204
4. Kelly (1958). Is pain due to pressure on nerves? *Neurology*, **6**, 32–36

5. Frickholm (1951). Cervical nerve root compression resulting from disc degeneration and root sleeve fibrosis. *Acta Chirugica Scand.*, **(Suppl.)** **160**, 11–49
6. Murphey (1968). Sources and patterns of pain in disc disease. *Clin. Neurosurg.*, **15**, 343–350
7. Loeser and Ward (1967). Some effects of deafferentiation on neurones of the cat's spinal cord. *Arch. Neurol.*, **17**, 620–636
8. Loeser and Ward (1968). Chronic deafferentiation of human spinal cord neurones. *J. Neurosurg.*, **29**, 48–50
9. Dykes and Terzis (1981). Spinal nerve distributions in the upper limb. The organisation of the dermatome and afferent myotome. *Phil. Trans. R. Soc. of London, Series B Biol. Sci.*, **293**, 529–554
10. Dubuisson (1983). In Wall and Melzack, op. cit., p. 594
11. Sterling and Kuypers (1967). Anatomical organisation of the brachial spinal cord of the cat. 1. The distribution of dorsal root fibres. *Brain Res.*, **4**, 115
12. Imai and Kusama (1969). Distribution of the dorsal root fibres in the cat. An experimental study with the nauta method. *Brain Res.*, **13**, 338–359
13. Wall and Werman (1976). The physiology and anatomy of long ranging afferent fibres within the spinal cord. *J. Physiol.*, **255**, 321–334
14. Brown and Culverson (1981). Somatotopic organisation of hind limb cutaneous dorsal root projections to cat dorsal horn. *J. Neurophys.*, **45**, 137–143
15. Wall (1977). The presence of ineffective synapses and the circumstances which unmask them. *Phil. Trans. R. Soc. London*, **278**, 361–372
16. Dubuisson *et al.* (1979). Amoeboid receptive fields of cells in laminae 1, 2 and 3. *Brain Res.*, **177**, 376–378
17. Dubuisson and Wall (1980). Descending influences on single units in laminae 1 and 2 of cat spinal cord. *Brain Res.*, **199**, 283–298
18. Kibler and Nathan (1960). Relief of pain and paraesthesiae by nerve block distal to the lesions. *J. Neurol., Neurosurg. Psychiatry*, **23**, 91–98
19. Wall and Cronly-Dylan (1960). Pain, itch and vibration. *Arch. Neurol.*, **2**, 365–375
20. Wall (1964). Presynaptic control of impulses at the first central synapse in the cutaneous pathway. In *Physiology of Spinal Neurones. Progress in Brain Research 12*, pp. 92–118. (Amsterdam: Elsevier)
21. Wall and Sweet (1967). Temporary abolition of pain in man. *Science*, **155**, 108–109
22. Willer *et al.* (1980). Human nociceptive reactions. Effects of spatial summation of afferent input from relatively large diameter fibres. *Brain Res.*, **201**, 465–470
23. Wall (1962). The origin of a spinal cord slow potential. *J. Physiol.*, **164**, 508–526
24. Coggeshall *et al.* (1975). Unmyelinated axons in human ventral roots, a possible explanation for the failure of dorsal rhizotony to relieve pain. *Brain*, **98**, 157–166
25. Hosobuchi (1980). The majority of unmyelinated axons in human ventral roots probably conduct pain. *Pain*, **8**, 167–180
26. Devor (1983). The pathophysiology of damaged nerves. In Wall and Melzack, op. cit., p. 51
27. Ochoa and Torebjork (1980). Paraesthesiae from ectopic impulse generation in human sensory nerves. *Brain*, **103**, 835–853
28. Wall (1983). Introduction. In Wall and Melzack, op. cit., pp. 6–9
29. Wynn-Parry and Withrington (1983). The management of painful peripheral nerve disorders. In Wall and Melzack, op. cit.
30. Wilkins and Brody (1969). Lasegue's sign. *Arch. Neurol.*, **21**, 219
31. Nachemson (1976). Lumbar spine. An orthopaedic challenge. *Spine*, **1**, 59
32. Cyriax (1981). *Illustrated Manual of Orthopaedic Medicine.* (London: Butterworth)
33. Bradford and Spurling (1945). *The Intervertebral Disc.* 2nd Edn. (Springfield, Ill.: Thomas)
34. Barr (1951). Protruded discs and painful backs. *J. Bone Jt. Surg.*, **33B**, 3
35. Friberg (1954). Lumbar disc degeneration in the problem of lumbago sciatica. *Bull. Hosp. Jt. Dis.*, **15**, 1
36. Rabinovitch (1961). *Diseases of the Intervertebral Disc and its Surrounding Tissues.* (Springfield, Ill.: Thomas)
37. Hirsch (1965). Efficiency of surgery in low back pain disorders. Pathoanatomical, experimental and clinical studies. *J. Bone Jt. Surg.*, **47A**, 991

38. De Palma and Rothman (1970). *The Intervertebral Disc.* (Philadelphia: Saunders) 3. cit.
39. Scott-Charleton and Roebuck (1972). The significance of posterior primary divisions of spinal nerves in pain syndromes. *Med. J. Aust.*, **2**, 945
40. Arnoldi (1972). Intravertebral pressures in patients with lumbar pain. A preliminary communication. *Acta Orthop. Scand.*, **43**, 109
41. Mooney and Robertson (1978). The facet syndrome. *Clin. Orthop. Rel. Res.*, **115**, 149
42. Weinstein, Ehni and Wilson (1977). *Lumbar Spondylosis. Diagnosis, Management and Surgical Treatment.* (London: Year Book Medical Publications)
43. Sunderland (1978). Traumatised nerves, roots and ganglia. Musculoskeletal factors and neuropathological consequences. In Korr (ed.) *The Neurobiological Mechanisms in Manipulative Therapy*, p.137. (London: Plenum Press)
44. Andersson (1982). Mechanisms of spinal pain. In Colt Symposium (London: National Back Pain Association)
45. O'Brien (1983). Mechanisms of spinal pain. In Wall and Melzack, op. cit.
46. Spangfort (1983). Disc surgery. In Wall and Melzack, op. cit.
47. Lewit (1985). *Manipulative Therapies in the Rehabilitation of the Motor System.* (London: Butterworths)
48. Lewis and Kellgren (1939). Observations related to referred pain, viscero-motor reflexes and other associated problems. *Clin. Sci.*, **4**, 47
49. Pederson *et al* (1956). The anatomy of lumbo-sacral posterior rami and meningeal branches of spinal nerves (sinuvertebral). *J. Bone Jt. Surg.*, **38A**, 377
50. King (1977). Randomised trial of the Rees and Shealy methods for the treatment of low back pain. In Buerger and Tobis (eds). *Approaches to the Validation of Manipulation Therapies*, p.70. (Springfield, Illinois: Thomas)
51. Kirkaldy-Willis and Hill (1979). A more precise diagnosis of low back pain. *Spine*, **4**, 102
52. Mcnab (1977). *Backache.* (Baltimore: Williams and Wilkins)
53. Sylvest, Hentzer and Cobayashi (1977). Ultrastructure of prolapsed disc. *Acta Orthop. Scand.*, **48**, 32
54. Bromage *et al.* (1963). Local anaesthetic drugs. Penetration from the spinal extradural space into the neuraxis. *Science*, **140**, 392–393
55. Cohen *et al.* (1968). The role of pH in the development of tachyphylaxis to local anaesthetic agents. *Anaesthesiology*, **29**, 994–1001
56. Drayer and Rosenbaum (1978). Studies of the third circulation. Amipaque CT cisternography and ventriculography. *J. Neurosurgery*, **48**, 946–956
57. Macnab (1971). Negative disc exploration. *J. Bone Joint Surg.*, **53A**, 891
58. Finneson (1978). A lumbar disc surgery predictive score card. *Spine*, **3**, 186–188
59. Spengler and Freeman (1979). Patient selection for lumbar discectomy. An objective approach. *Spine*, **4**, 129–134
60. Harkness *et al.* (1983). Osteoarthritis. In Wall and Melzack, op. cit., p. 215
61. Kellgren and Moore (1952). Generalised osteoarthritis and Heberden's nodes. *Brit. Med. J.*, **1**, 181–187
62. Peter *et al.* (1966). Erosive osteoarthritis of the hand. *Arthritis and Rheumatism*, **9**, 365–388
63. Ehrlich (1975). Osteoarthritis beginning with inflammation. *J. Am. Med. Assoc.*, **232**, 157–159
64. Huskisson *et al.* (1979). Another look at osteoarthritis. *Ann. Rheum. Dis.*, **38**, 423–428
65. Goldenberg *et al.* (1982). Inflammatory synovitis in degenerative joint disease. *J. Rheumatology*, **9**, 204–209
66. Cooper *et al.* (1981). Diagnostic specificity of synovial lesions. *Human Pathology*, **12** 314–328
67. Schumacher *et al.* (1981). Osteoarthritis, crystal deposition, and inflammation. *Seminars in Arthritis and Rheumatology*, **11**, 116–119
68. Bullough (1982). *Semin. Arthr. Rheum.*, (Suppl. 1) 11
69. Hart (1974). Pain in osteoarthritis. *Practitioner*, **212**, 244–250
70. Vernon-Roberts (1980). The pathology and interrelation of intervertebral disc lesions, osteoarthrosis of the apophyseal joints, lumbar spondylosis and low back pain. In Jayson (ed.) *The Lumbar Spine and Low Back Pain.* (London: Pitman Medical)

71. Hay (1974). The incidence of low back pain in Busselton. In Twomey (ed.). *Symposium. Low Back Pain*, p. 7. (Perth: Western Australian Institute of Technology)
72. Nachemson (1980). Lumbar intradiscal pressure. In Jayson (ed.) op. cit.
73. Kellgren (1978). In Copeman, *Textbook of the Rheumatic Diseases*, 5th Edn. (London: Pitman Medical)
74. Wyke (1980). The neurology of low back pain. In Jayson (ed.) op. cit.
75. Kellgren (1939). On the distribution of pain arising from deep somatic structures with damage of segmental pain areas. *Clinical Science*, 35, 193, 303
76. Frykholm (1951). Cervical nerve root compression resulting from disc degeneration and root sleeve fibrosis. *Acta. Chir. Scand.*, (Suppl.) 160
77. Cloward (1959). Cervical discography. *Ann. Surg.*, 150, 1052
78. Holt (1964). Fallacy of cervical discography. Report of 50 cases in normal subjects. *J. Am. Med. Assoc.*, 188, 799
79. Klafta and Collis (1969). The diagnostic inaccuracy of the pain response in cervical discography. *Clev. Clin. Court.*, 36, 35
80. Kirk and Denny-Brown (1970). Functional variations in dermatomes in the macaque monkey following dorsal root lesions. *J. Comp. Neurol.*, 139, 307
80a. Denny-Brown *et al.* (1973). The tract of Lissauer in relation to sensory transmission in the dorsal horn of the spinal cord of the macaque. *J. Comp. Neurol.*, 151, 175
81. Last (1978). *Anatomy, Regional and Applied.* 4th Edn., p. 27. (Edinburgh: Churchill Livingstone)
82. Wall (1983). In Wall and Melzack (eds.) op. cit., p. 81
83. Bourdillon (1973). *Spinal Manipulation.* 2nd Edn. (Lodon: Heinemann)
84. Wall (1983). In Wall and Melzack (eds.) op. cit., p. 80
85. Ibid., p. 85
86. O'Brien (1979). Anterior spinal tenderness in low back pain syndromes. *Spine*, 4, 85
87. Simons and Travell (1983). Myofascial pain syndromes. In Wall and Melzack (eds.) op. cit.
88. Froriep (1943). Ein beitrag zur pathologie und therapie des rheumatismus. (Weimar)
89. Simons (1975). Muscle pain syndromes. Part 1. *Am. J. Phys. Med.*, 54, 289
90. Copeman and Ackerman (1947). Oedema or herniations of fat lobules as a cause of lumbar and gluteal fibrositis. *Arch. Int. Med.*, 79, 22
91. Simons (1976). Muscle pain syndromes. Part 2. *Am. J. Phys. Med.*, 55, 15
92. Melzack *et al.* (1977). Trigger points and acupuncture points for pain. Correlations and implications. *Pain*, 3, 23
93. Wyke (1970). The neurological basis of thoracic spinal pain. *Rheum. Phys. Med.*, 10, 356
94. Vrettos and Wyke (1974). Articular reflexogenic systems in the costovertebral joints. *J. Bone Joint Surg.*, 56B, 382
95. Reading (1983). Testing pain mechanisms in persons in pain. In Wall and Melzack (eds.) op. cit.
96. Stoddard (1969). *Manual of Osteopathic Practice.* (London: Hopkinson)
97. Denslow, Korr and Krems (1947). Quantitative studies of chronic facilitation in human motoneuron pools. *Am. J. Physiology*, 150, 229–238
98. Fitzgerald (1983). Primary afferents. In Wall and Melzack (eds.) op. cit.

8
RELEVANT PATHOLOGY –
REGIONAL CONSIDERATIONS

The cervical spine

1. "It has to be kept in mind that there is no strict interdependence between clinical symptoms and radiological pathology in the cranio-vertebral region."[1]
2. It has been shown that the incidence of arthrosis in the upper cervical spine increases with age from 36% from the age of 41 to 50, to 68% from the age of 51 to 60, and to 88% at the age of 61 and above[2].
3. The frequency of incidence, in descending order, of spondylosis at successive segmental levels is[3,4]: C5/6 > C3/4 > C4/5 > C7/T1
4. Osteoarthritic encroachment into the intervertebral canal can also lead to compression of both artery and nerve roots[5].
5. Vascular compression can be shown to have far-reaching and extensive clinical consequences both above and below the level of compression[6]. These are given in detail in Relevant Anatomy (p. 13) and Clinical Presentations (p. 173).
6. The ligamentum flavum may buckle in the spinal canal[3].
7. Thickening of the dura mater can cause tethering of the spinal cord.
8. With regard to the basilar artery syndrome (well documented in other texts) arteriographic changes have only been shown in 30% of cases[7]. The remainder are due to distortion of neurological input due to degeneration of soft tissues, in turn leading to loss of nerve receptors.

Grisel's syndrome
It has been shown, and confirmed radiologically, that children with upper respiratory tract infections may develop a temporary laxity of the cranio-vertebral ligaments. This reverts to normal following appropriate treatment and given time. The time required is variable, resolution being judged by X-ray[8-10].

The rheumatoid neck
The cervical spine is involved in approximately 40% of rheumatoid arthritis[11] and atlanto-axial subluxation has been demonstrated as occurring in about 25%[12]. The criterion here employed is an anterior arch-odontoid separation

of more than 3 mm being demonstrated[13]. The reason for this is that rheumatoid arthritis has a predilection for the cranio-cervical ligaments, in particular the transverse ligament[14].

The lower cervical spine can also be severely affected[15].

There is no positive correlation between the degree of the radiological changes and the clinical features[16].

Atlanto-axial joint fixation

Rotatory deformity of this joint is usually short lived[17]. However, it can persist. In a series of 17 patients, 13 came to atlanto-axial arthrodesis[17]. The importance of recognizing atlanto-axial rotational deformity lies in the fact that it may indicate a compromised atlanto-axial complex, with the potential to cause neural damage or even death[17].

Clinical consequences of cervical problems

1. a. With regard to vertebrobasilar artery problems, manual therapy is strongly contraindicated.
   b. Even clinical testing has been known to cause fatal accidents and is therefore absolutely contraindicated.
2. With regard to Grisel's syndrome, manual therapy is again contraindicated, until such time as there remains no hypermobility.
3. Clearly, manipulation of the rheumatoid neck is potentially dangerous and is therefore again absolutely contraindicated.
4. With regard to atlanto-axial problems, the same considerations apply.

The thoracic spine

1. The incidence of arthrosis is common, with the highest incidence demonstrated both radiologically and at postmortem examination at the upper and lower ends of the thoracic spine[18,19].
2. In a series of 195 cadavers, it was found that degenerative changes involved the sympathetic trunks in 78.4% of cases[20].
3. The incidence of thoracic disc lesions is low[21]. In a series of 2948 cases of disc prolapse, only 7 occurred in the thoracic spine between the segments T8 and T12[22]. However, although these lesions are extremely rare, they are clinically important because surgical results are poor[22]. In a series of 17 cases, only 1 was improved by surgery, and none recovered completely.
4. Scheuermann's disease[23]. This occurs mainly in the second decade of life, its aetiology being unknown[24]. As a result of osteochondritis of the cartilaginous plate, the nucleus pulposus causes damage to the cancellous bone of the vertebral body. In minor cases this damage is trivial; in severe cases it may cause collapse of the vertebral body.
5. Gout is a rare cause of spinal pain, but when it does cause spinal pain it is

usually in the thoracic region[25].

6. a. Osteoporosis is five times more common in women than in men and is often asymptomatic, but back ache is its most frequent presenting symptom[26].

    b. Backache associated with osteoporosis is common. In a survey of 481 patients with backache, 31% were found to have osteoporosis[27].

7. Ankylosing spondylitis is also a not uncommon cause of thoracic pain.

Practical clinical consequences of thoracic problems
1. Degenerative changes are, once again, not necessarily related to pain.
2. Rheumatological factors should particularly be borne in mind.

The lumbar spine
Degenerative changes
1. These are universal. A recent study of 100 lumbar spines has shown that degenerative changes are present in the intervertebral discs of all subjects by middle age and are present in many spines by the age of 30[28].
2. It has been shown that in 90% of cadavers over the age of 40, interspinous ligaments between L1 and L5 have degenerated or completely ruptured[29].
3. However, there is no correlation between the severity of radiological signs of degeneration and clinical features[30].
4. Every pathological change and lumbosacral anomaly demonstrated in patients with backache have subsequently been found in pain-free populations[31].
5. Macnab[32] has summarized the possible causes of root entrapment syndrome as follows:
    a. Foraminal impingement of the emerging nerve root by a subluxated posterior zygoapophyseal joint.
    b. Kinking of a nerve root by a pedicle, and compression of the nerve root against the pedicle by a diffuse bulging disc.
    c. Entrapment of the nerve root in the subarticular gutter.
    d. Diffuse spinal stenosis.
    e. Segmental spinal stenosis.
    f. Iatrogenic (postfusion) spinal stenosis.
    g. Extradural tumours.
    h. Laminar impingement as in spondylolisthesis. Extraforaminal entrapment – the corporotransverse ligament; engulfment by a peripheral disc bulge.
6. However, "possibly the great majority of root compressions due to disc protrusion are asymptomatic". In a series of 300 patients having no symptoms referable to cervical or lumbar roots, myelography showed root sleeve deformities and other abnormalities characteristic of disc

protrusion in 110 (37%). Multiple defects were shown in 18%. The incidence of symptomatic root compression is not known[30].

7. The segmental incidence in a series of 2948 cases of disc prolapse was as follows[33]: L1/L2, 6; L2/L3, 14; L3/L4, 135; L4/L5, 1667; L5/S1, 1090.
8. "The multiple variety of degenerative changes in the lumbar region is well illustrated in an analysis of 227 patients whose pains and disabilities were sufficient to warrant surgery . . . only 70 had a simple prolapse of the nucleus pulposus, 65 had lumbar spondylosis, 5 had spinal stenosis. The remainder had a combination of 2 or more of these conditions, observed with myelography and confirmed at operation."[34]

Spondylolisthesis
1. The term spondylolisthesis means the forward slip of a vertebral body on its subjacent fellow, this being secondary to a defect in the pars interarticularis[35].
2. The incidence of the condition in the general population is not known, but it is frequently picked up radiologically and is often symptomless. It is at present not possible to give an accurate estimate of the percentage of all cases that do experience pain.

Spinal stenosis
1. This term is used to denote narrowing of the lumen of the spinal canal, but the shape of the canal is also important; a narrow canal of trefoil shape being a combination putting nerve roots at risk. It can be classified as being developmental or acquired[36].
2. Its study has been much enhanced by the work with ultrasound by Porter *et al.*[37]. This has considerable clinical significance. For example, if the measurement is above the mean, the cause of back pain may not be in the canal at all. It may help to answer the question as to whether the backache is mechanical or if the lesion is in the root canal. Detection of this condition will also help surgeons to plan operations. Thus a very narrow canal is likely to incline them to decompress the canal by removal of the laminae and spinous processes[37].
3. It is also an interesting example of the vagaries of clinical fashion. "Although there are several degenerative spinal diseases, not until 1960 was spondylotic caudal radiculopathy accurately diagnosed and properly treated. For nearly 20 years the syndrome was confused with that of a protruded disc. Medical opinion to the contrary was either disregarded or unpublished. Evidence suggests that compression of the cauda equina in a smaller than normal spine has long existed, but the clues leading to its discovery were repeatedly misinterpreted."[38]

144

Scoliosis
1. This has been shown to be variable. In a study of 545 X-rays it was shown that 45% of spines showed a convexity to one side, 32% to the other, while 23% showed a straight spine[24].
2. There is no positive correlation between scoliosis and pain[39–41].

Lateral pelvic tilt
1. "There is no detailed information on the effect on the spine of lateral pelvic tilt due to leg length discrepancy."[42]
2. In one series more than twice the number of patients presenting with backache had a short leg in comparison with a control group without backache, although 40% of the group with backache did not have leg length inequality. Therefore the association of these two factors is seen to be variable[24].
3. Moreover, there is disagreement with regard to the assessment of lateral pelvic tilt. "There is no one general agreement on the incidence of leg length inequality in otherwise normal subjects, or on how much this difference may be associated with symptoms. The recorded incidence of difference in leg length will depend upon the methods of assessment and the selection of patients. The smaller the unit of measurement, the greater will be the incidence, and the larger the unit of measurement, the greater will be the agreement between observers."[43]

Sagittal pelvic tilt
"Critical evaluation of all available investigative results makes it difficult to diagnose an abnormal lumbosacral angle, and it is even more difficult to consider it as a cause of pain."[44]

Practical clinical consequences of lumbar problems
Structural features: A study has been undertaken of a group of 150 people between the ages of 35 and 40 years. Subjects had been engaged in heavy work all their lives. Those of one group were under treatment for low back pain, those of the other group were pain free and denied any history of low back pain at any time. There was no statistical difference in anatomical variants seen on X-ray, and measurements for lumbar lordosis and lumbosacral angle were evenly distributed between the two groups. There was no correlation between anatomical variants and the degree of disc degeneration. The only correlation observed was that between disc degeneration and age[45].

Therefore, it is clear that lumbar or any other regional spinal abnormality is not necessarily the cause of pain.

Sphincter disturbances. It has been shown that, while the incidence of degenerative changes on X-ray has no positive correlation with sphincter disturbance, the size of the neural canal is a crucial factor[46].

The pelvis
The sacroiliac joints
Degenerative changes
1. "The normal life history of the sacroiliac joints conforms essentially to the same pattern of degenerative change as occurs in the peripheral joints."[47]
2. In examination of 257 cadavers, osteophyte formation was demonstrated as follows[48]:

    Ages 40–49: females 50%; males 85%
    Ages 50–59: females 85%; males 100%

Sacroiliitis
1. As long ago as 1930 it was noted that the joint is invariably involved in ankylosing spondylitis[48].
2. It is a common denominator of other seronegative arthritides as well, including psoriatic arthropathy, Reiter's disease and intestinal arthropathies, for example regional ileitis, ulcerative colitis and Behçet's syndrome[49].

Practical consequences of pelvic changes
If one considers the complexity of the relevant anatomy and the paucity of validated pathology, it is clear that current diagnosis of mechanical problems of the sacroiliac joints remains highly unsatisfactory. Nowhere in the whole field of musculoskeletal medicine is the mass of conjecture, assertion, opinion and hypothesis greater than with regard to these problems. Why this should be so is not clear, but there is no doubt that the vast scale of this material is daunting for those with a developing interest in this subject.

The reality is, however, that manual procedures used by clinicians in dealing with problems presumed to originate from these joints will be essentially the same as those employed for pain of lumbar origin, since diagnostic and therapeutic procedures applied to either inevitably involve both.

Therefore the pragmatic clinician can safely ignore this literature, without prejudice to his patients.

Clinical consequences of general and regional pathology

1. In general, all these factors, severally or together, may or may not cause pain.

2. The material we have presented in general and regional pathology shows that nerve and root pain are not understood. Their diagnosis is therefore difficult.

3. From a practical point of view, valid diagnosis of mechanical problems is in the majority of cases unattainable, and specificity often spurious and possibly dangerous, since it may mislead the clinician into a false sense of certainty; in the event of the deployment of major invasive procedures this may prove disastrous.

4. Nevertheless, the universally recognized physiological phenomena which may not accompany pain can be useful in case analysis, despite their acknowledged limitations.

References

1. Von Torklus and Gehle (1972). *The Upper Cervical Spine*. (London: Butterworth)
2. Olsson (1942). Arthrosis Deformans des Zahngelenkens. *Fortscher Roentgen*, **66**, 233
3. Brain, Lord and Wilkinson (eds.) *Cervical Spondylosis*. (London: Heinemann)
4. Friedenberg *et al.* (1959). Degenerative changes in the cervical spine. *J. Bone Jt. Surg.*, **41A**, 61
5. Finneson (1969). *Diagnosis and Management of Pain Syndromes*. 2nd Edn. (London: Saunders)
6. Keuter (1970). Vascular origin of cranial sensory disturbances caused by pathology of the lower cervical spine. *Acta Neurochirurg.*, **23**, 229
7. Wyke (1983). In *Proceedings of the Seventh Congress of the International Federation of Manual Medicine*, Zurich. (Unpublished)
8. Grisel (1930). Enucleation de l'atlas et torticollis nasopharyngien. *Press Med.*, **38**, 50
9. Bell (1830). *The Nervous System of the Human Body*, appendix P cxxvii. No. lxiiv. (London: Longman)
10. Gutmann (1970). X-ray diagnosis of spinal dysfunction. *Man. Med.*, **4**, 1973
11. Sharpe and Purser (1961). Spontaneous atlanto-axial dislocation in ankylosing spondylitis and rheumatoid arthritis. *Am. Rheum. Dis.*, **20**, 47
12. Conlon *et al.* (1966). Rheumatoid arthritis and the cervical spine. *Am. Rheum. Dis.*, **25**, 120
13. Matthews (1969). Atlanto-axial subluxation in rheumatoid arthritis. *Am. Rheum. Dis.*, **28**, 260
14. Ball and Sharpe (1971). Rheumatoid arthritis of the cervical spine. In *Modern Trends of Rheumatology*, p. 117. (London: Butterworth)
15. Whaley and Dick (1968). Fatal sub-axial dislocation of the spine in rheumatoid arthritis. *Br. Med. J.*, **2**, 31
16. Cregan (1966). Internal fixation of the unstable rheumatoid cervical spine. *Am. Rheum. Dis.*, **25**, 242
17. Fielding and Hawkins (1977). Atlanto-axial rotatory fixation. *J. Bone Jt. Surg.*, **59A**, 37
18. Nathan *et al.* (1964). The costo-vertebral joints. Anatomico clinical observations in arthritis. *Arthritis Rheum.*, **7**, 228
19. Shore (1935). On osteo-arthritis in the dorsal intervertebral joints. *Br. J. Surg.*, **22**, 833
20. Nathan (1968). Compression of the sympathetic trunk by osteophytes of the vertebral column in the abdomen. An anatomical study with pathological and clinical considerations. *Surgery*, **63**, 609

21. Epstein (1969). *The Spine. A Radiological Text and Atlas.* 3rd Edn. (Philadelphia: Lea and Febiger)
22. Simeone (1971). The modern treatment of thoracic disc disease. *Orthop. Clin. Am.*, 2, 453
23. Scheuermann (1921). Zur roentgensymptomatologie der juvenilen osteochondritis dorsi. *Z. Orthop. Clin.*, 41, 305
24. Stoddard (1969). *The Manual of Osteopathic Practice.* (London: Hutchinson)
25. Tkach (1970). Gouty arthritis of the spine. *Clin. Orthop. Res.*, 71, 81
26. Nassim (1959). Osteoporosis. In Nassim and Burrows (eds.) *Modern Trends in Diseases of the Vertebral Column*, p. 125. (London: Butterworth)
27. Devlin and Goldman (1966). Back ache due to osteoporosis in an industrial population. *Irish J. Med. Sci.*, 484, 141
28. Vernon-Roberts and Pirie (1977). Degenerative changes in the intervertebral discs and their sequelae. *Rheum. Rehabil.*, 16, 13
29. Rissanen (1964). Comparisons of pathological changes in intervertebral discs and intraspinous segments of the lower part of the lumbar spine. *Acta Orthop. Scand.*, 34, 54
30. Hitselburger and Witten (1968). Abnormal myelograms in asymptomatic patients. *J. Neurol. Surg.*, 28, 284
31. Troup (1975). The biology of back pain. *New Scientist*, 65, 17
32. McNab (1977). *Backache.* (Baltimore, Md: Williams and Wilkins)
33. Huwyler (1952). Hernias discales. *Rev. Orthop.*, 38, 219
34. Grieve (1981). *Common Vertebral Joint Problems*, p. 145. (London: Churchill Livingstone)
35. Newman (1963). The aetiology of spondylothesis. *J. Bone Jt. Surg.*, 45B, 39
36. Porter *et al.* (1980). The shape and size of the lumbar canal. In *Proceedings of the Conference on Engineering Aspects of the Spine*, p. 19. (London: Mechanical Engineering Publications)
37. Porter *et al.* (1978). The spinal canal in symptomatic lumbar disc lesions. *J. Bone Jt. Surg.*, 60B, 485
38. Weinstein *et al.* (1977). *Lumbar Spondylosis. Diagnosis, Management and Surgical Treatment.* (London: Year Book Medical Publications)
39. Nilsonne and Lundgren (1968). Long term prognosis in ideopathic scoliosis. *Acta Orthop. Scand.*, 39, 456–465
40. Nachemson (1968). Back problems in childhood and adolescence. *Lakartidningen*, 65, 2831–2843
41. Collis and Ponsetti (1969). Long term follow-up of patients with ideopathic scoliosis not treated surgically. *J Bone Jt. Surg.*, 61A, 425–455
42. Farfan (1973). *Mechanical Disorders of the Low Back.* (Philadelphia: Lea and Febiger)
43. Nicholls (1960). Short leg syndrome. *Br. Med. J.*, 2, 1863
44. Schmorl and Junghanns (1971). *The Human Spine in Health and Disease.* 2nd American Edn. (New York: Grune and Stratton)
45. LaRocca and Macnab (1969). Value of pre-employment radiographic assessment of the lumbar spine. *Can. Med. J.*, 101, 383
46. Robinson (1965). Massive protrusion of lumbar discs. *Br. J. Surg.*, 52, 858
47. Newton (1957). Clinical aspects of sacro-iliac disease. *R. Soc. Med.*, 50, 850
48. Sashin (1930). A critical analysis of the anatomy of pathological changes of the sacro-iliac joint. *J. Bone Jt. Surg.*, 12, 891
49. Moll and Haslock (1975). Associations between ankylosing spondylitis, psoriatic arthritis, Reiter's Disease. The intestinal arthropathies and Beçhet's Syndrome. *Excerpta. Med. (Section 19)*, 18, 216

Part II
CLINICAL APPLICATIONS

9
BASIC CASE ANALYSIS

Introduction
This chapter relates to musculoskeletal medicine, excluding malignant, inflammatory and metabolic disorders.

We use the term case analysis rather than diagnosis because of the unpredictablity of the phenomena of referred pain and referred tenderness, and because nociceptor systems are present in many sites, and therefore, "in the great majority of cases we do not know the tissue or tissues from which back pain is originating, or the cause of that pain."[1]

Basic considerations and case analysis
The basic considerations, epidemiology (p. 1 *et seq.*), anatomy (p. 11 *et seq.*), physiology (p. 30 *et seq.*), psychology (p. 88 *et seq.*) and pathology (p. 118 *et seq.*), all demonstrate the extreme difficulty of making a valid diagnosis. We give particular emphasis to those aspects of physiology and psychology that we find most helpful in basic case analysis.

Physiology
History
a. The problem of referred pain means that the site of perception of pain is not necessarily of diagnostic significance and is frequently misleading.
b. The 'hornet's nest' of physiological activity to be found at all levels of the neuraxis, periphery, dorsal horn, and cerebral cortex, means that symptoms are inevitably subject to modification on this count alone.

Examination
a. The phenomenon of referred tenderness mirrors that of referred pain.
b. The hornet's nest referred to above is as applicable to physical signs as it is to symptoms.
c. The physiological phenomena that may or may not accompany pain (see p. 129), can, with certain limitations, be used in case analysis.
d. On scientific grounds, physiological parameters cannot be used in case analysis, as a means of measurement of pain.

151

Psychology
It will be appreciated that any clinician dealing with the chronic pain patient who is unaware of the complexities of these problems, as of the possibilities and limitations of the methods of their assessment, is clearly at a disadvantage in effective case analysis.

We allocate primacy to behavioural indices in case analysis, because these are objective and therefore may be agreed by all clinicians, whatever their discipline (see p. 111). This greatly simplifies the complex question of patient assessment and, as has been shown, avoids the difficulties inherent in subject report. We choose to use these criteria in the knowledge that no single response channel can ever be the perfect method of evaluation, but that they afford the clinician a practical basis for case analysis. We do not favour this to the exclusion of all else, because, "if it is pushed too far, it (behavioural assessment) results in a rather farcical situation, where patients say, 'they will treat me, but they will not listen to me about my pain,' and that is no good."[2]

Other relevant factors
Reference to the case analysis record sheet (pp. 162, 163) will show that other administrative and historical data are familiar to the clinician and need no description. Of particular relevance to musculoskeletal practice are disturbances of gait (raising the question of myelopathy), saddle anaesthesia and problems with micturition (raising the possibility of sacral root compression) and symptoms of basilar artery insufficiency.

Additional clinical procedures
The basic case analysis we present is simple enough to be used readily by any clinician, and in particular in general practice, where these problems so commonly present.

The scientific reality is that further tests, which are legion, do not in any way add to diagnostic validity. For this reason the clinician may bypass them without prejudice to the patient, thereby further saving time and limiting confusion.

Traditional medical examination
Posture
Some may find it surprising that posture has not been shown to predispose to back pain in general[3]. We include it because it may be relevant.

Global movements
These are flexion, extension, sidebending and rotation. Owing to the wide normal variation in range of all these movements (with age, gender, build and habit) it will be appreciated that their value lies more in monitoring progress

than in contributing towards a diagnosis. (See Relevant Anatomy, pp. 15, 18, 22).

We have found no convincing evidence that the subjective estimation of passive and resisted movements adds anything of value to the initial assessment.

Reflexes

Contrary to what is commonly believed, diminished reflexes do not necessarily denote root involvement, since it has been shown that the injection of zygoapophyseal joints with hypertonic saline can abolish ankle reflexes, and that these may subsequently be restored by injecting the same joints with steroid. Diminished reflexes must therefore be viewed with some reservation as a diagnostic index[4].

Straight leg raising

There are considerable reservations to be expressed with regard to this test. First, many structures are involved, and further, either muscle spasm or hip pathology will restrict movement[5]. It is normal to observe a variation between individuals between 70 and 120°; there is commonly a 10% variation of normal between left and right legs in the same individual, and many people develop pain[6] at no more than 60°. It has been shown that the injection of hypertonic saline into the zygo-apophyseal joints can reduce the straight leg raise to less than 70°, which can be restored to a full range by the subsequent injection of steroid into those joints[4]. King has demonstrated that this is also the case on treating trigger points in the paravertebral musculature[7]. Thus the principal value of this test is seen to be as a measure of therapeutic progress, rather than as a diagnostic index.

These findings also illustrate the limitations of any test which involves concurrent movement of numerous structures. Therefore we do not include tests such as Piedallu's[8] since they add nothing to diagnostic certainty, but merely increase the complexity of the clinician's task and the demands on his time. This latter is, of course, of particular relevance to general practice.

Altered sensation

Search for this is a part of traditional examination. It has been observed that hyperaesthesiae may be associated with paraesthesiae[9]. In musculoskeletal practice such changes are seldom found. "Rarely a patient will experience nuchal or suboccipital pain with simultaneous paraesthesiae of the ipsilateral part of the tongue" . . . (in disorders of the cervical spine)[10]. In view of the physiological complexity, such signs are obviously of limited diagnostic value, but again they may be helpful in the monitoring of management.

However, saddle anaesthesia is a sign of cardinal importance, appropriately included in this category and demanding immediate surgical referral[11].

Additional signs
See note on case analysis data recording (p.160; Figure 9.1).

Muscle testing
We do not include this in our basic system of case analysis for the following reasons:

1. The complexity of muscle action and interaction is such as to make the clinical testing of individual muscle strength difficult. (See p. 69 *et seq.*).
2. "Difficulties of measuring back and abdominal muscle strength and the subject selection make assessment of possible correlations difficult."[3]
3. Clinical methods are of necessity crude and non-specific. For example, "Another project we have carried out is to measure the maximum voluntary strengths of the trunk muscle in various populations. To do this, we arranged to have the subject's pelvis supported, while the back was extended as forcefully as possible against a chest harness which was connected to a force measuring load cell."[12]
4. With regard to the traditional neurological examination, Magora *et al.* (1974) examined 57 patients with headache syndromes and found EMG evidence of neuropathic or spinal lesions in the semispinalis muscles in a high proportion of them[13]. Their second remarkable observation was the high incidence of neuropathic lesions disclosed by EMG, **even though a careful neurological examination had not revealed any pathological signs**. Reliance upon this form of clinical assessment must therefore provide a relatively insensitive audit.
5. "Manual muscle tests are currently the primary procedure for determining muscular strength and the progression or regression of strength. Yet these tests are subjective, and their accuracy depends on the training, skill and experience of the clinician performing the examination[14]. A relatively recent report, stated that there are no quantitative methods for measuring muscle function in clinical use today . . ."[15]
6. "When a muscle or group of muscles is weakened, there is a tendency for subtle shifts in the pattern of muscle activity to occur, to enable the synergistic muscles to generate the required force. This is known as muscle substitution, and it denies the impaired muscle the intended exercise. Muscle strength is difficult to test by current manual testing, which depends greatly on the experience of the clinician."[16]

Those who, in spite of the very real limitations indicated above, continue to find these tests of clinical value may enter such data under 'Additional signs'.

154

Investigations
Special investigations are surprisingly seldom required in musculoskeletal
practice. Such investigations as are from time to time regarded as necessary
by the clinician include the following:

Conventional radiology	Magnetic resonance imaging
Thermography	Transverse axial tomography
Myelography	Erythrocyte sedimentation rate
Electromyography	Scintography
Radiculography	Serum urea estimation
Electronystagmography/cupulo-	Interosseous spinal venography
graphy	Serum uric acid estimation
Epidurography	Vertebral artery angiography
Radioactive isotope studies	Rose–Waaler test
Discography	Intervertebral disc manometry
Ultrasonography	Latex test
Tomography	

This list is not intended to be comprehensive, rather is it offered to stress the
very considerable number of tests which may be found relevant in individual
cases. Details of these tests will be found in the appropriate texts.

Comment on special investigations
1. Conventional radiology
a. Attempts have also been made to relate back pain to skeletal defects, be
   they congenital or aquired. La Rocca and Macnab, in 1969, showed that
   many different defects exist without causing pain[17].
b. As the detection on palpation of segmental hyper- and hypomobility has
   been used to diagnose spinal lesions and monitor their treatment, so has
   conventional radiology. In fact radiological hyper- and hypomobility and
   their responses to manipulative treatment have never been conclusively
   demonstrated. The fact that Swezey and Silverman, in 1971, showed that
   the overriding of zygoapophyseal joints of 3 mm in the middle of the
   cervical spine and 3.5 mm at the level of L5 and S1 were not detectable on
   routine X-rays indicates the difficulty of such endeavours[18].
c. There is no positive correlation between degenerative changes shown by
   conventional radiology and pain. The clinical consequences of this are
   discussed on p. 129.

2. Myelography
a. Hitzelberger and Witten showed that 37% of pain-free subjects had
   positive myelograms[19].

b. Hudgins refers to the fact that at operation 20% of cases had operable space-occupying lesions in the absence of myelographic evidence[20].

c. Wright *et al.* showed that in 12 cases out of 150 coming to operation there were false positive myelograms[21].

These findings exemplify the difficulties of precise diagnosis met with in all special investigations.

Therefore in spite of the "impressive development of the technological investigative methods, it may still be an extremely difficult task to supply the necessary diagnostic foundation for decisions about the proper surgical treatment in the individual cases of lumbar pain syndromes."[22]

Local examination of the back

Introduction

The traditional methods of clinical examination and investigation we have outlined are, of course, essential. They do, however, as we have indicated, have limitations.

With regard to the cervical spine, "We early came to the conclusion, reinforced by long experience, that, contrary to the statements of many physicians on this topic, but in agreement with Brain et al (1952) neurological findings are of extremely limited use in the assessment of the precise level of cord and root involvement, and may be misleading."[23]

"In a series of 500 patients surgically treated for disc disease, correct preoperative clinical localisation was achieved in only 39.2%."[24]

Local examination is traditionally medically unorthodox. There are perhaps two exceptions to this; the search for trigger points, and, more recently, the emergence of the 'facet joint syndrome'.

However, local examination is an integral part of both osteopathic and chiropractic practice; for both of them mobility is of fundamental import-ance. For the chiropractor, "the first characteristic of the manipulable lesion is restricted joint motion. This is the so-called fixation or blockage. The diagnosis of restricted joint motion is through palpation of movement between vertebrae or by motion X-ray. For example, the palpation of flexion–extension motion can be achieved by placing the fingers between the spinous processes and having the patient flex and extend the spine."[25] The chiropractor seeks to find by palpation tissue changes, and in particular changes in mobility, at the segmental level assumed to be at fault.

For the osteopath, the keystone of his practice is the osteopathic spinal lesion, which is a condition of impaired mobility in an intervertebral joint. To quote Colin Dove, "what the osteopath aims to do is to restore the normal functions of tissues, particularly movement where it is perceived to be lacking. Even if his assessment leads him to assume that the symptoms are arising at the level of hypermobility, he will seek to improve mobility elsewhere."[26]

We have reservations regarding the use of mobility tests in local examination (see p. 26).

For these reasons we confine ourselves to the undisputed physiological phenomena, described by Kellgren, in Copeman's *Textbook of the Rheumatic Diseases*[32]. They may or may not accompany pain, but they are not quantifiable indices of the severity of that pain, nor are they reliable indicators of its site. For these reasons, the use of physiological changes to measure pain has invariably failed. "In general there would seem to be little basis for discrete physiological changes related to the pain experience."[27] Because of referred pain and referred tenderness, these signs cannot be used to identify a specific site of origin of that pain.

What is the point of seeking these signs? The answers are two.

1. As an indication of segmental level or levels to which local therapy may best be directed.
2. As a monitor of therapeutic progress (like global movements or the SLR test).

For these reasons they have clinical relevance.

Historical

These signs have been known to clinicians for a very long time. For example, Korr, in 1948[28], described, the 'spinal lesion' as being associated with:

a. Tenderness
b. Muscular changes
c. Autonomic changes
d. Alterations in pain description.

Items (a) and (b) are clearly relevant to this discussion, and appear in a paper entitled, "The emerging concept of the osteopathic lesion," in 1948[28]. Item (c) is discussed under Autonomic Nervous System (p. 135) and item (d) under Subject Report (p. 105).

These signs have been described in many varying and at times eccentric ways. Within the body of orthodox medicine many authors from different countries have seen fit to make use of these signs (e.g. Brugger[29] and Sutter[30]). In fact many doctors may share scientific bases to a greater extent than they realise. This is a matter from which bodies such as the Fédération Internationale de Médecine Manuelle might well profit.

More than twenty years ago, Maigne made (amongst others) two major contributions[31]; the first was to translate the description of these signs into terms both intelligible and acceptable to the medical profession in his country, the second was to use diagnostically the term which translates most readily into English as the 'painful segmental disorder'. By the latter he avoided the pitfall of making a specific diagnosis which, in the light of subsequent modification of understanding, would of necessity become untenable. This showed remarkable prescience, and has stood the test of time. Indeed the system we present is modelled closely upon his work.

Clinical tests

These are all unoriginal and, for reasons already given, are presented in terms as explicit and orthodox as possible.

They must be sought anteriorly as well as posteriorly (for example, as detailed elsewhere, spinal pain and tenderness can be referred to the anterior chest and abdominal wall).

In view of the difficulties we have emphasized already, local examination must be comprehensive. The whole spine should be examined.

1. Skin pinching

This is a test for tenderness of the skin and subcutaneous tissues. The examiner raises a fold of skin at paired sites either side of the midline and pinches as nearly symmetrically as he can. Because of the phenomenon of referred tenderness, this must be done widely, both posteriorly and anteriorly. Not infrequently the examiner will observe a difference in thickness of the skinfold between the two sides at the level the patient reports tenderness. This difference may be eliminated on resolution of the tenderness. There is currently no valid explanation for this phenomenon. A positive finding does not indicate the segmental level of dysfunction.

2. Muscle guarding

This test seeks to identify segmental levels at which there is a difference in muscle tone between the two sides. A positive finding, while clearly subjective, is well known to physicians and generally accepted by them, as in the case of guarding in acute abdominal pathology. This finding is commonly associated with tenderness.

3. Trigger points

Deep palpation seeks to elicit tenderness in trigger points. Since these may be found widely, they must be sought equally widely.

4. Segmental sagittal pressure

This test seeks to elicit pain on applying a midline sagittal force to the spinous processes at successive segmental levels. It serves to implicate either the vertebra to which it is applied, or the various joints above and below. Since the spinous processes in the cervical spine are (except for that of C7) so deep and small as to be in practice impalpable, this test is inapplicable to the cervical region. Of course, many more joints are moved by this test than those immediately adjacent to the vertebra pressed upon, but the force and resultant movement are concentrated in sequence at each segmental level.

5. *Lateral spinous process pressure*
This test produces a forced rotation of successive vertebrae, performed by pressing with the thumbs on the lateral aspect of each spinous process, alternately to the left and the right. Once more, it involves a **minimum** of **all** the joints between the vertebra pressed upon and its two neighbours, but many more joints must be affected, so rendering it pretty non-specific.

6. *Zygoapophyseal tenderness*
This test seeks to reveal any tenderness there may be of the zygoapophyseal joint capsules and adjacent structures, in an attempt to locate the site of origin of the symptoms. The examiner presses firmly over the joints at each segmental level in turn and asks the patient to report tenderness at any site. Apart from its use in determining a possible site of dysfunction, this test is of value in that it may reveal the potentially most suitable site for local treatment (e.g. injection). It is more specific than the previous two tests, in that it gives some indication of the side as well as the segmental level, to which attention may profitably be directed (e.g. in the case of the employment of local injections).

Conclusion
The practical features of this system of case analysis are:
1. It is based on the relevant anatomical, physiological, psychological and pathological facts, as they are currently understood.
2. Whatever its acknowledged shortcomings, it provides a rational basis for clinical assessment and management.
3. It is intended to be brief enough to be of use to every clinician.
4. To this scientifically orientated basis physicians may add whatever further symptoms and signs they may find useful in their individual practices (e.g. spinal joint mobility).
5. Because it is founded on scientific considerations, it will inevitably be subject to modification in the light of further knowledge and understanding.
6. It thereby avoids dogma, as baneful an influence in musculoskeletal medicine as in other fields.
7. The case analysis sheet provides a check list for the clinician, which aims at: (a) being comprehensive, and (b) affording comparability of data from different observers.

159

Notes to case analysis data sheet

1. General

We present a case analysis data recording form which we regard as a working compromise between the amassing of excessive information and the practical need of the clinician for brevity. The reasons for the omission of various symptoms and signs is to be found in the Introduction, p.151. Here we offer notes on the use of the form.

2. History

a. Subject report

Site and radiation of pain are entered by region, left or right, anterior or posterior, (as shown in the example in Figure 9.2). Intensity is recorded as being severe, moderate or slight, its duration in suitable shorthand. Also entered are items the patient thinks worsen or improve his pain. Altered sensation is treated similarly. Provision is made for entries on three dates.

b. Activities of daily living and pain behaviour

i. The number chosen is intended to be sufficient for their clinical purpose, yet too many to be manipulated by the patient. This is, of course, a compromise, and one which may readily be modified to suit the individual clinician.

ii. We suggest that entries be made as each activity constituting a major, moderate or minor disability for the patient, a nil entry meaning no problem. It should be noted that, if a patient complains of severe pain, but exhibits little objective disability, this is of substantial clinical significance and can be recorded. (See discussion of abnormal pain behaviour, p. 101).

iii. In pill taking we record the identity, quantity and frequency of medication, as this affords a measure of pain behaviour and illustrates the changes that may take place following therapy.

iv. With regard to other treatments, we have in mind (for example) a self-selected therapy such as acupuncture, which patients often deploy as an auxiliary treatment, and any change in the use of such an additional therapy is of value in the assessment of clinical progress.

v. With regard to bedrest, we record the number of hours spent in bed each day, for the same reasons that we record details of pill taking.

3. Investigations

This item appears on the form following history purely due to the demands of space. It is considered in the text in its conventional place, following traditional examination.

BASIC CASE ANALYSIS

MUSCULOSKELETAL CASE ANALYSIS SHEET

Patient's name..Serial No:..........
Address...Insurance..........
....Phone..............
Date of birth   /   /   Male.... Female....

Family doctor's name...........................
Address.......................................
..................................Phone..............NHS/Private......

HISTORY - Present episode.

Subject report

		/ /		/ /		/ /	
		L	R	L	R	L	R
Pain –	Site						
	Radiation						
	Intensity						
	Duration						
	Worsened by						
	Improved by						
Altered sensation							
	P & N						
	Numbness						

Activities of daily living

Hoovering			
Bedmaking			
Ablutions			
Cooking			
Ironing			
Putting on socks			
Shopping			
Gardening			
Sports.			
Sitting at desk			
Other work			
Road/rail travel			
Air travel			

Pain behaviour

Pill taking habit			
Other treatments			
Hours in bed per 24			
Forced absenteeism			
Litigation pending			

Previous episodes
        Year...... Site.......... Duration Days... Weeks... Months....
        Therapy........................... Outcome..................
        Year...... Site.......... Duration Days... Weeks... Months....
        Therapy..........................Outcome..................

Relevant medical history...

Investigations...

Figure 9.1 Case analysis sheet (front)

MUSCULOSKELETAL MEDICINE – THE SPINE

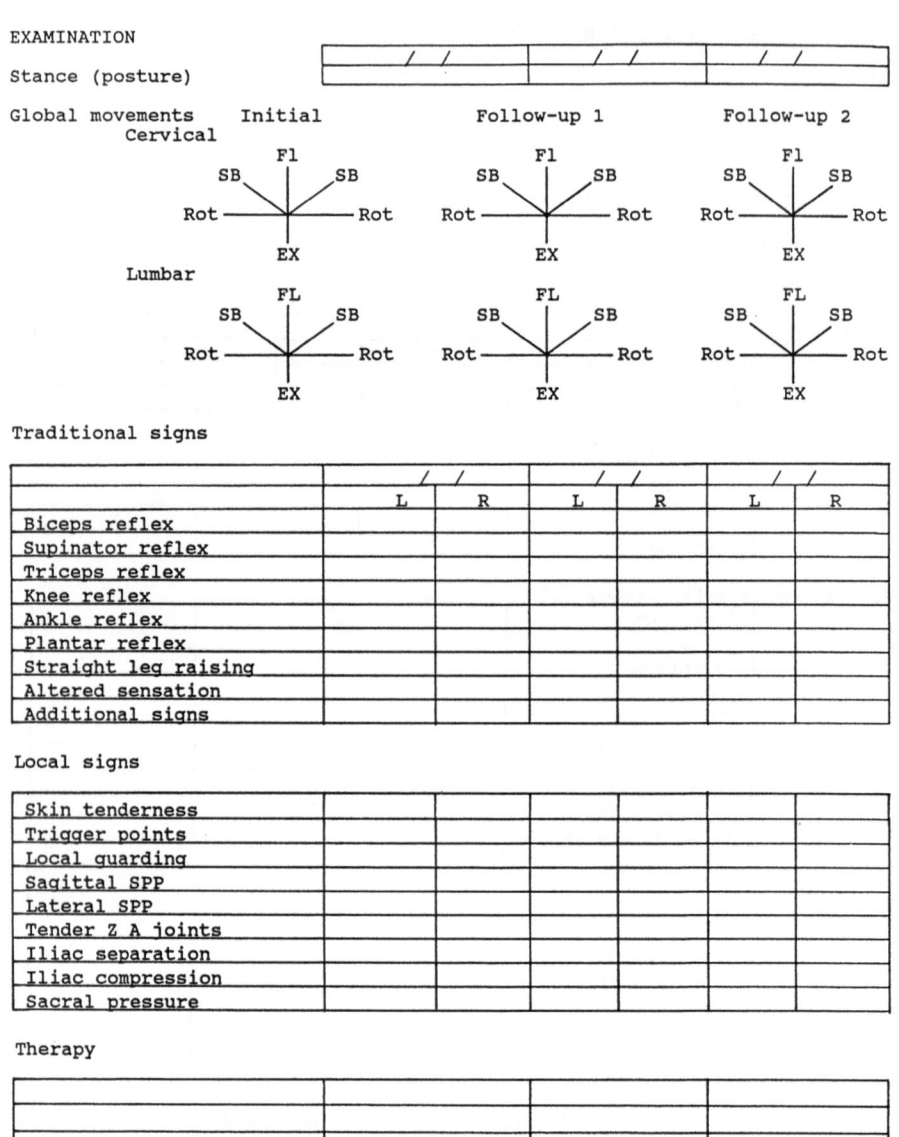

EXAMINATION

Stance (posture)

Global movements

Therapy

Figure 9.1 Case analysis sheet (back)

4. Examination

As with the activities of daily living and pain behaviour parts of the history, we allow for entries in relation to examination to be made on three separate occasions. A large tick indicates no abnormality found.

a. *Stance/posture*. We record this since it is an observable phenomenon which may alter with treatment. Its description is left to the clinician. This must include assessment of pelvic tilt, since this **may** be relevant to the patient's symptoms, albeit in an unpredictable proportion of cases.

b. *'Global' movements*. These are entered by marking the limbs of the 'star' with either dashes for apparent restriction of movement and crosses for pain provoked by that movement, in each case from 0 to 3. An example of this method of data entry (also illustrating the whole record for a fictitious case) is to be found in Figure 9.2. This system is not applicable to the thoracic spine.

c. *Traditional signs*. The limitations of these signs are discussed in some detail on p. 154. We record these by +, – or 0 in respect of reflexes (or a tick if within normal limits) as we do for altered sensation, and in approximate degrees from the horizontal in the case of straight leg raising.

d. *Additional signs*. This heading allows the clinician to enter data derived from the use of any signs which we have not included in this basic system, if he finds them useful.

e. *Local signs*
i. Entries are made by segmental level, left or right, anterior or posterior. (See example in Figure 9.2). It should be noted that segmental levels are here used as topographical indicators only, with no indication as to the aetiology of the pain.
ii. We use the three crude sacroiliac tests to elicit local pain and tenderness. The results are entered by + where pain is elicited. We do not use any of the numerous tests for sacroiliac mobility for the reasons given on p. 24.

It will be appreciated that the extensive use of figures and simple symbols rather than words greatly reduces the time required for entry of data and for its retrieval.

MUSCULOSKELETAL CASE ANALYSIS SHEET

Patient's name... *Mrs Rosemary BLOGGS* .... Serial No: *F. 5231*
Address... *3. Treelined Avenue* .... Insurance. *BUPA*
.... *West Homersham, Hants* .... Phone. *5290. 176921*
Date of birth *14 / 01 / 42*   Male....   Female. ✓

Family doctor's name... *H. Fernandez* ....
Address... *The Health Centre, High Street* ....
.... *West Homersham* .... Phone. *5290. 671426* ..NHS/Private. *N*...

HISTORY - Present episode.

Subject report		23 /01/ 89		30 /01/ 89		/ /	
		L	R	L	R	L	R
Pain -	Site	Head A					
	Radiation	Shoulder					
	Intensity	Severe					
	Duration	3/52					
	Worsened by	Moving					
	Improved by	Analg.					
Altered sensation							
	P & N	o					
	Numbness	o					

Activities of daily living

	Hoovering	Major					
	Bedmaking	Moderate					
	Ablutions	Moderate					
	Cooking	Minor					
	Ironing	.					
	Putting on socks	O					
	Shopping	Moderate					
	Gardening						
	Sports·						
	Sitting at desk	Minor					
	Other work						
	Road/rail travel						
	Air travel						

Pain behaviour

	Pill taking habit	Distalgesic x 2yds		o			
	Other treatments			o			
	Hours in bed per 24	7		7			
	Forced absenteeism	2/7					
	Litigation pending	No					

Previous episodes
    Year. *1969* . Site. *LBP* ..... Duration Days... Weeks *3*. Months....
    Therapy *Bed + Analgesics* .... Outcome *No recurrence since* ..
    Year...... Site......... Duration Days... Weeks... Months....
    Therapy..........................Outcome..................
Relevant medical history... *1969 - Heavy fall from horse* ....
Investigations... *o* ....

Figure 9.2 Case analysis sheet in use (front)

BASIC CASE ANALYSIS

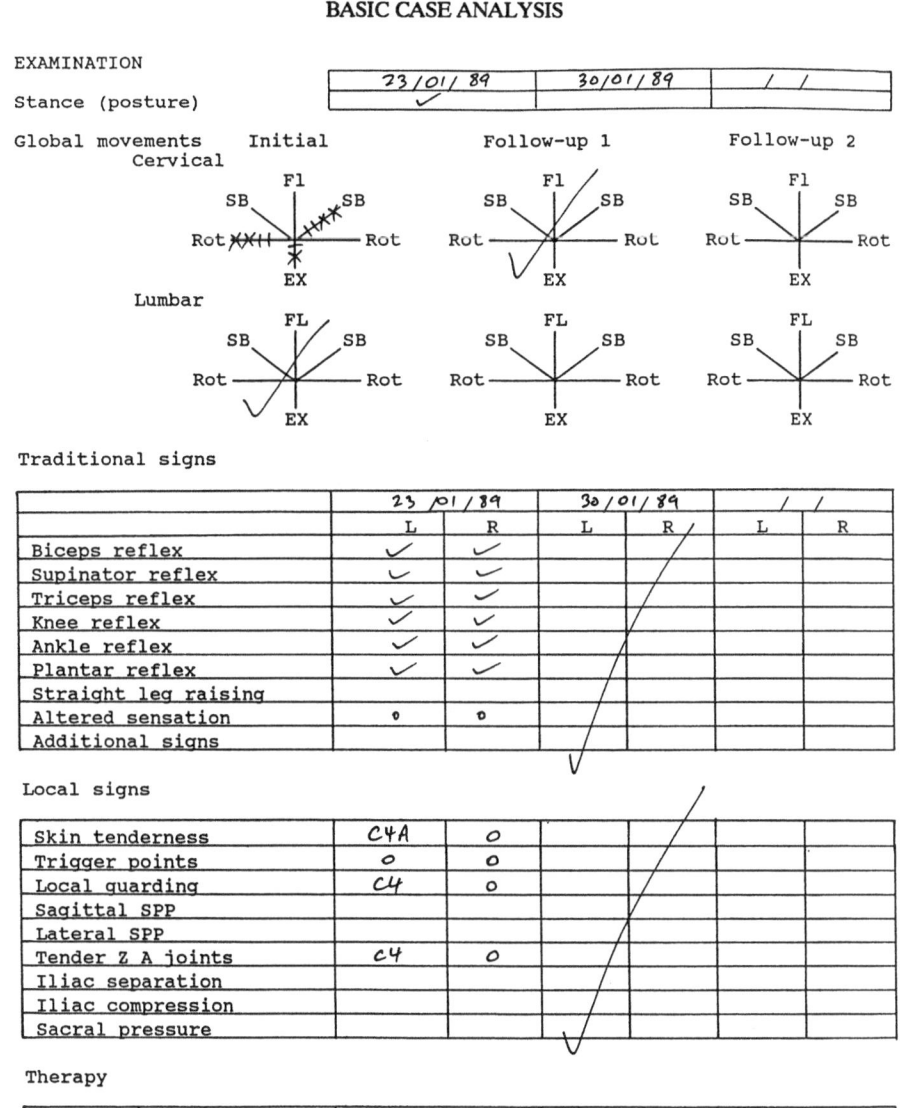

EXAMINATION

Stance (posture)

	23/01/89	30/01/89	/ /
	✓		

Global movements   Initial   Follow-up 1   Follow-up 2
        Cervical

Lumbar

Traditional signs

	23/01/89		30/01/89		/ /	
	L	R	L	R	L	R
Biceps reflex	✓	✓				
Supinator reflex	✓	✓				
Triceps reflex	✓	✓				
Knee reflex	✓	✓				
Ankle reflex	✓	✓				
Plantar reflex	✓	✓				
Straight leg raising						
Altered sensation	0	0				
Additional signs						

Local signs

Skin tenderness	C4A	0				
Trigger points	0	0				
Local guarding	C4	0				
Sagittal SPP						
Lateral SPP						
Tender Z A joints	c4	0				
Iliac separation						
Iliac compression						
Sacral pressure						

Therapy

Manipulation		✓	NIL		

Figure 9.2 Case analysis sheet in use (back)

165

References

1. Wyke (1983). In *Proceedings of the 7th FIMM Congress*, Zurich. (Unpublished)
2. Merskey (1982). Psychiatry. In *Proceedings of the Colt Symposium*, p. 82. (London: National Back Pain Association)
3. Andersson (1982). Occupational aspects of low back pain. In ibid.
4. Mooney and Robertson (1976). The facet syndrome. *Clin. Orthop. Ed. An. R. Res..* 115, 149
5. Pedersen *et al.* (1956). The anatomy of the lumbo-sacral posterior rami and meningeal branches of spinal nerves (sinuvertebral nerves). *J. Bone Jt. Surg.*, 38A, 377
6. Grieve (1981). *Common Vertebral Joint Problems.* (London: Churchill Livingstone)
7. King (1977). Randomized trial of the Rees and Shealy Methods for the treatment of low back pain. In Buerger and Tobis (eds.) *Approaches to the Validation of Manipulation Therapy*, p. 70. (Springfield, Ill.: Thomas)
8. Pièdallu (1952). Problemes sacro-iliaques. In Bière (ed.) *Homme Sain 2* (Bordeaux: Bione)
9. Glover (1960). Back pain and hyperaesthesia. *Lancet*, 1, 1165
10. Dubuisson (1983). In Wall and Melzack (eds.) *Textbook of Pain*, p. 437. (London: Churchill Livingstone)
11. Jennett (1956). A study of 25 cases of compression of the cauda equina by prolapsed intervertebral discs. *J. Neurol. Neurosurg. Psychiatry*, 19, 109
12. Schultz (1982). Biomechanics of the spine. In *Colt Symposium*, op. cit., pp. 20–24
13. Magora *et al.* (1974). An electro-myographic investigation of the neck muscles in headaches. *Electromyogr. Clin. Europhysiol.*, 14, 453
14. Kendall *et al.* (1971). *Muscles. Testing and Function*, 2nd Edn. (Baltimore: Williams and Wilkins)
15. Edwards and Hyde (1977). Methods of measuring muscle strength and fatigue. *Physiotherapy*, 65, 51–55
16. Basmajian and De Luca (1985). *Muscles Alive*, 5th Edn., p. 220. (Baltimore: Williams and Wilkins)
17. La Rocca and Macnab (1969). Value of pre-employment radiographic assessment of the lumbar spine. *Can. Med. Assoc. J.*, 101, 383
18. Swezey and Silverman (1971). Radiographic demonstration of induced vertebral facet displacement. *Arch. Phys. Med. Rehabil.*, 52, 244
19. Hitselburger and Witten (1968). Abnormal myelograms in asymptomatic patients. *J. Neurosurg.*, 28, 204
20. Hudgins (1977). The crossed straight leg raising test. *N. Engl. J. Med.*, 297, 1127
21 Wright *et al.* (1971). Some observations on the value and techniques of myelography in lumbar disc lesions. *Clin. Radiol.*, 22, 33
22. Spangfort (1983). Disc surgery. In Wall and Melzack (eds.) *Textbook of Pain*. (London: Churchill Livingstone)
23. Phillips (1975). Upper limb involvement in cervical spondylosis. *J. Neurol. Neurosurg. Psychiatry*, 38, 386
24. Lansche (1960). Correlation of the myelogram with clinical and operative findings in lumbar disc lesions. *J. Bone Jt. Surg.*, 48, 193
25. Haldeman (1982). Spinal manipulative therapy. In *Colt Symposium*, op. cit.
26. Dove (1982). Osteopathy. In ibid.
27. Reading (1983). Testing pain mechanisms in persons with pain. In Wall and Melzack (eds.) *Textbook of Pain*. (London: Churchill Livingstone)
28. Korr (1948). The emerging concept of the oesteopathic lesion. The collected papers of Irvin M. Kow. *Ann. Acad. Osteopathy*, (Colorado Springs, Col.) 18, 128
29. Brugger (1962). Pseudoradikulär Syndrome. *Acta Rheumatol.*, 19,
30. Sutter (1963). Versuch einer Wesensbestimmung pseudoradikulärer Syndrome. *Schweiz Rundsh Med. Praxis*, 842
31. Maigne (1968). *Douleurs d'Origin Vertebrale.* (Paris: Expansion scientifique)
32. Kellgren (1978). In Copeman (ed.) *Textbook of the Rheumatic Diseases.* (London: Butterworths)

10
CLINICAL PRESENTATIONS

In this chapter we present illustrations of musculoskeletal problems of vertebral origin commonly presenting in clinical practice. To these we add relevant clinical consequences.

Cervical
Headache
Pain taxonomy is a particularly pressing problem in headache research[1]. Although generally accepted, the belief that tension of the frontalis muscle reliably causes muscle contraction headache is not supportable. That this view is erroneous is well documented[2-7].

The symptoms most frequently diagnostic of migraine (prodrome, unilateral onset and nausea) occur together little more frequently than by chance[8].

Analysis of headache symptoms yields factors that are not congruent with current diagnostic opinion[9].

"The preponderance of inverted commas in any list of the nomenclature of head pain reveals the degree of uncertainty in this ubiquitous clinical feature."[10]

"The aetiology of many cases of headache remains unknown and treatment remains empirical."[11]

Migraine
It has been stated that classical migraine occurs in approximately 10% of patients with migraine[12].

This is illustrated by the analysis of a series of 109 patients who had been diagnosed as having migraine. The ultimate diagnoses were:
1. Cervico-occipital syndrome, 67,
2. Intracranial aneurysm, 15,
3. Brain tumour, 11,
4. Cerebrovascular disease, 4,
5. Hypertensive disease, 3,
6. Aneurysm + cervico-occipital syndrome, 2,
7. Aneurysm, cervico-occipital syndrome + subdural haematoma, 3.
   The significance of the spine in this series will be noted[13].

"In my experience, cervical migraine is the type of headache most frequently seen in general practice and also the type most frequently misinterpreted. It is usually erroneously diagnosed as classical migraine, tension headache, vascular headache, hypertensive encephalopathy or post-traumatic encephalopathy. Such patients have usually received inadequate treatment and have often become neurotic and drug dependent."[14]

For these reasons, this diagnosis must be regarded with some suspicion by the musculoskeletal clinician. Clinical assessment of the cervical spine seems essential, and, on the detection of abnormal local signs, the deployment of local therapy of one sort or another is rational and often effective.

These considerations indicate the difficulty of specific diagnosis in many cases.

Cervical headache

Pain in the head and facial regions is a frequent complaint in cervical spine disorders. Experimental work from as long ago as 1939 (Kellgren)[15] and 1944 (Campbell and Parsons)[16] has shown that stimulation of paravertebral tissues in the cervical region can cause headache.

Local signs in the C2 and C3 segments have been shown to be associated in unilateral supraorbital headaches. In a series of 50 cases deemed to be of cervical origin, local treatment by injection and/or manipulation relieved the headache in 43 cases (i.e. 86%)[17].

"Perhaps the most common form of headache is that related to muscular contraction occurring around the head and neck . . . . . in treating this type of pain, a search should be made for painful and tender areas of the head and neck, as well as significant arthritis of the spine. Post-traumatic headache is included in this group."[18]

"Many patients with cervical spondylosis have significant posterior headaches, particularly in the occipital region."[19]

The incidence of these problems is put by some authorities as being 1 in 3. Therefore routine analysis of any headache must involve examination of the cervical spine. The topography of these conditions is given as being 75% supraorbital, 20% occipital, 5% radiating to the ear and in up to 5% to the vertex[20].

Pain known to be of upper cervical origin has been recorded as radiating to:
1. The vertex
2. The temporal region
3. The occiput
4. The ear
5. The mastoid
6. The underside of the jaw

7. The neck
8. The interscapular region.

Pain may be unilateral or bilateral[21]. Therefore the existence of headache of cervical origin seems to be beyond dispute and is held by many to be common.

ENT symptoms of cervical origin

In the work of Campbell and Parsons already referred to[16], not only was headache produced, but also a number of other symptoms, including giddiness, pallor, sweating, nausea and sometimes tinnitus. A strong resemblance between these symptoms produced in experimental subjects and what they described as the "post-traumatic head syndrome" was noted.

In another series of 80 patients, the combination of abnormal electronystagmographic recordings with neck movement, together with normal routine audiological and vestibular findings, was regarded by the authors as specifically diagnostic of true cervical vertigo[22].

In a further series of 57 patients suffering from headache with involvement of the cervical spine, clinical features were:

1. Occipital hemicranial pain, hemicranalgia or more widespread head pain.
2. Vertigo, dysphagia, tinnitus and nystagmus.
3. These features therefore may mimic tension, ophthalmological headache or migraine, and may be superimposed on these.
4. A major finding was the high incidence of EMG evidence of nerve involvement in the headache syndrome[23].

From this it appears beyond doubt that many bizarre problems suggesting ENT involvement can be of cervical spinal origin. However, this is still insufficiently widely appreciated by many clinicians.

Post-traumatic headaches

In an analysis of 5500 cases cervical spine disorder of which more than 85% resulted from trauma, headache was one of the most frequent complaints[24].

Patients with cervical spine trauma frequently present symptoms apparently out of proportion to objective findings, and in one series further audiovestibular invesigation revealed tangible abnormalities in about 50% of cases. Tinnitus, high-frequency sensory neural loss, semicircular canal weakness and positional nystagmus were observed[25].

In a series of 15 patients studied after whiplash injury, ocular manifestations occurred, including blurred vision, strain, fatigue, diplopia, photophobia and inability to read[26].

Because degenerative and traumatic conditions of the cervical spine can mimic so many syndromes, such as migraine or vertigo, these diagnoses should not be arrived at without the cervical spine having been considered.

Torticollis

This condition can be defined as a postural deformity with the head in flexion and side bending away from the painful side. It is not a specific diagnosis[27].

It has been noted that, in a series of 103 case, 80% could not localize their pain[28].

Upper limb pain

"Upper extremity pain can be an enigma to physicians as it may be related to many different conditions. The process of degeneration of the cervical spine, the variations of the affected joint, traumas to the cervical spine or affected joint, vascular compromise, nerve impingement, thoracic or abdominal pathology or any combination of those elements."[29]

"A thorough screening to determine probable aetiology of upper extremity pain usually begins with a routine evaluation of head, neck and cervical spine."[29]

"The importance of cervical investigation in any patient with head, neck, chest, shoulder and arm pain cannot be over emphasized."[30]

With regard to pain of cervical root origin, the complexity of the neurophysiology may be illustrated by the work of Murphey[31]. In a large number of cervical discectomies under local anaesthetic, touching the damaged root produced severe pain in the arm, whereas touching the normal cervical roots produced only electrical sensations. When an involved root was blocked with local anaesthetic and retracted, it was sometimes possible to reproduce pain in the neck, shoulder, chest and scapular region by pressing on the posterior longitudinal ligament and the torn annulus fibrosus[31].

Neck problems may also be associated with peripheral changes in the upper limb, and these may have 'labels', such as periarthritis, bicipital tendinitis, lateral epicondylitis and medial epicondylitis. All these conditions are ill-understood[32].

A series of interest in this connection is that of 50 patients who had been diagnosed as having tennis elbow, and who had failed to respond to 4 weeks of conservative local treatment. The author then directed treatment to the patient's neck (but not manipulation). They used mobilization, cervical traction, isometric exercises and heat and/or ultrasound. 47% patients responded and of these 44 who were reassessed at three months and six months remained symptom free[33].

With regard to the 'shoulder/hand syndrome':
1. In a group of over 200 patients, precipitating factors were reported in 146 case and 75% of the cases were idiopathic[34] post-infarctional, cervico-discogenic or intraforaminal spurring and trauma.
2. In a further group of 139 patients, 23% of cases were ascribed to cervicoarthrosis or discogenic disease[35]. Here then is a condition with

peripheral changes, where aetiology can be shown to be either spinal or visceral. Or, as remarked elsewhere, a combination of the two.

A further example of cervical spinal problems associated with peripheral changes which has long been well established is the so-called 'cellulo-tendino-myalgic syndrome'[36].

Posterior thoracic radiation

It has been clearly demonstrated that cervical problems can not only radiate pain into the arm, but also into the interscapular region.

Referred tenderness, usually interscapular, frequently accompanies this phenomenon[36].

Anterior chest pain

This can also be of cervical origin[37]. When severe, it may imitate the pain of angina or myocardial infarction[38]. In patients whose attacks of substernal, precordial pain closely resembled the events of coronary insufficiency, it was shown that all the symptoms could be reproduced by manipulation of the neck[39]. Firm pressure over the lower cervical and upper thoracic vertebrae can cause excruciating pain in the chest[39].

Complex cervical presentations

In some cervical problems the picture may be extremely confusing. The pain may be diffuse or bilateral. There may be numbness in both ulnar and radial aspects of the forearm and hand. Weakness and alterations of brachial reflexes may be present. A spastic gait and increased reflexes in the leg may indicate cord involvement. Pain and paraesthesiae may be referred to the legs in a non-radicular pattern. Occipital pain may be present, thus presenting a picture of a patient with pain 'everywhere'[38]. In vascular lesions associated with lower cervical pathology, symptoms and signs are at considerable distances from the site of the lesion. For example, one patient showed partial analgesia and dimished temperature sense of the left hemicranial area, head-aches, vertigo and dysaesthesia in the territory of the 6th 7th and 8th cervical nerves in the distal left upper limb. In another case, involving occipital headache, giddiness, disturbances of vision and facial numbness which had lasted 4 years, relief was obtained for a further 4 years by removal of a bony spur between C6 and C7[39].

Uncommon symptoms and signs in cervical clinical presentations

Although signs both orthodox and local are described in case analysis, we mention some points of particular interest with regard to the cervical spine.

Although dysaesthesiae are rare, in the so-called 'neck–tongue syndrome' head or neck pain may be associated with simultaneous paraesthesiae of the ipsilateral half of the tongue[21].

Hyperaesthesiae in the occipital or mastoid regions are sometimes reported in upper cervical neuralgia[21].

Paraesthesiae in the scalp may also be associated with upper cervical problems[21].

Trigger points
These are commonly found in the soft tissues of the head and neck in association with cervical problems[21].

With regard to the so-called muscle contraction headache, pressure on trigger points may not only augment headache intensity but may elicit tinnitus, vertigo or lachrymation[19]. This provides an interesting correlation with the work of Campbell and Parsons[16] (see p. 169).

Rheumatological considerations
Rheumatoid arthritis, the seronegative arthritides, polymyalgia rheumatica and Scheuermann's disease must be borne in mind.

Practical clinical consequences of cervical presentations
The difficulties of taxonomy with regard to headache, so like those of back pain, and the complexities of symptoms and signs discussed make specific diagnosis a matter of some difficulty.

We have shown that the manifestations of cervical problems are extraordinarily varied.

It is undeniable that within orthodox medicine the spine is neglected and many labels are attached to various syndromes without the cervical spine being considered at all.

The clinical consequence of this is that, "often the pains are erroneously assumed to originate in structures where they are felt, for instance in the eyes, the ears, the tongue, the gums and the lips (orolingual paraesthesiae.) In the effort to discover the underlying cause of craniofacial pains, dentists, otolaryngologists, ophthalmologists and other specialists are consulted. The skull, the sinuses, the orbits, the jaws and the teeth are X-rayed and many types of treatment are employed, including surgery, but to no avail. Eventually some patients, despairing of relief, become neurotic and resort to narcotic drugs to alleviate their suffering. Finally, physicians, unable to discover signs of organic pathology, make an ultimate diagnosis of psycho-somatic pain. Such a mistake may be serious, with harmful consequences."[40]

Thoracic
Pain referred from the cervical spine
(See above.)

Chest pain of visceral origin

"Muscular tenderness following the onset of this pain (that of myocardial infarction) varies from a few hours to half a day. It mainly involves the pectoralis major, deep muscles of the interscapular region, the muscles of the forearm and less frequently the trapezius and the deltoid muscles."[41]

Patients with cardiac disease frequently have well-known pectoral and periscapular trigger points which, when firmly pressed, will severely exacerbate existing pain for many hours. They often respond well to the injection of local anaesthetic[42].

This was observed as long ago as 1955[42]. In this series the authors evolved a points system for differentiating between the two forms of chest pain, musculoskeletal and cardiac. They wrote, "It is entirely possible that somatic anterior chest wall pain is pathologically analogous to the shoulder/hand syndrome."[42]

Chest pain of spinal origin

Many authors have noted cases in which pain felt in the chest wall was musculoskeletal in origin and had nothing whatsoever to do with cardiac problems[43-45].

Fossgreen, observing admissions for chest pain to Årrhus Hospital in Denmark over a period of two years, found that in 20% of cases the pain was musculoskeletal[46].

Other cases have been described of people with chest pain of musculoskeletal origin, this being demonstrated because it was brought on by movement of the thoracic spine, such as twisting, bending or turning in bed[47].

Abdominal pain of spinal origin

In 1962 a series of cases was presented[48] which had been operated on due to an error of diagnosis; the pain being in fact of spinal origin. One patient had been operated on no fewer than three times. "The resultant abdominal manifestations can usually be traced to stem from irritation of one or more of the thoracic spinal roots . . . in this group of syndromes we are concerned with the entire abdominal wall supplied by the sensory and motor roots from about T6 down to about L1 level."[48]

In 1977 a series of 73 patients with abdominal pain of spinal origin was studied and treated with nerve blocks[49]. "Spinal root or referred pain often arise synchronously and in the same segment as visceral abnormalities, either because of summation or through visceroparietal reflexes."[49] The possibility of vertebral problems and the need for examination, including local examination, is therefore essential. "An acute abdomen may be simulated by aching from skeletal structures in febrile illnesses."[49]

Situations in which visceral and spinal features may be difficult to differentiate
Since reflex muscle spasm and tenderness may accompany both visceral disease and abdominal pain referred from the spine, it has been suggested that physical signs may be unhelpful in resolving this diagnostic dilemma[50]. (See also Relevant Pathology – General Considerations, p. 137).

"Frequently heart pain can be confused with pain arising from other structures (angor coronariens intriguîs). For instance, myocardial ischaemia may be concommitant with cervicothoracic osteoarthritis, with chest fibromyalgias or with many diseases of the gastrointestinal tract, such as hiatus hernia, gastroduodenitis, peptic ulcer, calculous and non-calculous cholecystitis . . . in these cases algogenic summation from different organs probably occurs."[41]

Inferior referral of pain of thoracic spinal origin
It was shown in 1972 that:
1. Apophyseal lesions between T10 and L2 can refer pain to the low back and upper buttock.
2. Tenderness over the iliac crest can be elicited.

In the opinion of the author, up to 60% of low back pain may have this origin. Anterior radiation to the abdominal wall can also take place[36].

Rheumatological considerations
Ankylosing spondylitis and other seronegative arthropathies, polymyalgia rheumatica and osteoporosis should be borne in mind.

Practical clinical consequences of thoracic presentations
The wide referral of pain of thoracic origin will be noted.

We emphasize the difficulty of discriminating between problems of visceral and somatic origin, with the important clinical consequences which may ensue.

The reader will note the neglect of the spine in current medical teaching.

Lumbar
Cervical and thoracic pain referred to the lumbar region
See sections above.

Referred pain of lumbar spinal origin
All the essential features of renal colic, pain diffused from loin to scrotum, iliac and testicular tenderness and cremasteric retraction can be provoked by a stimulus confined to the somatic structures of the spine[51].

Lower abdominal and scrotal pain from upper lumbar disc herniations is not infrequently confused with renal or ureteric disorders[52].

Patterns of referred pain from experimental injection of interspinous tissues at the L1 and L2 segments indicate that unilateral loin pain is likely to be more frequent than groin pain, but that the latter will certainly occur[53].

In certain situations, pressure on the spinous processes and over the facet joints of L1 and/or L2 elicit marked tenderness and sometimes reproduce the loin and groin pains[54].

Pain from the lumbar spine can also be referred down the lower limbs. An example of the latter is the 'sacro-cellulo-tendino-myalgic syndrome', which emphasizes not only the referral of pain down the leg but also peripheral changes and trigger points in the lower limb[20].

Referred backache

Pain may be experienced in the lower back although the causative lesion lies either with the tissues in which the pain is felt or along the course of the afferent nerves that innervate these tissues, but instead involve some tissue or organ whose innervation is segmentally related to that of the superficial tissues of the lumbosacral spine. This constitutes referred backache[55].

The development of a primary visceral or peritoneal disorder may be accompanied by pain (and often tenderness) in one or more sections of the skin in the lumbosacral area in which reflex motor changes may also occur, and this is frequently associated with reflex spasm of segmentally related portions of the spinal musculature[55].

Clinically referred back or pelvic pain are commonly encountered gynaecologically in dysmenorrhoea, in lesions of the ovaries or in ectopic pregnancy, or with uterine prolapse or retroversion, and finally in carcinoma of the uterine cervix[55].

Patients with diseases of the urinary tract often experience referred backache, particularly with pyelitis, pyelonephritis and renal calculus. It may also occur in lesions of the renal pelvis, in the presence of a retrocaecal appendix and in various forms of prostatitis[55].

Bladder symptoms

The chief symptom is incontinence, but the diagnosis is often obscure because neurological features are commonly absent[56].

Myelography is frequently negative or equivocal[57].

Out of 25 cases, 24 had objective sensory loss in the sacral area, but some patients had not noticed this[58].

The great clinical importance of the early detection of these problems and their prompt surgical treatment revolves around the poor prognosis if therapy is delayed. "Recovery from cauda equina lesions is slow, but it is doubtful if it is realised just how unsatisfactory it can be."[59] It has been reported that in a series of 18 patients 11 still showed abnormal bladder function on follow-up examination, and a review of the literature indicates only a small proportion of patients show signs of clearing of bladder symptoms[59].

Neurogenic claudication

In this syndrome, first described by Verbiest in 1954[60], paraesthesiae often appear when the patient is standing still and are commonly relieved by flexion, but they are typically brought on by walking[60]. These points help to distinguish the syndrome from peripheral vascular claudication, in which cramps affect the leg muscles after exercize, regardless of posture[61].

Complex lumbar problems

Weinstein showed in 1977[62] that, of patients with spinal stenosis:
1. 66% had back pain.
2. 36% had unilateral leg pain.
3. 36% had bilateral leg pain.
4. Muscle spasms and cramps were common,
    a. in the back,
    b. in the legs.
5. Pain localization was inconsistent and diagnostically unhelpful. Of 227 cases,
    a. 25 had pain in the buttock or hip,
    b. 22 had pain in the thigh,
    c. 9 had pain in the groin or genitalia.
6. The series included 20 cases of neurogenic claudication.
7. Objective sensory abnormalities
    a. were present in half the cases,
    b. did NOT obey dermatomal patterns.
8. Knee or ankle reflexes were decreased or absent in 70% of cases.
9. 10% had bladder involvement or impotence.
10. There was a positive straight leg raising test in 30% of cases.

Under these circumstances, specific diagnostic certainty is far from easy.

Trigger points

As long ago as 1938, in a review of 451 cases of low back pain with pain referred to the leg, on palpation around the lumbosacral region in 228 cases a point was located where needle contact produced both local and referred pain; both were relieved by the injection of local anaesthetic[63].

Referral of pain is often confusing. For example it has been found that pressure at a low thoracic sacrospinalis trigger point may refer pain to the lower buttock, while an upper lumbar point may refer pain to an area over the upper buttock[64].

Rheumatological considerations
Thought should be given to Scheuermann's disease, polymyalgia rheumatica, ankylosing spondylitis and other seronegative arthritides, as well as Paget's disease and osteoporosis.

Practical clinical consequences of lumbar presentations
1. Pain is commonly referred both into the region and out of it.
2. Pain can be referred both anteriorly and posteriorly, and this may have serious consequences. Missed diagnoses occur commonly, and major surgery has been inappropriately deployed, sometimes on more than one occasion.
3. Weinstein's series shows yet again the extreme difficulties of accurate diagnosis[62].

The pelvis
The sacroiliac joints
Pain can undoubtedly be referred into the region of the pelvis from both thoracic and lumbar spines.

Pain can undoubtedly be referred from the sacroiliac joints, but evidence for this is currently very limited. However, it has been shown that abdominal pain can be relieved on certain occasions by injection of local anaesthetic into the sacroiliac joint[65].

Sacroiliitis is commonly associated with low back pain and frequently exhibits tenderness on sacral pressure[66].

The coccyx
Again, valid material relating to this structure is limited. However, in one series of 112 cases of coccygeal tenderness, 22 patients had pain in the coccyx and another 79 in the low back[67].

Symphysis pubis
This structure is undoubtedly the source of pain and referred pain, but material is again limited. For example, in one series it was described as radiating pain to the pubic, inguinal and abdominal areas[68]. However, the diagnostic criteria were radiological, and therefore some doubt must be cast on the validity of this work, since one of the relevant criteria was simple sclerosis of the pubic margins, which is a degenerative change, and there is no proven correlation between such changes and the incidence of pain.

Practical clinical consequences of pelvic presentation
1. The paucity of validated material is remarkable and most surprising.
2. Objective diagnoses are at present in most cases unobtainable in mechanical problems, while conjecture and hypothesis abound.
3. In terms of management, this is of little moment. The reason for this is that any local mechanical treatment will inevitably also involve the lumbar spine and therefore many other structures. Thus such treatment is unavoidably empirical and will have widespread effects.

Practical clinical consequences of vertebral pain presentations
1. Although pain may be experienced relatively local to its source, referred pain may be experienced at a distance, in an unpredictable manner.
2. With regard to visceral pain, this can be very confusing. For example, "Pain from somatic structures may closely simmulate visceral disease, faithfully reproducing the character and distribution of visceral pain, of angina with breathlessness, abdominal pain with nausea and vomiting, the flatulence of cholecystitis and the frequency of renal disease. Additionally, the other visceral signs, such as abdominal tenderness and abdominal rigidity, are often produced."[69]
3. The complexity, unpredictability and constant variability of both the symptoms and signs of vertebral problems make comprehensive and thorough assessment and reassessment essential. (See Relevant Physiology, p. 53).
4. The clinical consequences of abdominal and chest pain caused by vertebral problems not being appreciated can be serious.
5. The sheer scale of incidence of pain of vertebral origin surely suggests that greater emphasis needs to be given to it, clinically and in both undergraduate and postgraduate medical education.

References

1. Bakal (1975). A biophysical perspective. *Psychol. Bull.*, **82**, 369–382
2. Haynes *et al.* (1975). Electromyographic biofeedback and relaxation instructions for the treatment of muscle contraction headaches. *Behav. Therap.*, **6**, 672–678
3. Philips (1977). The modification of tension headache pain using EMG biofeedback. *Behav. Res. Ther.*, **15**, 119–129
4. Epstein *et al.* (1978). The relationship between frontalis muscle activity and self-reports of headache pain. *Behav. Res. Ther.*, **16**, 153–160
5. Gray *et al.* (1980). Electrode placement, EMG feedback, and relaxation for tension headaches. *Behav. Res. Ther.*, **18**, 19–23
6. Nuechterlein and Holroyd (1980). Biofeedback in the treatment of tension headaches. *Arch. Gen. Psychiatry*, **37**, 866–873
7. Andrasik and Holroyd (1980). A test of specific and non-specific effects in the biofeedback treatment of tension headache. *J. Consult. Clin. Psychol.*, **48**, 575–586
8. Walters (1973). The epidemiological enigma of migraine. *Int. J. Epidemiol.*, **2**, 189–194

9. Zeigler *et al.* (1972). Headache syndromes suggested by factor analysis of symptom variables on a headache prone population. *J. Chronic Dis.*, **25**, 353–363
10. Lance (1969). *Mechanisms and Management of Headache.* (London: Butterworth)
11. Mehta (1973). *Intractable Pain,* p. 147. (London: W.B. Saunders)
12. Friedman (1975). Migraine. *Psychiatr. Ann.*, **5**, 29
13. Sheldon (1967). Headache patterns and cervical nerve root compression. A 15 year study of hospitalisation for headache. *Headache*, 180
14. Frykholm (1971). Clinical picture. In Hirsch and Zotterman (eds.) *Cervical Pain*, p. 5. (Oxford: Pergamon Press)
15. Kellgren (1939). On the distribution of pain arising from deep somatic structures with charts of segmental pain areas. *Clin. Sci.*, **4**, 35
16. Campbell and Parsons (1944). Referred head pain and its concomitants. *J. Nerve Ment. Dis.*, **99**, 544
17. Maigne (1976). Un signe evocateur et inattendu de cephalee cervicale. La douleur au pince-roule du sourcil. *Ann. Med. Physique*, **19**, 416
18. Dalessio (1983). Headache. In Wall and Melzack (eds.) *Textbook of Pain*, p. 278. (London: Churchill Livingstone)
19. Dalessio (1983). Headache. In Wall and Melzack, op. cit., p. 289
20. Maigne (1972). *Douleurs d'Origine Vertebrale et Traitements par Manipulations.* 2nd Edn. (Paris: Expansion Scientifique)
21. Dubuisson (1983). In Wall and Melzack, op. cit.
22. Wing and Hargrave-Wilson (1974). Cervical vertigo. *Aust. NZ. J. Surg.*, **44**, 275
23. Magora *et al.* (1974). An electromyographic investigation of the neck muscles in headache. *Electromyogr. Clin. Physiol.*, **14**, 453
24. Jackson (1967). Headaches associated with disorders of the cervical spine. *Headache*, **6**, 175
25. Kosay and Glassman (1974). Audiovestibular findings with cervical spine trauma. *Text Med.*, **70**, 66
26. Roca (1972). Ocular manifestations of whiplash injury. *Am. Opth.*, **4**, 63
27. Cavaziel (1977). Acute torticollis. Clinical features and treatments. *Man. Med.*, **4**, 58
28. Spisak (1972). Bedentung des Segments C2C3 im klinischen Bild des akuten Tortikollis. *Man. Med.*, **6**, 87
29. Sola (1983). Upper extremity pain. In Wall and Melzack, op. cit.
30. Jackson (1966). *Cervical Syndrome.* 3rd Edn. (Springfield, Ill.: Thomas)
31. Murphey (1968). Sources and patterns of pain in disc disease. *Clin. Neurosurg.*, **15**, 343–350
32. Huskisson and Hart (1973). *Joint Diseases. All the Arthropothies.* (Bristol: Wright)
33. Gunn and Milebrandt (1976). Tennis elbow and the cervical spine. *Can. Med. Assoc. J.*, **144**, 803
34. Steinbrocker (1947). The shoulder-hand syndrome. Associated painful humero-lateral disability of shoulder and hand with swelling and atrophy of the hand. *Am. J. Med.*, **3**, 402
35. Steinbrocker and Argyios (1958). The shoulder-hand syndrome. Present status as a diagnostic and therapeutic entity. *Med. Clin. Ed. Am.*, 15–33
36. Maigne (1972). La semiologie clinique des derangements intervertebraux mineurs. *Ann. Med. Physique*, **15**, 275
37. Dubuisson (1983). In Wall and Melzack, op. cit.
38. Ibid., p. 440
39. Keuter (1970). Vascular origin of cranial sensory disturbances caused by pathology of the lower cervical spine. *Acta Neuro. Chirug.*, **23**, 229
40. Ederling (1975). The abandoned headache syndrome. In *Proceedings of the Golden Jubilee Congress SA Physio. Assoc.*, Johannesburg.
41. Procacci and Zoppi (1983). Heat pain. In Wall and Melzack, op. cit.
42. Prinzmetal and Massumi (1955). The anterior chest wall syndrome. Chest pain resembling pain of cardiac origin. *J. Am. Med. Assoc.*, **159**, 177
43. Eckerson *et al.* (1928). Thoracic pain persisting after coronary thrombosis. *J. Am. Med. Assoc.*, **90**, 1780
44. Allison (1950). Pain in the chest wall simulating heart disease. *Br. Med. J.*, **1**, 332

45. Edwards (1955). Musculo-skeletal chest pain following myocardial infarction. *Am. Heart J.*, **49**, 713
46. Fossgreen (1985). In *BAMM Symposium*. (Unpublished)
47. Grant and Keegan (1958). Rib pain. A neglected diagnosis. *Ulster Med. J.*, **37**, 162
48. Marinacci and Courville (1962). Radicular syndromes simulating intra-abdominal surgical conditions. *Am. Surg.*, **28**, 59
49. Ashby (1977). Abdominal pain of spinal origin. *Ann. R. Coll. Surg. Eng.*, **59**, 242
50. Leading article (1977). Abdominal pain of spinal origin. *Lancet*, **1**, 1190
51. Lewis and Kellgren (1939). Observations relating to referred pain, viscero-motor reflexes and other associated problems. *Clin. Phys.*, **4**, 47
52. Kirkaldy-Willis and Hill (1979). A more precise diagnosis of low back pain. *Spine*, **4**, 102
53. Feinstein (1977). Referred pain from paravertebral structures. In Buerger and Tobis (eds.) *Approaches to the Validation of Manipulative Therapy*, p. 139. (Springfield, Ill.: Thomas)
54. Sunderland (1975). Anatomical perivertebral influences on the intervertebral foramen. Research status of spinal manipulative therapies, p. 129. (Bethesda, Md: US Dept of Health) NINCDS Monograph no. 15
55. Wyke (1980). The neurology of pain. In Jayson (ed.) *The Lumbar Spine and Low Back Pain*, 2nd Edn., p. 310. (London: Pitman Medical)
56. Sharr *et al.* (1976). Lumbar spondylosis and neuropathic bladder. Investigation of 73 patients with chronic urinary symptoms. *Br. Med. J.*, **1**, 695
57. Emmett and Love (1971). Vesical dysfunction caused by protruded lumbar disc. *J. Neurol.*, **105**, 86
58. Jennet (1956). A study of 25 cases of compression of the cauda-equina by prolapsed intervertebral discs. *J. Neurol. Neurosurg. Psychiatr.*, **19**, 109
59. Aho *et al.* (1969). Analysis of cauda-equina symptoms in patients with lumbar disc prolapse. *Acta Chir. Scand.*, **135**, 413
60. Verbiest (1954). A radicular syndrome from developmental narrowing of the lumbar vertebral canal. *J. Bone Joint Surg.*, **36B**, 230–237
61. Dubuisson (1983). In Wall and Melzack, op. cit.
62. Weinstein *et al.* (1977). *Lumbar Spondylosis.* (Chicago: Year Book)
63. Steindler and Luck (1938). Differential diagnosis of pain low in the back. *J. Am. Med. Assoc.*, **110**, 106
64. Simons (1975). Muscle pain syndromes. Part 1. *Am. J. Phys. Med.*, **54**, 289
65. Norman (1968). Sacro-iliac disease and its relationship to lower abdominal pain. *Am. J. Surg.*, **116**, 54
66. Davis and Lentle (1978). Evidence for sacro-iliac disease as a common cause of low back ache in women. *Lancet*, **2**, 496
67. Lewit (1967). The coccyx and lumbago (sacral pain). *Man. Med.*, **4**, 2
68. Durey and Rodineau (1976). Les lesions pubiennes des sportifs. *Am. Med. Physique*, **3**, 232
69. Kellgren (1940). Somatic simulating visceral pain. *Clin. Psychiatr.*, **4**, 303

11
INTRODUCTION TO MANAGEMENT

In this section of the book, we lean heavily on the relevant chapters in Wall and Melzack's *Textbook of Pain*[1].

Basic considerations and management
Diagnostic problems
These have been dealt with elsewhere (see Case Analysis, p.151).
"In the absence of a valid diagnosis, controlled therapy is not possible."[2]

Chronic pain
With regard to chronic pain, "Similarly to other chronic pain syndromes, temporomandibular pain and dysfunction is a complex entity, and both pain and dysfunction are associated with behavioural changes, secondary psychological gains, changes in mood and attitudes to life and drug abuse. Consequently, it is very important to consider that alleviation of pain and dysfunction, although primary goals of therapy, cannot be the only objectives of treatment. The complex aetiology necessitates a combination of therapeutic approaches, and the mode of therapy should be tailored individually for each patient, based on a careful . . . . evaluation of that patient."[3]

Management assessment
This of itself provides formidable problems, as shown by Jessup[4].

Causes of management failure
These have been summarized by Bonica[5] as:
1. Inadequate knowledge of pain syndromes.
2. Inadequate evaluation of patients.
3. Lack of knowledge of other therapeutic modalities which might better be used in individual patients.
4. Lack of appreciation of the specific indications, limitations and possible complications of the procedures.

Practical application

We review 30 therapies applicable to musculoskeletal problems, compared and contrasted in a Management Chart (p. 285). Our intention is to identify a scientific basis, if any, for their individual deployment.

References

1. Wall and Melzack (eds.) (1983). *Textbook of Pain*. (London: Churchill Livingstone)
2. Wyke (1983). Presentation at FIMM Congress, Zurich. (Unpublished)
3. Sharav (1985). In Wall and Melzack (eds.) *Textbook of Pain*, pp. 344–345. (London: Churchill Livingstone)
4. Jessup (1983). Biofeedback. *J. Pain*, 776 *et seq.*
5. Bonica (1983). Local anasthesia and local blocks. *J. Pain*, 541 *et seq.*

12
INDIVIDUAL THERAPIES

Therapy 1 – non-narcotic analgesics

Introduction
The prescription of 'pain-killer' is the commonest form of treatment used for
pain in so-called 'western medicine'. These drugs are of particular interest to
practitioners of musculoskeletal medicine.

The narcotics, because of their addictive properties, and the systemic
steroids, are not discussed in this text.

Non-narcotic analgesics are broadly classified into two groups, the
analgesics and the non-steroidal anti-inflammatory drugs (NSAIDs).
1. Analgesics are believed only to relieve pain.
2. NSAIDs are also pain killers, but additionally have further actions related
   to their effect upon inflammation, reducing stiffness, swelling and
   tenderness.

Anti-inflammatory drugs "work in any inflammatory disease, and analgesics
relieve any sort of pain". But "there are undoubtedly patients who do not
respond to any of the currently available anti-inflammatory drugs"[1].

The prescription of non-narcotic analgesics
"The clinician choosing a drug for his rheumatic patient is presented with a
bewildering array of analgesic, anti-inflammatory, immunosuppressive and
other medicines, the same drug also appears under different names in
different dosages, combinations and formulations."[1]

"There is a particular requirement for education of the medical profession
in the face of evidence that prescribing habits leave much to be desired[2]. The
accumulating evidence that anti-rheumatic drugs may be associated with
iatrogenic mortality as well as morbidity confers urgency on the problem."[3,4]

"It can not be over-emphasised that the prescription of any drug to a
patient is not an automatic progression from the diagnosis of a disease."[5]

Mode of action
"The mode of action of anti-rheumatic drugs is completely unknown, and too
often authorities have produced evidence 'validating' a particular mechanism,

rather than attempting to find evidence which is disconcordant."[5]

No 'unifying hypothesis' currently extant explains with any conviction why or how anti-rheumatic drugs work, and in particular there is a dearth of evidence suggesting any degree of specificity[6]. While narcotic analgesics act on the endorphin system in the central nervous system, non-steroidal anti-inflammatory drugs act peripherally at the site of pain.

The biochemistry of pain remains unknown, and problems at the periphery (see Relevant Physiology, p.34), in the dorsal horn (see Relevant Physiology, p.51) and with the endorphin-mediated analgesic systems (EMASs) make progress difficult.

Clinical pharmacology and pharmacokinetics
In most cases, plasma level profile, protein binding and the mode of excretion are not relevant to the action of these drugs in man. The most striking example of this is that, if indomethacin is given at night, it produces a peak pain relief the following morning, at a time when the drug has disappeared almost entirely from the plasma[7]. Therefore "great caution should be exercised in the interpretation of plasma levels of analgesics which do not necessarily reflect clinical changes."

"In fact, none of the known biological effects of the anti-rheumatic drugs can be produced in support of any existing theory which would explain why these drugs relieve the symptoms of many thousands of patients."[5]

The simple analgesics
The analgesics seem to be primarily centrally acting. There are several agonist/antagonist compounds available, including pentazocine, butorphanol and buprenorphine. These compounds, like codeine, dihydrocodeine and dextropropoxyphene, are all presumed to act on the morphine receptors.

Combinations are frequently used because they are not only popular, but also appear to be effective.

Dextropropoxyphene
This is a weak analgesic and is frequently prescribed on its own. In overdose it may cause respiratory depression.

A combination of dextropropoxyphene and paracetamol (Distalgesic) is very popular, and is as effective as aspirin. It is also dangerous in overdose[8].

Codeine and dihydrocodeine
Codeine is hardly ever used as an analgesic, but dihydrocodeine can be and causes less constipation than does codeine, although it can cause nausea and vomiting. It is also used in various combinations.

Pentazocine
This is much more effective given by injection than orally. It is quite potent, but it has several side-effects, including nausea, dizziness and light-headedness, in addition to mental changes, including euphoria, dysphoria, feelings of disorientation, hallucination, depersonalization and other strange and usually unpleasant sensations.

Nephopam (= Nefopam)
This is a centrally acting analgesic which acts at a different site. It is as effective as aspirin and does not cause CNS depression.

Aim of treatment
Relief of pain.

Diagnosis
Seldom possible.

How do they work?
Unknown.

Indications
Pain, including that of vertebral origin.

Contraindications
None.

Dangers
Overdosage, possibly attempted suicide. Their ready availability may be of significance.

Complications
None.

Predictability of outcome
Unknown, either in the short term or the long term.

Similar therapies
Non-steroidal anti-inflammatory drugs.

References

1. Huskisson (1974). *Recent Drugs and the Rheumatic Diseases. Report on Rheumatic Disease 54.* (London: Arthritis and Rheumatism Council)
2. Lee *et al.* (1974). Observations on drug prescribing in rheumatoid arthritis. *Br. Med. J.*, **1**, 424–426
3. Lee *et al.* (1973). Adverse reactions in patients with rheumatoid diseases. *Ann. Rheumatic Dis.*, **32**, 565–573
4. Girdwood (1974). Death after taking medicaments. *Br. Med. J.*, **1**, 501–504
5. Carson Dick (1978). In Copeman (ed.), *Textbook of the Rheumatic Diseases*, 2nd Edn. (London: Churchill Livingstone)
6. Rooney *et al.* (1975). A short term double blind control of prenozone (DA 2370) in rheumatoid arthritis. *Curr. Med. Res. Opin.*, **2**, 43–50
7. Huskisson (1976). Chronopharmacology of anti-rheumatic drugs with special reference to Indomethacin. In Huskisson and Velo (eds.) *Inflammatory Arthropathies*, pp. 99–105. (Amsterdam: Excerpta Medica)
8. Carson and Carson (1977). Fatal dextro-propoxyphene poisoning in Northern Ireland. Review of 30 cases. *Lancet*, **1**, 894–897

Therapy 2 – non-steroidal anti-inflammatory drugs

Classification

Table 12.1 shows the great number of these preparations and the variety of their various dosage schemes. Clearly, in view of their number alone, some form of classification would be helpful. Various attempts have been made.

Chronological: The first was aspirin, followed by phenylbutazone and indomethacin. Since then there have been very many additions.

Safety: Propionic acid derivatives are far safer than aspirin, and since their introduction, the motto 'safety first' has been the priority in drug prescription. Classification by lack of side-effects is possible.

Convenience: For example, pyroxicam can be given once a day and achieve relief of symptoms over a 24-hour period. It is possible to use this as a basis for classification.

Chemistry: This has been found to bear little or no relationship to the clinical action of NSAIDs.

Anti-inflammatory drugs: Indomethacin is an example of a major anti-inflammatiory drug, ibuprofen a minor one. "The large number of compounds which is now available probably represents all shades of analgesic and anti-inflammatory potency. Between the extremes – and there is no clear-cut distinction between them – such a sub-classification is no longer useful."

Table 12.1 A selection of non-steroidal anti-inflammatory drugs with appropriate doses

Approved name	Trade name	Dosage
Aspirin	(various)	600–900 mg.q.d.s.or 600 mg as required for pain
Azapropazone	Rheumox	600 mg b.i.d.
Benorviate	Benoral	10 ml(4g)b.i.d.of suspension or 1.5g t.i.d.using tablets
Choline magnesium trisalicylate	Trilisate	1g b.i.d.for osteoarthritis.1.5g b.i.d. for rheumatoid
Diclofenac	Voltarol	50 mg made 100 mg nocte or 50 mg t.i.d.
Dilfunisal	Dolobid	500 mg stat then 250 or 500 mg b.i.d.
Fenbufen	Lederfen	300 mg mane 600 mg nocte. Night dose only may be enough
Fenclofenac	Flenac	300 mg b.i.d.
Fenoprofen	Fenopron	600 mg t.i.d. or 300 mg as required for pain
Feprazone	Methrazone	200 mg b.i.d.
Flurbiprofen	Froben	50 mg mane 100 mg nocte
Flufenamic acid	Meralen	200 mg t.i.d.
Ibuprofen	Brufen	400 mg t.i.d. or 400 mg as required for pain
Indomethacin	Indocid	25 mg t.i.d. 75–100 mg at night for night pain/morning stiffness
Indomethacin (slow release)	Indocid R	75 mg nocte or b.i.d.
Indoprofen	Flosint	200 mg t.i.d. or 200 mg as required for pain
Ketoprofen	Orudis	100 mg b.i.d.
Meclofenamate sodium	Meclomen	50–100 mg t.i.d. or q.i.d.
Mefenamic acid	Ponstan	500 mg t.i.d. or 500 mg as required for pain
Naproxen	Naprosyn	500 mg b.i.d.
Phenylbutazone	Butazolidin	100 mg t.i.d. Not more than 7 days
Piroxicam	Feldene	20 mg o.d. morning or night
Sulindac	Clinoril	200 mg b.i.d.
Tolmetin sodium	Tolectin	400 mg t.i.d.
Zomepirac	Zomax	100 mg t.i.d. or 100 mg as required for pain

Specific use: "Several attempts have been made to offer a more practical classification in the choice of which drugs are particularly suitable for any particular situation, such as chronic disease, night time use for night pain or morning stiffness, and once a day drugs. This, though possible, is complex."[1]
Side-effects: The use of these has also been attempted as a basis for classification. For example, there are some drugs which should not be given to patients with peptic ulcers and others to persons taking anticoagulants.

From the foregoing, it can be seen that there is no classification for this great variety of drugs which is of prima facie practical value to the clinician.

Actions
1. These drugs have in common the relief of pain and stiffness.
2. They act peripherally and, save for paracetamol, they reduce the signs of inflammation and swelling.
However, it should be remembered that their mode of action remains unknown.

Side-effects
These are significant, and in a recent publication it was suggested that, before starting therapy, every patient should be asked the following:
1. Have you ever had (or been suspected of having) a gastric or duodenal ulcer?
2. Have you ever had a barium meal? If so, what did it show?
3. Have you ever had an allergic or toxic reaction to aspirin or any other pain killer?
4. Have you ever had a skin reaction or rash when taking any other pain killer?
5. Are you now taking any medicines for any other disorder? If so, what[1]?
This is important, because few patients volunteer this information, and it has to be elicited from them.

The most common side-effects demanding cessation of NSAID therapy are gastrointestinal, dermatological or cerebral (such as headache, dizziness or tinnitus).

"On the whole, this class of drugs is very safe. It appears in mortality statistics only in respect of aplastic anaemia due to phenylbutazone and oxyphenbutazone, and gastrointestinal bleeding, particularly related to aspirin and indomethacin."[1]

However, "the most important factor which determines both response and side-effects is individual variation[2] . . . individual variation is probably also the most important factor determining the occasional incidence of gastrointestinal side-effects. This was investigated in relation to flurbiprofen, and other factors, such as dosage and formulation did not appear to be important. Flurbiprofen was a very effective drug, but some patients could not take it. Occasional intolerance is also predictable."[3]

The clinical implication of this must be twofold. First the onset of side-effects requires immediate withdrawal of the particular drug. Second to choose an alternative drug is rational.

Since withdrawal from prescription in general practice of the more dangerous drugs (such as phenylbutazone) and with increasing knowledge of the other NSAIDs, side-effects are of much less importance than they were. Nevertheless, despite the most careful of histories, it is clear that such side-effects remain, at times, unpredictable. Thus, in selecting what treatment or treatments to use in a given situation, these matters must be borne firmly in mind.

Efficacy

"The difference between the most effective drug in the class and the least effective is relatively small. They are all more or less similarly effective, differences between them are overshadowed by individual variation in response."

This has been clearly demonstrated in the study of four propionic acid derivatives. "Overall differences between these compounds in a large group of patients with rheumatoid arthritis were small. However, individual patients showed large differences, and it was possible to identify groups of patients who responded well to all four drugs. Experience in practice confirms the importance of this phenomenon. Some patients respond well to one drug, and some respond to another. Unfortunately, response is unpredictable. It is not related to plasma level or pharmokinetics."[1] The only currently available way of selecting appropriate non-steroidal anti-inflammatory drugs for the individual patient is therefore to try a succession of different agents.

Empiricism in drug prescription is thus as important, and indeed as unavoidable, as it is in any other treatment in musculoskeletal medicine.

Aspirin
Prescription

It has been shown that 3–6 g is the lowest dose at which aspirin may exert an anti-inflammatory effect[4]. It should be prescribed with caution in the elderly and in children, since side-effects may occur insidiously and at low doses in these patients.

Side-effects

These, while unquestionably significant, should be seen in proportion. In Britain over 4000 million aspirin tablets are taken every year[5]! In view of this enormous consumption, the incidence of side-effects seems remarkably low.

Gastrointestinal discomfort or pain: This is the commonest reason for stopping aspirin therapy. It is dose related, but individually unpredictable.

Gastrointestinal bleeding: Over 70% of patients taking aspirin in high doses will suffer from minor gastrointestinal bleeding, which will continue as long as they take the drug[6], the average blood loss being less than 5 ml per day[7]. In those losing persistently more than 10-15 ml per day, iron deficiency anaemia may ensue. Major haemorrhage can occur[8] but it is extremely rare, and there is no relationship between major bleeding and either minor bleeding or dyspepsia[9].

Peptic ulceration: A close correlation has been demonstrated between aspirin ingestion and peptic ulceration, making it likely that aspirin is a predisposing factor[10].

Pregnancy: Aspirin, like all other NSAIDs, should be avoided in pregnancy[11].

Haematological: Aspirin can very rarely cause reversible pancytopenia[12] and it should never be given to patients taking anticoagulants[13,14].

Hypersensitivity: Occasional deaths from hypersensitivity have been reported on the administration of even minute amounts of aspirin. Once a patient has been found to be aspirin sensitive, no other antirheumatic drug can be prescribed with complete impunity[15].

Aspirin variants: Because of aspirin side-effects, particularly of the gastrointestinal tract, a number of variants has been developed. Enteric coating, micro-encapsulating and the use of aspirin as an aluminium derivative have all proved as effective as aspirin, with far fewer gastrointestinal side-effects[16-19].

Indomethacin
Prescription
This is usually started at a dose of 25 mg three times a day, and it is increased to that dose at which patient symptoms are controlled, without intolerable side-effects. This ranges from 75 mg to over 200 mg per day.

It may also be given in the form of a suppository of 100 mg, a matter of individual patient preference. It may be given in sustained release formulation, as Indocid-R 75 mg. Indomethacin is an effective drug and is particularly useful for patients with night pain.

Side-effects
Unfortunately, these are several. About one third of patients will suffer side-effects on conventional doses[5].

Gastrointestinal: Dyspepsia is the most common complaint, but both perforation and acute gastrointestinal haemorrhage have been reported. Therefore blood loss may produce iron deficiency anaemia[20]. It is wise to avoid the use of this drug in patients with peptic ulceration.

Central nervous system: Headaches, drowsiness and loss of concentration are common in patients on high dosage of indomethacin, and side-effects include severe depression and even psychosis. Loss of concentration and headache may be sufficiently troublesome as to impair driving skills[21].

Miscellaneous:.Other rarer side-effects include increased bleeding time[13] and skin rashes[21]. Blood dyscrasias, including agranulocytosis, throbocytopenia and aplastic anaemia, have been reported rarely with indomethacin alone, more often when other drugs were being taken at the same time[22].

Propionic acid derivatives
These include ibuprofen (Brufen) flurbiprofen (Froben) phenoprofen (Phenopron) and naproxen (Naprosyn). "The propionic acid derivatives introduced to the clinician and entirely different order of incidence of side-effects. The difference between a drug like phenoprofen and full doses of aspirin is enormous. There are far fewer side-effects and patients are seldom withdrawn from treatment because of these."[1]

Amongst the newer drugs, differences in the incidence of side-effects are relatively small. Ibuprofen is very well tolerated, and probably causes no more side-effects than an inert placebo tablet. Other very well-tolerated drugs include sulindac, naproxen and pyroxicam.

Paracetamol
Although this drug appears to act peripherally, it has not been shown to have any anti-inflammatory effect and therefore, strictly, it is not an NSAID. In therapeutic doses, paracetamol seldom causes any side-effects. There has been some suspicion as to its rôle in renal capillary necrosis; however, few such cases have been reported.

Psychological aspects of non-narcotic analgesics
Pain behaviour: The indiscriminate over-prescription of these drugs in general practice is not only 'bad medicine', but can lead to becoming in itself a pain behaviour. Thus in any cognitive behavioural regime, almost the first

item in the order of business is the elimination of drug therapy. In these admittedly extreme circumstances, this has been found essential, if the patient is to benefit from the programme.

Non-analgesic properties: It has been shown by the use of the McGill pain questionnaire that these drugs can moderate the severity of affective distress, leaving sensory qualities relatively unaffected[23]. This shows that, in common with all other therapies, response is complex, but, because of its unpredictability, this phenomenon is of little practical value to the clinician.

Practical clinical consequences
Biochemistry: Since the biochemistry of pain is not understood, the production of a specific analgesic is currently not possible. (See Relevant physiology, pp. 34, 43).

Mode of action: This remains unknown, as is the case in all other forms of management, save at least in part for massage, manipulation and TNS.

Choice of drug: In view of the unpredictability of the efficacy of these drugs, this is a matter for therapeutic empiricism.

Over-prescription: Over-prescription of any of these drugs is to be deplored, as is the over-prescription of any other treatment (e.g. manipulation, acupuncture or local injections).

Side-effects: These have been described in detail, but on the whole, these drugs are very safe. Furthermore, it seems sensible to warn the patient of the possibility of the occurrence of side-effects. For example, with indomethacin, it is true that 20–30% of patients will develop symptoms: if, however, they are warned of possible side-effects and are advised to stop therapy immediately should these occur, these problems may be minimized.

Comparison with other treatments: The almost invariable lack of a specific diagnosis in this field adds to the unpredictability of outcome of therapy, as does individual variation in response (see Drugs, p.189).

Ease of delivery: This is unique, by comparison with other forms of treatment, to the advantage of both patient and clinician.
1. For example, prescribed bedrest involves major disruption of the patient's life, including enforced unemployment.
2. Drug therapy is relatively non-invasive, by comparison with surgical techniques.

3. It is less time-consuming than acupuncture, exercises, psychological treatment programmes or physiotherapy (such as ultrasound or traction, masssage or even manipulation).
4. It is less painful than the use of injections.

It follows that drug therapy must be at the forefront of the management of pain in musculoskeletal medicine, provided:
1. It is realistically deployed in the sense that the clinician is aware of the side-effects (such as they are) and the unpredictability of outcome, and
2. That it must must at all times be considered in the context of all the many therapies available in this field.

Treatment time
The convenience for the patient of taking oral medication is obvious. There is virtually no disturbance of his working or domestic habit.

References

1. Hart (1987). *Eular Bulletin*, 16(3), 91
2. Huskisson *et al*. (1976). Four new anti-inflammatory drugs. Responses and variations. *Br. Med. J.*, 1048–1049
3. Huskisson (1980). Flurbiprofen. Efficacy, side effects, dosage and formulation. *Br. J. Chem. Pract.*, **(Suppl) 9**, 95–96
4. Multz *et al*. (1974). A comparison of intermediate dose aspirin and placebo in rheumatoid arthritis. *Clin. Pharm. Ther.*, **15**, 310–315
5. Carson Dick (1978). In Copeman (ed.), *Textbook of the Rheumatic Diseases*, 2nd Edn. (London: Churchill Livingstone)
6. Leonards, Levy and Niemczura (1973). Gastrointestinal blood loss in prolonged aspirin administration. *N. Engl. J. Med.*, **289**, 1020–1022
7. Scott *et al*. (1961). Studies of gastrointestinal bleeding caused by cortico steroids, salicylates and other analgesics. *Q. J. Med.*, **167**,
8. Levy (1974). Aspirin use in patients with major upper gastrointestinal bleeding and peptic ulcer disease. *N. Engl. J. Med.*, **290**, 1158–1162
9. Emmanual and Montgomery (1971). Gastric ulcer and the anti-arthritic drugs. *Post Grad. Med. J.*, **47**, 227–232
10. Cameron (1975). Aspirin and the gastric ulcer. *Mayo Clin. Proc.*, **50**, 565–570
11. Collins and Turner (1975). Maternal effects of regular salicylate ingestion in pregnancy. *Lancet*, **1**, 335–339
12. Winja, Snijder and Nieweg (1966). Acetylsalicylic acid as a cause of pancytopenia from bone marrow damage. *Lancet*, **2**, 768–780
13. O'Brien *et al*. (1970). A comparison of the effect of different anti-inflammatory drugs on human platelets. *J. Clin. Pathology*, **23**, 522–525
14. Mills *et al*. (1974). The effects of in vitro aspirin on blood platelets of gastrointestinal bleeders. *Clin. Pharmacol. Ther.*, **15**, 187–192
15. Szczekalk, Gryglewski and Czerniawska-Mysik (1975). Relationship of inhibition of prostaglandin biosynthesis by analgesics to asthma attacks in aspirin sensitive patients. *Br. Med. J.*, **1**, 67–69
16. Leonards and Levy (1972). Gastrointestinal blood loss from aspirin and sodium salicylate tablets in man. *Clin. Pharmacol. Ther.*, **14**, 62–66
17. Pierson *et al*. (1961). Aspirin and gastrointestinal bleeding. *Am. J. Med.*, **31**, 259–265

18. Champion *et al.* (1975). Salicylates in rheumatoid arthritis. In Pierson and Carson Dick (eds.) *Clinics in the Rheumatic Diseases*, pp. 245–265. (London: W.B. Saunders)
19. Maneksha (1973). Safapryn and benorylate. A comparative trial of two new preparations of aspirin and paracetamol in the treatment of rheumatoid arthritis and osteoarthritis. *Curr. Med. Res. Opin.*, **1**, 563–568
20. Hart and Boardman (1965). Indomethacin and phenylbutazone. A comparison. *Br. Med. J.*, **2**, 1281–1284
21. Healey (1967). An appraisal of indomethacin. *Bull. Rheum. Dis.*, **18**, 483–486
22. Fowler (1975). Indomethacin and phenylbutazone. In Pierson and Dick (eds.) *Clinics in Rheumatic Diseases*. (London: W.B. Saunders)
23. Graceley *et al.* (1978). Narcotic analgesia. Fentanyl reduces the intensity but not the unpleasantness of painful tooth pull sensation. *Science*, **203**, 1261–1263

PSYCHOTROPIC DRUGS

Psychotropic drugs have often been used:
1. Because "human pain is an experience with an affective element, and it is not surprising that these substances have been used as part of the therapeutic approach to this complex problem"[49].
2. Whether or not they have an analgesic effect has also been extensively studied.
3. There are three major groups of these drugs, antidepressants, neuroleptics and tranquilisers, which will be considered in sequence.
4. In all cases, their aim is pain relief.

Therapy 3 – antidepressants – tricyclics and monoaminase oxidase inhibitors

Diagnosis
This is unknown in the great majority of cases.

How they work
A number of modes of action has been proposed to explain how these drugs work.
Antidepressant action
1. The use of these drugs is supported by the finding that the great majority of patients with co-existing chronic pain and depression have gained relief from both disorders when responding to monoaminase oxidase inhibitor (MAOI) or tricyclic antidepressant (TCAD) therapies[1-9].
2. The presence of a depressive disorder preceding or accompanying the onset of a chronic atypical pain complaint predicts a much better response to TCAD or MAOI than if depression followed the onset of pain[10].

194

Separate analgesic effect
1. There is evidence that this takes place. The onset of analgesia with TCADs in chronic pain states is more rapid than the usual onset of an antidepressant effect in clinically depressed patients: 3 to 7 days, as compared with 14 to 21 days[11].
2. Pain relief has been noted despite a lack of antidepressant response[5,9,12] and improvement has been demonstrated in patients without detectable depression. This means that pain relief may be obtained in some instances without altering psychological features[3,9,12,13].

Neurotransmitter alteration
It has been proposed that the action of these drugs is due to their effect on central neurotransmitter functions[14-19]. Much of the supporting evidence is based upon animal experimentation[20].

Opiate effects
Much of the existing evidence is either on animals, or is described as "preliminary"[14,15,21-24]!

Indication
Pain of vertebral origin.

Contraindications
None.

Dangers
Overdose.

Complications
The complications of the TCADs are:
1. Anticholinergic effects,
2. Allergic and hypersensitivity reactions,
3. Cardiovascular and central nervous system problems,
4. Drug interactions,
5. Drug withdrawal effects,
6. Weight gain.

Those of the MAOIs are:
1. Urinary retention,
2. Orthostatic hypotension,
3. Severe parenchymatous hepatotoxic reactions,
4. Central nervous system effects,

5. Hypertensive crises,
6. Drug interaction,
7. Interactions with inappropriate diets.

Predictability
TCADs
In an extensive review published in 1981, 48 papers were surveyed, describing 52 trials in this field[11]. Most of them suffered from inadequacies of various sorts. However, in every case, except for 2 out of 3 trials for low back pain, the TCAD produced clinically significant pain relief, superior to placebo.

In the 2 low back pain studies TCAD and comparative placebo both produced clinically significant pain relief.

In the case of imipramine, studies have been undertaken for the relief of pain in chronic osteoarthritis and rheumatoid arthritis, and these are supported by two control studies each, all regarded as adequate[25,26].

With regard to TCADs, statistical evidence was available only for a correlation of positive outcome with depression onset preceeding or accompanying pain onset[10,11].

Of the adequate controlled trials, in 41 out of 46 studies which gave sufficient details, more than 50% of patients obtained moderate to total relief and a decrease in or cessation of analgesic use. The defect of all these trials was the length of follow-up; in 50% of them less than 1 month, in 73% of them less than 3 months.

A subsequent trial, not included in this series, gave details of a 21 to 28 month questionnaire follow-up of 104 patients systematically treated with TCADs for chronic pain without significant somatic findings. At 9–16 months, 57% had improved significantly, while 31% had dropped out. At 21–28 months, about one quarter of the patients were improved or free of pain and still on TCADs[27].

MAOIs
Phenelzine has been reported to be effective in chronic pain of psychological origin in 1 uncontrolled and 1 adequately controlled trial. In spite of these reasonably encouraging figures, it is not possible to predict which patient will benefit from these drugs.

Similar treatments
Neuroleptics and tranquillizers.

References
See p.200.

Therapy 4 – neuroleptics

Aim of treatment
Pain relief.

Diagnosis
Unknown.

How they work
Because neuroleptics have numerous central and peripheral effects, they have been much studied, both in the laboratory and clinically.

The analgesic properties of phenothiazines and morphine are comparable for acute pain in mice, and for acute and chronic pain in man[28-31].

They have been shown to vary in the strength of their analgesic action[32,33].

It has been suggested that the basis of analgesia with some phenothiazines may be their adrenolytic action. On the evidence offered, this remains a proposal[34].

Indications
Twenty trials have been reviewed (although no trials on low back pain). Phenothiazines were found to be most appropriate for those psychiatric illnesses which caused pain. However, it must be noted that these are extremely rare, in particular schizophrenia.

The main indication for the use of phenothiazines in chronic pain is in patients with recognizable organic lesions that are not amenable to treatment by any other conservative means. Because of the adverse effects of the phenothiazines, they should not be used until other modalities of treatment (such as TNS) have been attempted and failed to help. They are strongly indicated in the control of pain that wakes patients from sleep, and are also helpful in cases of nerve lesion, including various neuralgias and some instances of back pain, if there is clear evidence of associated damage to nerves or nerve roots.

Contraindications
Apart from the reservations given above, there are none.

Dangers
Overdosage.

Complications
1. Drowsiness and some dysphoria.

2. Dry mouth.
3. Blurred vision.
4. Constipation.
5. Retention of urine.

Predictability
In summarizing 18 papers, reporting 20 trials, it was found that none was controlled[11]. However, in 2 controlled trials of single-dose efficacy in mixed groups of acute and chronic pain disorders, the neuroleptics were found to provide pain relief equal to that of the usual analgesic doses of narcotics[29,31]. Unhappily, the majority of trials lasted less than 3 months. The importance of this limitation is demonstrated in the case of chronic post-herpetic neuralgia, where both trials lasting more than 6 months reported almost total failure after initial impressive relief[35].

Despite the lack of controlled trials, evidence for neuroleptic-induced pain relief is strongly supported by a series of anecdotal single-patient experiments, and by uncontrolled group reports[36-40]. Patients with very chronic stable baseline neurological pain disorders refractory to many interventions responded rapidly (in less than 4 days) frequently had total pain relief, and suffered relapse rapidly on placebo substitution or on stopping the neuroleptics.

Combined neuroleptic/antidepressant therapy
1. A small number of anecdotal case reports or uncontrolled group studies has been reported on the combined use of these drugs in chronic pain conditions[41-43]. Good to total pain relief was reported in more than 50% of patients in 8 out of 9 studies, and total pain relief in 5 out of 7 studies. However, reported pain follow-up was less than 2 weeks in 4 out of 9 studies, and 5–6 months in 3.
2. Comparison of neuroleptics with TCAIDs or MAOIs is not possible, as no relevant trials have been found.

Once again, the evidence upon which prediction might be established is sadly lacking.

Similar treatments
The antidepressants and tranquillizers.

References
See p.200.

Therapy 5 – tranquillisers

Aim of treatment
Pain relief and anxiolysis.

Diagnosis
Unknown.

How they work
Benzodiazepines are often given to diminish anxiety and insomnia, commonly felt to contribute adversely to acute and chronic pain states[44-46]. The mechanism of any such action they may have is unclear.

Indications
Pain of vertebral origin.

Contraindications
None.

Dangers
Overdosage.

Complications
Physical dependency and withdrawal symptoms can occur with prolonged, moderate to high dose usage. Such problems are seldom encountered at normal therapeutic dose levels[47].

Predictability
There is suggestive evidence that short-term benzodiazepines may help to diminish pain associated with a number of conditions, and, from the musculoskeletal point of view, in particular acute and chronic intervertebral disc problems, with muscle spasm[48]. (With regard to the difficulties in arriving at these particular diagnoses see The Prolapsed Intervertebral Disc, p.124. This difficulty must greatly diminish the validity of this work.)

In the treatment of chronic pain, benzodiazepines have been compared with TCADs in a number of studies, in particular on pain of psychological origin and chronic tension headaches[11,13]. They were found to be definitely inferior to TCADs. Again, the taxonomy of tension headache is notoriously difficult.

Once more, the only conclusion to be drawn from examination of the available evidence is that prediction of outcome of this therapy is not possible.

Practical clinical consequences
The mode of action of all these drugs remains unknown. Although much work has been done in trying to assess the proper rôle of the psychotropic drugs, its limitations mean that it is of little clinical value. The problems of assessing pain management are illustrated here more clearly, perhaps, than in any other form of treatment.

From the analgesic point of view, tricyclics and neuroleptics seem to have a definite place, but, because of their potential adverse effects, the latter need to be used with care. Mild tranquillizers seem to be less effective from the analgesic point of view, to which is added the risk of potential addiction. Since 10% of pain clinic patients suffer clinical depression, this group should be identified and treated appropriately.

"It is important to recognise that the use of psychotropic drugs is only one of the adjunctive measures available in the comprehensive approach to many pain problems, especially those of more chronic duration."[49] For this reason they are used as analgesic agents – as a 'reserve therapy'.

Treatment time
These drugs share with all oral therapies the considerable advantage of making minimal demands upon the patient.

References

1. Couch et al. (1976). Amitriptyline in the prophylaxis of migraine. Effectiveness and relationship of anti-migraine and anti-depressant effects. *Neurology*, **26**, 121–127
2. Evans et al. (1973). The effects of antidepressant drugs on pain relief and mood in the chronically ill. *Psychosomatics*, **14**, 214–219
3. Jenkins et al. (1976). Imipramine in treatment of low back pain. *J. Int. Med. Res.*, **4 (Supp. 2)**, 28–40
4. Johannsen et al. (1979). A double blind controlled study of a serotonin uptake inhibitor (Zimelidine) versus placebo in chronic pain patients. *Pain*, **7**, 69–78
5. Lascelles (1966). Atypical facial pain and depression. *Br. J. Psychiatry*, **122**, 651–659
6. Okasha et al. (1973). A double blind trial for the clinical management of psychogenic headache. *Br. J. Psychiatry*, **122**, 181–183
7. Turkington (1980). Depression masquerading as diabetic neuropathy. *J. Am. Med. Assoc.*, **243**, 1147–1150
8. Ward et al. (1979). The effectiveness of tricyclic antidepressants in the treatment of co-existing pain and depression. *Pain*, **7**, 331–341
9. Watson et al. (1982). Amitriptyline versus placebo in post-herpetic neuralgia. *Neurology*, **32**, 671–673
10. Bradley (1963). Severe localised pain associated with the depressive syndromes. *Br. J. Psychiatry*, **109**, 741–745
11. Monks (1981). The use of psychotropic drugs in human chronic pain. A review. In *Proceedings of the Sixth World Congress of the International College of Psychosomatic Medicine*, Montreal, Canada. Sept. 15
12. Couch and Hassanein (1976). Migraine and depression. Effect of amitriptyline prophylaxis. *Trans. Am. Neurol. Assoc.*, **101**, 14
13. Lance and Curran (1964). A treatment of chronic tension headache. *Lancet*, **1**, 1236–1239

14. Fuentes *et al.* (1977). Potentiation of morphine analgesia in mice after inhibition of brain type B monoamine oxidase. *Neuropharmacology*, 16, 857–862
15. Lee and Spencer (1977). Antidepressants and pain. A review of the pharmacological data supported in the use of certain tricyclics in chronic pain. *J. Int. Med. Res.*, 5 (Supp. 1), 146–156
16. Messing and Lytle (1977). Serotonin containing neurones. Their possible role in pain and analgesia. *Pain*, 4, 121
17. Murphy *et al.* (1978). The current status of the indolamine hypothesis of the affective disorders. In Lipton, Mascio and Killam (eds.) *Psychopharmacology. A Generation of Progress*, pp. 1235–1247. (New York: Raven Press)
18. Shildkraut (1978). Current status of the catechol-amine hypothesis of affective disorders. In Lipton, Mascio and Killam (eds.), idem., pp. 1223–1224
19. Sternbach *et al.* (1976). The effects of altering brain serotonin activity on human chronic pain. In Bonica and Albe-Fessard (eds.) *Advances in Pain Research Therapy 1*, pp. 601–606. (New York: Raven Press)
20. Dennis and Melzack (1980). Pain modulation by 5-hydroxytryptaminergic agents and morphine as measured by 3 pain tests. *Exp. Neurol.*, 69, 260–270
21. Contreras *et al.* (1977). Effects of tricyclic compounds and other drugs having a membrane stabilizing action on analgesia. Tolerance to, and dependence on morphine. *Arch. Int. Psychodyn.*, 228, 293–299
22. Gonzalez *et al.* (1980). Antinociceptive activity of opiates in the presence of the antidepressant agent Nomifensine. *Neuropharmacology*, 19, 613–618
23. Tofanetti *et al.* (1977). Enhancement of propoxyphene induced analgesia by Doxepin. *Psychopharmacology*, 51, 213–215
24. Johanssen *et al.* (1980). Changes in endorphins and 5-hydroxy-indole acetic acid in cerebro spinal fluid as a result of treatment with a serotonin re-uptake inhibitor (Zimelidine) in chronic pain patients. *Psychiatry Res.*, 2, 167–172
25. McDonald Scott (1969). The relief of pain with an antidepressant in arthritis. *Practitioner*, 202, 803–807
26. Thorpe and Marchant-Williams (1974). The role of an antidepressant, Dibenzepine (Novoril), in the relief of pain in chronic arthritis states. *Med. J. Austr.*, 1, 264–266
27. Blumer and Heilbron (1981). Second year follow-up study on systemic treatment of chronic pain with antidepressants. *Henry Ford Hosp. Med. J.*, 29, 67–68
28. Maxwell *et al.* (1961). A comparison of the analgesic and some other central properties of Methotrimeprazine and morphine. *Arch. Int. Pharmacodyn.*, 132, 60
29. Bloomfield *et al.* (1964). Comparative analgesic activity of Levomepromazine and morphine in patients with chronic pain. *Can. Med. Assoc. J.*, 90, 1155–1159
30. Lasagna and De Kornfeld (1961). Methotrimeprazine. A new phenothiazine derivative with analgesic properties. *J. Am. Med. Assoc.*, 178, 887–890
31. Montilla *et al.* (1963). Analgesic effect of methotrimeprazine and morphine. *Arch. Intern. Med.*, 111, 91–94
32. Moore and Dundee (1961). Alterations in response to somatic pain associated with anaesthesia. 7. The effects of nine phenothiazine derivatives. *Br. J. Anaesth.*, 33 (9), 422–431
33. Dundee *et al.* (1963). Alterations to response in somatic pain associated with anaesthesia. 15. Further studies with phenothiazine derivatives and similar drugs. *Br. J. Anaesth.*, 35 (10), 597–609
34. Moore and Dundee (1961). Alterations in response to somatic pain associated with anaesthia. 7. The effects of nine phenothiazine derivatives. *Br. J. Anaesth.*, 33 (9), 422–431
35. Nathan (1978). Chlorprothixene (Taractan) in post herpetic neuralgia and other severe chronic pains. *Pain*, 5, 361–367
36. Cavenar and Maltbie (1976). Another indication for Haloperidol. *Psychosomatics*, 17, 128–130
37. Gade *et al.* (1980). Diabetic neuropathic cachexia. *J. Am. Med. Assoc.*, 243, 1160–1161
38. Maltbie and Kavenar (1977). Haloperidol and analgesia. Case reports. *Military Med.*, 142, 946–948

39. Margolis and Gianascol. (1956). Chlorpramazine in thalamic pain syndrome. *Neurology*, **6**, 302–304
40. Taub (1973). Relief of post herpetic neuralgia with psychotropic drugs. *J. Neurosurg.*, **39**, 235–239
41. Bourhis *et al*. (1978). Pain informity and psychotropic drugs in oncology. *Pain*, **5**, 263–274
42. Duthie (1977). The use of phenothiazines and tricyclic antidepressants in the treatment of intractable pain. *Med. J.*, **51**, 246–247
43. Kocher (1976). In Bonica and Albe-Fessard (eds.) *Advances in Pain Research Therapy*, pp. 57–9582. (New York: Raven Press)
44. Lasagna (1977). The role of the benzodiazepines in non-psychiatric medical practice. *Am. J. Psychiatry*, **134**(6), 656–658
45. Hollister *et al*. (1981). Long term use of diazepam. *J. Am. Med. Assoc.*, **46**(14), 1568–1570
46. Shimm *et al*. (1979). Medical management of chronic cancer pain. *J. Am. Med. Assoc.*, **241**(22), 2411
47. Marks (1980). The benzodiazepines. Use and abuse. In Leder (ed.) *New Perspectives in Benzodiazepine Therapy*. *Arzneimittel forsch (Drug Research)*, **31**, 898–901
48. Greenblatt and Shader (1974). Benzodiazepines. Parts I and II. *N. Engl. J. Med.*, **251**, 1011–1015; **291**(23), 1239–1245
49. Monil and Merskey (1983). In Wall and Melzack (eds.) *Textbook of Pain*, p.526. (London: Churchill Livingstone)

Therapy 6 – bedrest

Aim of treatment
Relief of pain.

Diagnosis
In the great majority of cases, this remains unknown.

How it works
This, too, is unknown, except for the fact that, as even skin touch may provoke the action of A fibre stimulation, there is inevitably a measure of A on C inhibition. With skin pressure spread so widely over much of the painful area, this may be relevant. This point, of course, also has relevance with respect to the use of collars and corsets.

Indication
Pain of vertebral origin.

Contraindications
There are no strict contraindications.

Dangers
Prolonged bedrest may increase the risk of deep vein thrombosis of the legs.

Complications
The only significant complication is the reinforcement of pain behaviour, leading to abnormal pain behaviour. This may prove a difficult problem to eradicate. Indeed, so important a behaviour is bedrest, that we include it as an integral part of case analysis.

Prediction of outcome
In the short term, it has been shown by Deyo *et al.* that there is no advantage in terms of pain relief in enforced bedrest for seven days as compared with two days[1]. Clinicians advising this form of therapy should bear this in mind, because the assumption that bedrest is beneficial in pain of vertebral origin is clearly open to question. In the long term, prediction of outcome is not possible.

Similar treatments
There are none.

Therapy time
The inconvenience factor in confining a patient to bed is substantial. In most cases it means that he is unable to work, with possible financial disadvantage to him and his family, and it also involves others in his care. It is frequently prolonged from days into weeks. Apart from the complication mentioned above, we have found no evidence supporting various ideas as to other disadvantages.

Comments
"Our data support a recent trend toward earlier mobilisation of patients with back pain. Not only are brief periods of bed rest apparently safe for selected patients, but they may reduce the potential adverse effects of bed rest, including physical deconditioning. Finally there are many who believe that an early return to work may help to prevent the emergence of chronic back pain syndromes, with their enormous human and monetary costs."[1]

We note the astonishing discrepancy between the frequency with which this treatment is prescribed and the almost complete lack of evidence which might justify its use.

Reference

1. Deyo *et al.* (1986). How many days of bed rest for acute low back pain? *N. Engl. J. Med.*, **315**, 1064–1070

Therapy 7 – heat and cold (including ultrasound, short-wave diathermy and microwave therapy)

Heat and cold are commonly used in the management of pain in painful disorders of the musculoskeletal system. This is particularly applicable to the treatment of muscle spasm.

Selection of treatment
Deep heating devices. These include:
1. Short-wave diathermy (a high-frequency electromagnetic current operating at a frequency of 2712 MHz),
2. Microwave (an electromagnetic radiation of the frequency of 2456 to 915 MHz),
3. Ultrasound (a high-frequency acoustic vibration at a frequency of 0.8 to 1 MHz).

Superficial agents: These include:
1. Hot packs,
2. Paraffin wax baths,
3. Radiant heat.

Some of these modalities permit non-thermal effects, for example exercises in hydrotherapy.

Tissue selection
Skin and superficial subcutaneous tissues are selectively heated by infrared, visible light, hot packs, paraffin baths and hydrotherapy.

Deeper subcutaneous tissues and superficial musculature are selectively heated by short-wave diathermy with condenser application, and by microwaves at a frequency around 2456 mHz.

Deeper musculature is heated preferentially by short-wave diathermy using induction coil applicators.

Deep-seated joints and fibrous scars within soft tissues are selectively heated by ultrasound, as are myofascial interfaces, tendon sheaths and nerve trunks.

Cold application
Dry: This is most commonly applied using a rubber bag containing ice cubes, as a compress.
Wet: The use of a terry cloth, dipped into a mixture of ice shavings with water, is applied to the body part.

Soaking: The part is immersed in iced water.

The use of ice massage: A block of ice is rubbed over the skin surface. (See Ice massage, p.235).

Cooling with ethyl chloride spray: This is done by spraying the skin from a distance of about 1 m applied with a 'stroking' motion[1]. It is most often used as a counter-irritant.

Aim of treatment
This is simply pain relief.

Diagnosis
This is almost always unknown.

How it works
Physiological basis
"The physiological basis for the relief of muscle spasm is incompletely understood."[19]

Much work has been done on the effects of temperature on muscle spindles, but the outcome is unclear. For example, "one could speculate, assuming that secondary muscle spasm is to a large degree a tonic phenomenon, that the selective cessation of stimuli from secondary endings may reduce the muscle tone."[2]

There is evidence that skin heating may produce muscle relaxation[3]; on the other hand there is evidence that selective cooling of the skin increases spindle excitability[4-6].

It is proven beyond doubt that heat increases blood flow, and that cold decreases this[7-9]. Again, the clinical relevance of this is not so certain. "The increase in vascularity and blood flow due to heating may play a rôle in obtaining relief from painful conditions such as myofibrositis, a poorly defined syndrome, which responds to heating the tender muscular nodes. In the same fashion, a resolution of painful inflammatory reactions may be achieved."[19]

Counter-irritant effects
1. It was shown as long ago as 1945 that cold applied with ethyl chloride spray for 20 seconds to the skin covering the tibia increased the pain threshold of tooth pulp, as measured by electrical stimulation[10].
2. In 1941 it was shown that heat producing a significant temperature elevation resulted in the same analgesic affect as cold application[11].
3. The effects produced by this mechanism seem to be of the same magnitude as those obtained by transcutaneous electrical nerve stimulation[12].

Effects on nerve and nerve endings
1. It has been shown in animal experiments that cold decreases nerve conduction first in the small myelinated fibres which include the A-δ fibres[13].
2. Unfortunately, this work is species dependent, and may involve counter-irritant effect.
3. Only tentative clinical conclusions may be drawn from this, "therefore it can be assumed that pain sensation may be markedly reduced by significant local coolling, through an indirect effect on nerve fibres and free endings."[14,15]

Heat application
This produces a large number of different responses, including changes in:
1. Neuromuscular activity,
2. Blood flow,
3. Capillary permeability,
4. Enzyme activity,
5. Pain threshold.
Vigorous local responses may be produced.

Distant heating
This produces a limited number of reflexogenic physiological responses. The consequence of this is that, "when vigorous responses are required, local heat is strongly preferred"[19]. The factors which determine the intensity of the physiological reaction locally are:
1. The level of tissue temperature elevation (to approximately 40–50°C).
2. The duration of tissue temperature elevation (approximately 5–30 min).
All these proposals remain hypothetical.

Indications
Pain of vertebral origin.

Contraindications
Heat:
1. Because it is not yet possible (particularly with deep heating modalities) to control temperature accurately, it is essential that treatment be stopped the moment pain commences.
2. Therefore, heat treatment to anaesthetic areas is contraindicated.
3. This is also the case in tissues with inadequate vascular supply, since ischaemic necrosis is a possibility.
4. It is contraindicated in the presence of a haemorrhagic problem, since the increase in blood flow and vascularity may increase bleeding.

206

Short-wave diathermy: This is contraindicated if an appreciable amount of energy can reach the site of a metal implant. This includes cardiac pacemakers and other electrophysiological apparatus.

Microwave therapy: Sensitive organs should not be exposed to any significant amount of radiation, and this includes the skull[16].

Ultrasound: It is important to avoid the occurrence of gaseous cavitation, which may occur in such fluids as cerebrospinal fluid and joint effusions. This is avoided under therapeutic conditions by using adequate equipment with adequate uniformity in the spatial and temporal distribution of the intensity of the beam. However, ultrasound can be applied to the intervertebral joints without significant exposure of the cerebrospinal fluid and spinal cord because of the intervening tissues such as bone, ligaments and muscles, and the beam can be aimed at the zygoapophyseal joints.

Complications
Cold: There are a number of hypersensitivity syndromes that may occur. The first is cold urticaria, with skin manifestations of itching and erythema. In some cases there may even be shock[17].

Heat: These have been dealt with under contraindications.

Practical clinical consequences
With regard to these therapies in pain of vertebral origin, either heat or cold may be used. Short-wave diathermy may be applied with either induction coil or condenser pads. Treatments should be given once or twice daily, for 20 to 30 minutes per session. In microwave, direct contact applicators can be used. Superficial heating agents, may be used, such as hot packs, hydrocollator packs or radiant heat with lamp or cradle, treatment usually being given for 20 to 30 minutes per session. Ice packs or ice massage can be used. It was shown in 1967 that in 117 patients with back pain heat and cold applications were equally effective[18]. Trigger points can be treated with both hot and cold applications, or with ethyl chloride spray. Ultrasound in low doses was also found to be effective.

"Precautions should be used when microwaves are applied over bony prominences, since the reflection of the wave at the bone interface may produce increased absorption in the tissue superficial to the bone. Burns have been observed under these circumstances."[19]

The mode of action and predictability of these treatments are unknown.

Treatment time

It must be remembered that 20–30 minutes therapy may often involve the patient in losing half a day's working time.

References

1. Bierman (1955). Therapeutic use of cold. *J. Am. Med. Assoc.*, **157**, 1189–1192
2. Mense (1978). Effects of temperature on the discharges of muscle spindles and tendon organs. *Pfulgers Archiv.*, **374**, 159–166
3. Fischer *et al.* (1965). Physiological responses to heat and cold. In Licht (ed.) *Therapeutic Heat and Cold*. 2nd Edn., pp. 126–169. (Waverley Press)
4. Knutsson and Mattsson (1969). Effects of local cooling on monosynaptic reflexes in man. *Scand. J. Rehab. Med.*, **1**, 126–132
5. Hartviksen (1962). Ice therapy in spasticity. *Acta Neurol. Scand.*, **38**, 79–84
6. Miglietta (1973). Action of cold on spasticity. *Am. J. Phys. Med.*, **52**, 198–205
7. Guy *et al.* (1974). Therapeutic applications of electromagnetic power. *Proc. Inst. Electron. Eng.*, **62**, 55–75
8. Lehmann *et al.* (1979). A comparison of patterns of stray radiation from the therapeutic microwave applicators measured near tissue substitute models and human subjects. *Radio. Science*, **14**, 271–283
9. Sekins *et al.* (1980). Muscle blood flow changes in response to 915 mhz. diathermy as simultaneously measured and numerically predicted. *Arch. Phys. Med. Rehabil.*, **61**, 105–113
10. Parsons and Goetzl (1945). Effect of induced pain on pain threshold. *Proc. Soc. Exp. Biol. Med.*, **60**, 327–329
11. Gammon and Starr (1941). Studies on the relief of pain by counter irritation. *J. Clin. Invest.*, **20**, 13–20
12. Melzack *et al.* (1980). Ice massage and transcutaneous electrical stimulation. Comparison of treatments for low back pain. *Pain*, **9**, 209–217
13. Douglas and Malcolm (1955). The effect of localising cooling on conduction in cat nerves. *J. Physiol.*, **130**, 53–71
14. Lehman *et al.* (1964). Modification of heating patterns produced by microwaves at the frequencies of 2456 and 900 Mc. by physiological factors in the human. *Arch. Phys. Med. Rehabil.*, **45**, 555–563
15. Hardy *et al.* (1940). Studies on pain. A new method for measuring pain thresholds. Observations on spatial summation of pain. *J. Clin. Invest.*, **19**, 649–657
16. Johnson *et al.* (1972). Non-ionizing electromagnetic wave effects in biological materials and systems. *Proc. Inst. Elect. Electron. Eng.*, **66**, 692–718
17. Juhlin *et al.* (1961). Role of mast and basophil cells in cold urticaria with associated systemic reactions. *J. Am. Med. Assoc.*, **117**, 371–377
18. Landon (1967). Heat or cold for the relief of low back pain? *Phys. Ther.*, **47**, 1126–1128
19. Lehmann and De Latuer (1983). Ultrasound, shortwave, microwave, superficial heat and cold in the treatment of pain. In Wall and Melzack (eds.), *Textbook of Pain*, p.717. (London: Churchill Livingstone)

Therapy 8 – collars and corsets

Aim of therapy
Pain relief.

Diagnosis
In the great majority of cases, this is unknown.

How they work
As with bedrest, there is inevitably a measure of 'A on C' effect in wearing a collar or corset. We have found nothing of note in the literature regarding the physiological effects of wearing collars. With regard to corsets, the degree of confusion which exists may be indicated by the fact that in 1970, Perry described more than 30 different designs[1]. More information is at hand than is the case with collars, and some of this is disconcerting. For example, Nachemson and Lindt, in 1969, proved that wearing a lumbar supprt for up to 5 years does not 'weaken the muscles'[2]. This conclusion was arrived at by a study of motor unit activity. Walters and Norris, in 1970, showed that there was no effect on lumbar musculature on standing and slow walking, but that during fast walking the support actually increased muscle activity[3]. Van Leuven and Troupe, in 1969, showed that the range of sagittal movement was the same whether a healthy symptom-free subject wore an instant corset, a tailored lumbar corset or no support at all[4]. Thus elaborate corsets may make some movements uncomfortable, but they do little to prevent such movements. Norton and Brown, in 1957, inserting Kirschner wires into the lumbar spinous processes of a normal subject, found that commonly used low back braces and plaster of Paris jackets failed to limit lumbar movements[5]. These actually appeared to increase lumbosacral movement, by restricting motion in the rest of the spine. Hence the basis of the prescription of corsets for many years, i.e. that it restricted spinal movement, is shown to be untrue. Further, Nachemson, in 1964, found that a tight lumbar support reduced intradiscal pressures by about 30%[6]. This led Macnab to write in 1977, "The most important component of the spinal brace is the abdominal binder"[7]. This evidence has led to the increasing popularity of abdominal strengthening exercises in the treatment of low back pain. While this is certainly reasonable, there is as yet no evidence as to how effective such exercises may be. Otherwise, their mode of operation remains obscure.

Indications
Pain of vertebral origin.

Contraindications
Collars are contraindicated in cases where there are proprioceptive problems:
1. For drivers of cars, as the collar will distort the cervical reflexes and may thereby cause loss of manual dexterity, with the resulting risk of disaster. Clearly this is most important, and it is astonishing how few clinicians are aware of this fact[8].
2. For the elderly, on entering a dark room from one well illuminated, when the dependence upon visual input may be revealed only on the patient falling, with possible resultant injury[9].

There are no contraindications to the wearing of a corset.

Dangers
These are traumatic, as indicated above.

Predictability
This is not possible.

Similar treatments
There are none.

Therapy time
Although there is some inconvenience in wearing either a collar or a corset, the actual time required on the part of the patient for putting them on or taking them off is minimal in all but the most complicated models.

References

1. Perry (1970). The use of external support in the treatment of low back pain. *J. Bone Jt. Surg.*, **52A**, 14–40
2. Nachemson and Lindt (1969). Measurement of abdominal and back muscle strength with and without low back pain. *Scand. J. Rehabil. Med.*, **1**, 60
3. Walters and Norris (1970). The effects of spinal supports on the electrical activities of the trunk. *J. Bone Jt. Surg.*, **52A**, 51
4. Van Leuven and Troup (1969). The 'instant' lumbar corset. *Physiotherapy*, **31**, 201
5. Norton and Brown (1957). The immobilising effect of back braces: their effect on the posture and motion of the lumbosacral spine. *J. Bone Jt. Surg.*, **39A**, 111
6. Nachemson (1964). In vivo measurement of intradiscal pressure. *J. Bone Jt. Surg.*, **46A**, 1077
7. Macnab (1977). *Backache.* (Baltimore: Williams and Wilkins)
8. Wyke (1965). Comparative analysis of proprioception in left and right arms. *Q. J. Exp. Psychol.*, **17**, 149
9. Lee and Lishman (1975). Vision in movement and balance. *New Sci.*, **65**, 69

Therapy 9 – traction

Aim of treatment
Relief of pain.

Diagnosis
This is almost invariably unknown.

How it works
Once again, the only mechanism known to operate is 'A on C'. While several theories are currently canvassed as to how traction achieves its undoubted (if unpredictable) proportion of good results, there remains no evidence as to their veracity. This applies equally to the various modalities of traction, sustained, intermittent or pulsed. There seems little to commend turning the patient upside down!

Indications
Pain of vertebral origin. In the light of the points made as to diagnosis and how it works, it is clear that a more precise indication is not valid.

Contraindication
The only contraindication is if the treatment increases pain.

Dangers
There are none.

Complications
There are none.

Predictabililty
This is not possible, either in the short term or in the long term.

Comment
Because such studies as that of Weber[1] have demonstrated the unpredictability of traction, its value has been diminished in the eyes of many UK rheumatologists. However, if it is compared with other treatments, it is not alone in its unpredictability of outcome and, in view of its safety, its trial seems reasonable, as many physiotherapists would agree[2].

Similar treatments
On account of its known mode of operation, it has similarities to manipulation, massage, TNS and acupuncture.

Therapy time
While a single session of traction usually lasts for about half an hour, it is likely to be deployed on a number of occasions, and the patient may well suffer considerable inconvenience in attending hospital or clinic for treatment. This latter aspect may be reduced by the employment of domiciliary traction, which has the added advantage of being available to the patient at a time which is convenient to him[3].

Reference

1. Weber (1973). Traction therapy in sciatica due to disc prolapse. *J. Oslo City Hosp.*, **23**, 167
2. Paterson and Burn (1985). *An Introduction to Medical Manipulation*, pp. 50–52. (Lancaster: MTP Press)
3. Idem, pp. 180–181

Therapy 10 – massage

Aim of treatment
Relief of pain.

Diagnosis
Unknown. Numerous syndromes have been described, purported to be amenable to massage, but all lacking validation.

How it works
'A on C'. But see comment on Therapy 6 – Bedrest. Any treatment involving contact with the patient **must** have this as a part of its mode of action. A number of techniques is employed, details of which are to be found in the appropriate literature.

Indication
Pain of vertebral origin.

Contraindication
Massage is contraindicated if it causes pain.

Dangers
None.

Complications
None.

Predictability
No valid prediction may be made in respect of outcome of massage, other than that it is commonly comforting.

Similar treatments
In respect of the known mode of action, massage has similarities with both TNS and manipulation.

Therapy time
This must take into account both the time of actual treatment and the time required to be away from work in order to receive it. Generally it involves a matter of hours.

Therapy 11 – manipulation

Aim of treatment
Relief of pain. We appreciate that, within orthodox medicine, world-wide, manipulation is perhaps the most controversial treatment for pain of musculoskeletal origin. However, when compared with other therapies for this group of conditions, it has its place, its advantages and its disadvantages. We therefore present it here amongst others, as being worthy of consideration. This treatment is more fully discussed in our companion volume[1].

Diagnosis
This is unknown in the great majority of cases.

How it works
A on C. But other mechanisms may be at work, although they have not been identified with any certainty. As with massage, many techniques are taught, and it is clear that there is no 'right' or 'wrong' technique to be employed; individual variations are wide, and indeed manipulative techniques are

customarily very personally evolved procedures, based on the broadest of outlines and adapted to the individual needs of patient and clinician.

Indications
Pain of vertebral origin.

Contraindications
General: Fracture, neoplasm, infection, inflammatory disease and vascular problems are all absolute contraindications for manipulation. Their identification may demand the use of laboratory or radiological investigations. However, the great majority of cases seen in musculoskeletal practice do not exhibit any of these features.

Cervical: Because of the predilection of rheumatoid disease for the odontoid process and the transverse ligament, this disease is an absolute contraindication for manipulation, which could endanger life by posterior dislocation of the odontoid process, either due to its fracture or due to the laxity of the damaged transverse ligament[1].

Drop attacks and vertigo are also important, as these may be the result of vascular insufficiency, and there is a risk of basilar artery thrombosis.

Recent (and even not very recent) upper respiratory tract infections in children may be a part of Grisel's syndrome, in which the transverse ligament may again be weakened[1].

Because of the rare possibility of cervical myelopathy, any suggestion of inadequacy of blood supply to the cervical cord must be regarded as a contraindication to maniulation[1].

Thoracic: The last item applies equally to the thoracic spine.

Lumbar: Sphincter problems and saddle anaesthesia are not only strong contraindications to manipulation, but demand immediate referral to the orthopaedic surgery department.

The contraindications and dangers are discussed more fully in *An Introduction to Medical Manipulation*, pp. 17–19[1].

Dangers and complications
These follow from the points made above. They are:
1. Death from 'pithing' the patient in rheumatoid arthritis.
2. Death or serious damage from ischaemia in cardiovascular problems.
3. Damage from ischaemia due to myelopathy.
4. Irreversible neurogenic bladder problems.

Similar therapies
1. Clearly related are massage and TNS.
2. More remotely related are bedrest, collars and corsets and traction.

Therapy time
This requires qualification. Strictly from the patient's point of view, it is comparable with massage, in that it is to be had at the hands of a professional. Although it takes no more than three to five minutes for actual treatment, as compared with thirty minutes, it is likely that treatment will involve travelling to the appropriate hospital or clinic. This means that it will probably require hours of the patient's time. However, from the clinician's point of view, it is very much quicker, and it is this factor which so commends itself to the musculoskeletal physician; if it works, it works with great speed. It is for this last reason that it is also well suited to use in general practice.

Reference

1. Paterson and Burn (1985). *An Introduction to Medical Manipulation*. (London: MTP Press)

Therapy 12 – local anaesthetic block

Local anaesthesia has been in use for nearly a century, and it is of great value in the treatment of acute and chronic pain[1].

General principles concerning anaesthetic agents
Thorough knowledge of the pharmacology and optimal concentrations of these materials is necessary.

High concentrations, such as 1% procaine or 1% lidnocaine, are unnecessary, because a lower concentration is sufficient to block A-δ and C fibres, while a higher concentration may block somatic motor fibres[2-5].

For diagnostic and prognostic purposes, short-acting agents are appropriate, but for therapeutic action the longer acting ones are to be prefered.

Technique
It is necessary to have:
1. High-quality equipment,
2. High-quality local anaesthetics,
3. Other drugs and equipment necessary for the prompt treatment of complications of therapy.

Prior to the block, details of the procedure should be explained to the patient.

If a neurological examination has not been carried out, it should be done in order to determine the patient's clinical status prior to treatment. Sterile technique nust be used, with appropriate antiseptics. If large needles are to be used, the skin should first be anaesthetized, raising a skin wheal.

Basic principles of application
According to Bonica[1], failure in the past was often due to:
1. Inadequate knowledge of pain syndromes.
2. Inadequate evaluation of patients.
3. Lack of knowledge of other therapeutic modalities which might be better used in individual patients.
4. Inadequate patient management before, during and after the block.
5. Lack of appreciation of the specific indications, limitations and possible complications of the procedures.

Aim of treatment
Pain relief.

Diagnosis
Unknown in the great majority of cases.

How it works
The basis for the use of local anaesthesia is as follows:
1. Either the interruption of nociceptive input at source, or the blocking of nociceptive fibres in peripheral nerves.
2. Blockade may also interrupt the afferent limb of abnormal reflex mechanisms which contribute to the pathophysiology of some pain syndromes.
3. It may also block sympathetic fibres, since sympathetic hyperactivity often contributes to certain pain syndromes.
4. Low concentrations of local anaesthetic may block the unmyelinated C and B fibres and small myelinated A-δ fibres, without blocking somatic motor functions.
5. At the same time it is possible to block somatic fibres on occasion, to relieve muscle spasm.

Any of these effects, alone or in combination, can produce relief of pain, which may last for varying periods of time, often outlasting by hours, days or weeks the transient pharmacological action of the local anaesthetic. It is thought that they may act by blocking off the input and thereby ending the self-sustaining activity which seems to be responsible for some chronic pain syndromes[1,6].

From the above it will be seen that the mode of action remains unknown.

Indications

Pain of vertebral origin.

Contraindications

The only real contraindication is known hypersensitivity to the anaesthetic drug.

Dangers

The chief danger is that of systemic toxic reaction.

Complications

Pneumothorax. This is in relation to thoracic injections. We do not believe that musculoskeletal physicians should undertake procedures that run this risk unless they have been adequately trained to do so.

Neurological complications do not occur with 'local' block.

Mild systemic toxic reactions may occur, characterized by palpitation, metallic taste, dryness of the mouth and throat, tinnitus, vertigo or confusion, but these are extraordinarily rare.

Preventative measures

Using the lowest concentration and volume of local anaesthetic reduces the risk of complications.

The use of adrenaline 1:200,000 in the solution, retards the rate of local anaesthetic absorption.

Aspiration prior to each injection reduces the risk of the needle point inadvertently entering and remaining in a blood vessel, which might otherwise result in intravenous injection.

Injecting about 3 ml of solution as a test dose (if large amounts are to be injected) reduces the risk of toxic reactions. The adrenaline (if the injection has been made intravenously) will cause transient tachycardia, of about 30 to 90 seconds duration[7,8].

Predictability

Accurate prediction of outcome, short term or long term, is not possible.

Treatment time

This is quite short, apart from the need to attend the doctor's surgery or the hospital outpatient department. It is this factor which converts the therapy from requiring minutes to requiring hours.

Practical clinical consequences
Local nerve block
In our companion volume, *An Introduction to Medical Manipulation*, we describe in detail techniques for trigger points, attachment tissues, and injections in the vicinity of the posterior vertebral joints, as also for nerve block restricted to the greater occipital nerve and the lateral femoral cutaneous nerve. All these extremely useful procedures are suitable for use in the general practice environment. Other spinal and cranial nerve blocks are not suitable, (a) because of the skills required to undertake these procedures, and (b) because of the possibility of severe complications necessitating both appropriate training and the availability of adequate resuscitatory equipment.

Trigger points
a. Patients with pain associated with tender 'fibrositic' areas in muscles and ligaments frequently have their symptoms relieved if these nodules are infiltrated with local anaesthetic[1,9-14].
b. "One of the most poorly understood phenomena related to the chronic pain syndromes is the focal hyper-irritability of tissues related to painful areas in the body . . . by a poorly understood mechanism local injections with anaesthetic provide relief at a distant location far longer than can be explained by the pharmacological action of the drug."[15] This observation is supported by the work of Mehta in 1973[16].
c. Usually 5–10 ml of dilute solution of a long-lasting anaesthetic is used, such as 0.5% bupivacaine.
d. If complete relief from pain is not achieved within 3–5 minutes it is likely that the trigger point was not injected and may require another attempt.
e. A fan-like approach is made, by inserting the needle at different angles until the most sensitive region is contacted.
f. Needle point stimulation or saline injection has been found to be as effective as the use of local anaesthetics in many instances[17].
g. The relief of pain, tenderness and spasm may long outlast the pharmacological life of the material used.
h. Whereas in acute cases one or two injections are usually sufficient, in chronic cases injections may need to be repeated every second, third or fourth day, depending on the severity of the condition and the rate at which it subsides.
i. Adjunctive therapy, such as massage, application of ice or coolant spray, may be used. Indeed, the latter is regarded by some as being an equivalent method of therapy[13].

Infiltration into muscles
a. This is sometimes useful in trauma, e.g. in some cases of low back pain or sudden muscular strain[1,2,16,18].
b. It may be used as an adjunct to heat, massage and other therapies.

Ligamentous strains
a. There are many instances of the use to which this may be put in pain of vertebral origin. These include the lumbosacral, sacroiliac, sacro-coccygeal, interspinous and supraspinous ligaments.
b. Injection of 5–10 ml of local anaesthetic and steroid into the most tender areas commonly produces relief for many hours, and this may be repeated as necessary.

Attachment tissue problems
a. Like ligaments, these are common, easily recognized by local examination, and commonly respond well to local anaesthetic injections. Common examples of these are the various rotator cuff syndromes, tennis and golfer's elbow, Tietze's disease and tender pyriformis insertion.
b. A mixture of steroid and anaesthetic is most commonly used, but the effect of the anaesthetic may wear off after a few hours and that of the steroid may not begin to work for some days. The patient should be warned of this phenomenon.

Zygoapophyseal injections
It is now realised that these joints are a common source of pain, and if so are likely to respond to injections of local anaesthetic and/or steroid[18,19].
Two further points are worthy of note:
a. The materials used are a matter of choice of the clinician; most often they are a mixture of local anaesthetic and some steroid.
b. Apart from their obvious use in the so-called facet joint syndrome in the cervical, thoracic and lumbar spine, these injections may also be used as a prognostic procedure prior to rhizotomy.

References

1. Bonica (1953). *The Management of Pain*. (Philadelphia: Lea and Febiger)
2. Bonica (1959). *Clinical Applications of Diagnostic and Therapeutic Blocks*. (Springfield, Ill.: Thomas)
3. Covino and Vassallo (1976). *Local Anaesthetics. Mechanisms of Action and Clinical Use*. (New York: Grune and Stratton)
4. De Jong (1977). *Local Anaesthetics*, 2nd Edn. (Springfield, Ill.: Thomas)
5. Scott and Cousins (1980). Clinical pharmacology of local anaesthetic agents. In Cousins and Bridenbaugh (eds.) *Neural Blockade in Clinical Anaesthesia and Management of Pain*. (Philadelphia: J.B. Lippincott)

6. Melzack (1971). Phantom limb pain. Indications for treatment of pathologic pain. *Anaesthesiology*, **35**, 409–419
7. Bonica *et al.* (1971). Circulatory effects of peridural block. 2. Effects of epinephrine. *Anaesthesiology*, **34**, 514–522
8. Moore and Batra (1981). The components of an effective test dose prior to epidural block. *Anaesthesiology*, **55**, 393–396
9. Bonica (1957). Management of myofascial pain syndrome in general practice. *J. Am. Med. Assoc.*, **165**, 732–738
10. Kraus (1970). *Clinical Treatment of Back and Neck Pain.* (New York: McGraw Hill)
11. Simons (1975). Muscle pain syndromes. Part 1. *Am. J. Phys. Med.*, **54**, 289–311
12. Sola (1981). Myofascial trigger point therapy. *Resident Staff Physician*, **57**, 38–45
13. Travell (1976). Myofascial trigger points. In Bonica and Albe-Fessard (eds.) *Advances in Pain Research and Therapy 1. Proceedings of First World Congress on Pain.* (New York: Raven Press)
14. Travell and Rinzler (1952). The myofascial genesis of pain. *Post Graduate Med.*, **11**, 425–434
15. Mooney and Cairns (1978). Management in the patient with chronic low back pain. *Orth. Clin. N. Am.*, **9**, 543
16. Mehta (1973). *Intractable Pain.* (Philadelphia: W.B. Saunders)
17. Melzack *et al.* (1977). Trigger points and acupuncture points for pain. Correlations and implications. *Pain*, **3**, 223
18. Finneson (1973). *Low Back Pain.* (Philadelphia: J.B. Lippincott)
19. Sedzimir (1980). Lumbo-sacral root pain. In Lipton (ed.) *Persistent Pain. Modern Methods of Treatment*, vol. 2. (London: Academic Press)

Therapy 13 – caudal epidural anaesthesia

This is by no means a new therapy: Caussade and Chauffard used the technique in the treatment of sciatica as long ago as 1909[1].

Solutions employed

Cyriax concluded that the addition of steroid to the local anaesthetic was of no assistance[2].

Yates, comparing four different solutions, showed that the addition of steroid carried a significant advantage in the restoration of mobility[3].

This discrepancy of view reinforces our statement as to the difficulty in establishing any clear preference regarding the materials to be used in these and other vertebral injections.

Volume injected

Again teaching is variable. Cyriax recommended the use of 50 ml; few practitioners now employ so large a quantity. We favour a volume between 10 ml and 20 ml.

Value
Harley, in 50 successive cases of sciatica, using one or two injections, achieved complete relief in 20 cases, improvement in 13 and no change in 17[4].

In 1961 Coombs investigated two groups of 20 patients with severe sciatica. One group was treated by caudal epidurals, the other by bedrest[5]. Symptoms before treatment were similar in duration, an average of 37 days for the group having epidurals and 31 days for those having bedrest. The solution used was 50 ml 0.5% procaine. The average recovery time for the group having bedrest was 31 days, compared with 11 days for the group having epidurals.

Aim of therapy
Pain relief.

Diagnosis
Unknown in the great majority of cases.

How it works
Regardless of any claims that may be made, this remains unknown.

Indications
It is indicated in severe lumbago and in sciatica.

Contraindications
It is contraindicated in cases of known sensitivity to local anaesthetics.

Dangers
These are minimal: (a) technical errors resulting in injection into the cerebrospinal fluid or the blood stream, and (b) sensitivity of the individual patient to the drug.

Complications
These are those of any other injection.

Predictability
This is impossible, both in the short term and in the long term.

Practical clinical consequences
Relatively recent work is of great theoretical and practical importance to the practitioner of musculoskeletal medicine. It is summarized as follows:

1. It used to be thought that the dura mater was impermeable to local anaesthetics, and that epidural anaesthesia occurred at the mixed nerve dorsal root ganglia, beyond the dural sheath surrounding each pair of anterior and posterior spinal roots.
2. Radioactive tracer studies have shown that the dura mater is not impermeable, and that subarachnoid and epidural anaesthetics act at precisely the same sites, namely the spinal roots, mixed spinal nerves and the surface of the spinal cord to a depth of a millimetre or more, depending on the lipid solubility of the anaesthetic[6,7].
3. In both techniques the local anaesthetic enters the CSF and remains there until taken up by the lipids of the cord and spinal roots, or until it is washed out by vascular uptake into the blood vessels of the region.
4. The lipid-soluble narcotics behave in the same way.
5. Cousins and his colleagues have shown that high concentrations of meperidine are found in the CSF of man within a few minutes of epidural injection[8].
6. Poorly lipid-soluble drugs may remain in the water phase of the CSF for long periods of time, and may float rostrally for great distances.
7. Water-soluble contrast materials reflect this behaviour, and myelographic studies show that contrast agents such as metrizamide can travel from the lumbar region to the basal cistern in a matter of minutes and to the lateral ventricles within an hour[9].

The caudal epidural and the prolapsed intervertebral disc
1. It is important to be quite clear about this matter, because the idea that the dura mater is impermeable to local anaesthetic was at one time widespread, and it is of ideological significance to the field of musculoskeletal medicine. In the light of the knowledge available at the time, the success of a caudal epidural injection was used quite reasonably as conclusive proof of the diagnosis of a prolapsed intervertebral disc. The more recent work cited shows that local anaesthetics penetrate so far and so fast that the disc and the dura are but two of the many structures involved, and therefore this procedure cannot be used as a diagnostic tool.
2. It follows that the caudal epidural is far more powerful and non-specific a treatment than has hitherto been appreciated. Its therapeutic value in pain relief is thereby greater than has been realised, and this is something to be borne in mind by every clinician.

References

1. Yates (1978). A comparison of the types of epidural injection commonly used in the treatment of low back pain and sciatica. *Rheum. Rehabil.*, **17**, 181

2. Cyriax (1975). *Textbook of Orthopaedic Medicine*, 6th Edn., vol. 1. (London: Baillière Tindall)
3. Yates (1978). A comparison of the types of epidural injection commonly used in the treatment of low back pain and sciatica. *Rheum. Rehabil.*, **17**, 181
4. Harley (1966). Extradural cortico-steroid infiltration. *Am. Phys. Med.*, **9**, 22
5. Coombs (1961). A comparison between epidural anaesthesia and bed rest in sciatica. *Br. Med. J.*, **1**, 20
6. Bromage *et al.* (1963). Local anaesthetic drugs. Penetration from the spinal extradural space into the neuraxis. *Science*, **140**, 392–393
7. Cohen *et al.* (1968). The role of pH in the development of tachyphylaxis to local anaesthetic agents. *Anaesthesiology*, **29**, 994–1001
8. Cousins *et al.* (1979). Selective spinal analgesia. *Lancet*, **1**, 1141–1142
9. Drayer and Rosenbaum (1978). Studies of the third circulation. Amipaque CT cisternography and ventriculography. *J. Neurosurg.*, **48**, 946–956

Therapy 14 – transcutaneous nerve stimulation

Peripheral nerve stimulation by the transcutaneous route has been found to relieve acute pain in 60% of all patients, and chronic pain in 30% of all cases. This confirms one of the predictions of the spinal gate theory, that α-fibre stimulation could inhibit C-fibre transmission in the dorsal horn. In 1967, Wall and Sweet demonstrated that prolonged stimulation of peripheral nerves with percutaneous needle electrodes modified the reaction of healthy human volunteers to acute noxious stimuli, without any ill-effects[1].

Techniques
Non-painful paraesthesiae can be used by four means:
1. TNS,
2. Nerve stimulation through subcutaneously implanted electrodes,
3. Electrodes implanted directly on nerves, and
4. Antidromic activation of primary afferent collaterals by stimulation of the dorsal columns, either directly or through the dura.

Stimuli
A typical range for a TNS stimulator is:
1. Current, 0–50 mA.
2. Frequency, 0–100 Hz.
3. Pulse width 0.1–0.5 ms.
The wide range of both frequency and amplitude that may be found clinically effective is of great interest. Once more empiricism is the key to discovering a satisfactory setting for these.

Mechanism

The aim of peripheral stimulation techniques is to activate large, sensory myelinated fibres without producing muscle contraction or pain". As will be discussed later, TNS can also be used as a hyperstimulation (painful) form of analgesia.

Positioning of electrodes is usually made over the course of a peripheral nerve innervating the site of pain, usually proximal to it, but not always so (e.g. in spinal root pain).

The most effective site for application of TNS is often impossible to predict, so that time and patience are essential to find the duration, strength and placement of electrodes. Hospital admission for up to a week may be necessary[2].

The appropriate stimulation parameters are a matter for empiricism, based on maximum comfort and pain relief for the patient (used as a painless procedure). Usual parameters are a frequency of between 40–50 Hz, with a pulse width of 0.1–0.5 ms.

Induction time (the time it takes to work) varies, usually about 20 minutes. However, it may vary from immediate to several hours. Therefore, to admit failure after a trial of only 30 minutes is quite inadequate[3].

Duration of stimulation varies from intermittent, at once or twice a day, to continuous.

Results vary from analgesia being established while treatment continues to some patients finding considerable periods of post-stimulation relief. The reasons for these differences is unknown[4,5].

Aim of treatment
Pain relief.

Diagnosis
Seldom known.

How it works
A on C inhibition, at least in part, but see p.226.

Indications
While implanted electrodes are invasive and are accompanied by additional problems, TNS itself is not invasive. It may be applied in any localized somatic or neurogenic pain.

Acute pain
Traumatic
1. Sports injuries. These are relevant to TNS, but it is seldom used because

of the cost of the equipment and the availability of other treatments which are equally effective.
2. Major trauma. Pain may be too severe for TNS to be employed, and other therapies, such as systemic analgesics, may have to be employed. However, in the treatment of fractured ribs, TNS is extremely helpful[6] being without the potential complications of:
  a. Non-narcotic analgesics,
  b. Narcotic analgesics,
  c. Intercostal blocks,
  d. Strapping of the rib-cage.

Postoperative pain

TNS may be used effectively after abdominal and thoracic surgery[7,8] and following hip replacement[9] and spinal surgery[10]. It has several advantages over narcotics:
1. The analgesia is continuous.
2. There is no respiratory depression.
3. There are no bowel problems.

Chronic pain

In the treatment of chronic pain, TNS has moved from being almost the 'final court of appeal' to, in many cases, the first line of attack. It is particularly useful in neurogenic pain resulting from:
1. Peripheral nerve lesions,
2. Causalgia,
3. Intercostal neuritis[1,5,11–13],
4. Chronic low back pain,
5. Radiculopathies[14,15],
6. Spinal injuries[16,17].

It is less likely to prove helpful in pain states where the pain is widespread and poorly localized, or where it is primarily psychogenic[18].

Generally speaking, it is indicated in any case of pain of vertebral origin.

Contraindication

An absolute contraindication is the presence in the patient of a pacemaker or other electrical device which might be affected by the field generated by the stimulator.

A possible contraindication, in the case of its use by the patient, is the failure of the patient to understand the controls.

Dangers

None – provided the absolute contraindication above is adhered to.

Complications
Allergic dermatitis, from the adhesive tape holding the electrodes in position.

Predictability
TNS is effective by comparison with placebo. In a study on postoperative pain in 50 patients, placebo was 33% effective and TNS was 77% effective, and there are many similar results from other studies[8]. Indeed, in osteoarthrosis, TNS was initially 50% effective, falling to 28% over one year. Even despite the phenomenon of 'attrition' (the fact that TNS becomes less effective with time) a stable long-term success rate with chronic pain of 20–30% can be achieved[19].

Nonetheless, this treatment remains unpredictable, both in the short-term and in the long term.

Similar treatments
These include acupuncture, needle effect, auriculotherapy and ice massage.

Treatment time
If TNS is used as a clinic therapy, then it must remain subject to the disadvantages of necessitating the patient complying with the clinic timetable, even to the extent of possible admission. However, if it is employed in the relatively mobile patient, enabling him to return to work and regulate his own therapy, then its 'nuisance value' is reduced to the barest minimum – electrode placement once a day and switching the machine on and off from time to time. Clearly, in the latter context, it has a real appeal for the patient.

Practical clinical consequences
It is clear that TNS is a remarkably multifaceted form of treatment; if its use by A on C inhibition fails, frequency and amplitude can be increased, independently of each other, until it becomes an example of hyperstimulation therapy, in which latter rôle it may also be effective.

TNS is quite harmless, and it can be used (commonly) by the patient himself, without interference with his domestic or business activities. In this latter respect, it compares favourably with treatments such as traction.

Finally, "Some clinicians find that admitting patients to a rehabilitation unit for a week or more is the only way to ensure an adequate trial of TNS"[20]. "In our hands, TNS has proved of inestimable value, and we are convinced that reports of its lack of success are due to failure to appreciate that it must be used intensively for many hours per day, for weeks or months at a time."[21] In these circustances, A on C inhibition and hyperstimulation can only be partial factors in its success. It must therefore be inextricably entangled with other forms of therapy which cannot specifically be identified.

Any form of treatment, pursued over a period of time, must be subject to similar considerations.

This shows that, the longer any treatment is pursued, the more difficult is it to identify outcome with any particular element of treatment being given. Any form of treatment (for example, acupuncture, TNS or manipulation) becomes less and less clearly correlated with therapeutic outcome, the longer that therapy continued.

References

1. Wall and Sweet (1967). Temporary abolition of pain in man. *Science*, **155**, 108–109
2. Wynn-Parry (1981). Pain in avulsion lesions of the brachial plexus. *Pain*, **9**, 41–53
3. Wolf *et al.* (1981). Examination of electrode placements and stimulating parameters in treating chronic pain with conventional transcutaneous electrical nerve stimulation (TENS). *Pain*, **2**. 37–47
4. Andersson *et al.* (1976). Evaluation of the pain suppressant effect of different frequencies of peripheral electrical stimulation in chronic pain conditions. *Acta Orthopaed. Scand.*, **47**, 149–157
5. Meyer and Field (1972). Causalgia treated by selected large fibre stimulation of peripheral nerves. *Brain*, **95**, 163–167
6. Myers *et al.* (1977). Management of acute traumatic pain by peripheral transcutaneous electrical stimulation. *S. Afr. Med. J.*, **52**, 309–312
7. Ali *et al.* (1981). The effect of transcutaneous electrical nerve stimulation on post-operative pain and pulmonary function. *Surgery*, **89**, 507–512
8. Cooperman *et al.* (1977). Use of transcutaneous electrical stimulation in control of post operative pain. Results of a prospective randomised controlled study. *Am. J. Surg.*, **133**, 185–187
9. Pyke (1978). Transcutaneous electrical stimulation. Its use in the management of post-operative pain. *Anaesthesia*, **33**, 165–171
10. Solomon *et al.* (1980). Reduction of post operative pain and narcotic use by transcutaneous electrical nerve stimulation. *Surgery*, **87**, 142–146
11. Loeser *et al.* (1975). Relief of pain by transcutaneous stimulation. *J. Neurosurg.*, **42**, 308–314
12. Nathan and Wall (1974). Treatment of post-herpetic neuralgia by prolonged electrical stimulation. *Br. Med. J.*, **3**, 645–647
13. Bates and Nathan (1980). Transcutaneous electrical nerve stimulation for chronic pain. *Anaesthesia*, **35**, 817–822
14. Cauthen and Renner (1975). Transcutaneous and electrical nerve stimulation for chronic pain states. *Surg. Neurol.*, **4**, 102–104
15. Eriksson *et al.* (1979). Long term results of peripheral condition stimulation as an analgesia measure in chronic pain. *Pain*, **6**, 335–347
16. Bannerjee (1974). Transcutaneous nerve stimulation for pain after spinal injury. *N. Engl. J. Med.*, **251**, 796
17. Richardson *et al.* (1980). Neurostimulation in the modulation of intractable paraplegic and traumatic neuroma pain. *Pain*, **8**, 75–84
18. Nielsen *et al.* (1982). Psychiatric factors influencing the treatment of pain with peripheral conditioning stimulation. *Pain*, **13**, 365–371
19. Taylor *et al.* (1981). Treatment of osteoarthritis of the knee with transcutaneous electrical nerve stimulation. *Pain*, **2**, 232–246
20. Wynn Parry (1980). Pain in avulsion lesions of the brachial plexus. *Pain*, **9**, 41–53
21. Wynn Parry (1983). Peripheral nerve injury. In Wall and Melzack (eds.) *Textbook of Pain*, p.393. (London: Churchill Livingstone)

Therapy 15 – acupuncture

The technique of 'fighting pain with pain' is as old as man and common to all cultures. These methods are generally known as 'counter-irritation' and, because they involve painful or near-painful levels of stimulation to relieve pain, they have also more recently been labelled, 'hyperstimulation analgesia[1]'.

Acupuncture involves "the insertion of fine needles made of steel, gold or other metals, through specific points at the skin, and then twirling them for some time at a slow rate. The needles may also be left in place for varying periods of time."[2]

Chinese theory is remarkably complex, and traditionally they chart 361 'acupuncture points', lying on 14 meridians. Much study has recently gone into the scientific validation of this form of treatment.

Acupuncture points

Stimulation of these has been compared, and it has been concluded that stimulation of sites close to the painful area is more effective than that of distant ones[3-5]. The latter, however, frequently produces analgesic effects greater than a placebo. It has been shown that stimulation need not be applied at the precise points indicated on acupuncture charts. It is possible, for example, to achieve as much control over dental pain by stimulating an area between the fourth and fifth fingers, which is not designated on acupuncture charts as being related to facial pain, as by stimulating the 'hoku point' between the thumb and index finger, which is so designated[6].

Results suggest that the site which can be effectively stimulated is not a discrete point, but a large area. This has been confirmed by other studies[7].

A study examining the correlation between trigger points and acupuncture points for pain showed that "every trigger point reported in Western medical literature has a corresponding acupuncture point. Furthermore, there is a close correspondence, 71%, between the pain syndromes associated with the two kinds of points. This close correlation suggests that trigger points and acupuncture points for pain, although discovered independently and labelled differently, represent the same phenomenon, and can be explained in terms of similar underlying neural mechanisms." This study has been confirmed[8].

It is the intense stimulation rather than the precise site that appears to be the crucial factor[9,10]. That acupuncture pain relief is not simply a placebo effect is also indicated by the fact that partial analgesia can be produced in animals such as monkeys and mice, and that acupuncture stimulation inhibits or otherwise changes the transmission of pain-evoked nerve impulses at several levels of the central nervous system[11-14].

These effects are produced not only by acupuncture, but also by other sources of intense sensory input, such as electrical stimulation, heat, and a variety of other inputs[15]. Therefore acupuncture may be properly regarded as no more than one method of hyperstimulation analgesia.

Aim of treatment
Relief of pain.

Diagnosis
Almost always unknown.

How it works
The precise mode of action of acupuncture is unknown, but current thinking on the question is that, "such high intensity conditioning stimuli, similar to those used in hyperstimulation analgesia, could operate in two ways.
1. One possibility is that they block the afferent fibres carrying the nociceptive pain information, or
2. They activate a system of inhibitory circuits in the spinal cord different from that activated by A delta afferent activity."[16-18]

Indications
Pain of vertebral origin (in so far as it concerns the musculoskeletal physician) but of course it has wider applications.

Contraindications
None.

Dangers
None.

Complications
Local sepsis is a possibility. It rarely occurs.

Predictability
Comparison with placebo: A review paper examined 24 controlled studies on acupuncture analgesia for the relief of pain produced experimentally by radiant heat, electrical stimulation of tooth pulp, induced ischaemia and other procedures. Of the 24, 3 reported unequivocally negative results, 4 contained equivocal results and 17 demonstrated significant analgesic effects during electrical or manual stimulation at acupuncture loci. Most studies utilized manual stimulation, DC electrical stimulation or very low frequency

AC stimulation (usually 2 Hz). An induction time of about 20 minutes for full analgesia was reported in some of these studies[19].

Comparison with TNS: Studies have been carried out comparing the relative efficacy of these two forms of treatment on low back pain. Results show that both forms of stimulation at the same points produce a substantial decrease in pain intensity, but neither procedure is statistically more effective than the other. Most patients were relieved of pain for several hours, some for one or more days. Statistical analyses also failed to reveal any difference in the duration of pain relief between these two procedures[2,20,21].

Other studies have confirmed these findings, and have practical implications:

a. The chief advantage of acupuncture is that the procedure is of short duration, and intense level stimulations sometimes last a few minutes. The method, however, is invasive, and requires a practitioner with specialized training.

b. TNS, on the other hand, is non-invasive, and once the appropriate points are located it can be administered by other personnel, including the patient.

The difference between using TNS as electro-acupuncture (low-frequency intense stimulation applied to the skin) and electrical stimulation through a needle that has penetrated the skin into deeper tissues are obvious. The results are the same; that is to say, relief of pain in a substantial proportion of patients. Nor is there any statistical difference between manual twirling of acupuncture needles and electrical stimulation through the needles. Both are equally successful.

As with almost all other treatments, however, the identification of those individuals who will benefit from acupuncture remains beyond our reach at the present time.

Similar treatment
TNS is discussed in the previous section.

Treatment time
This therapy demands time of the patient as well as of the clinician; this of the order of at least an hour or so from work for each treatment.

Practical clinical consequences
Acupuncture is safe, and it often works!

References

1. Melzack (1973). *The Puzzle of Pain*. (New York: Basic Books)
2. Melzack (1983). Acupuncture and related forms of folk medicine. In Wall and Melzack (eds.) *Textbook of Pain*, p.691 (London: Churchill Livingstone)
3. Andersson and Holmgren (1975). On acupuncture analgesia and the mechanism of pain. *Am. J. Chinese Med.*, 3, 311–334
4. Chapman *et al.* (1980). Evoked potential assessment of acupuncture analgesia. Attempted reversal with naloxone. *Pain*, 9, 183–197
5. Jeans (1979). Relief of chronic pain by brief, intense transcutaneous electrical stimulation. A double blind study. In Bonica, Lieberskind and Albe-Fessard (eds.) *Advances in Pain Research and Therapy 3*, pp. 601–606. (New York: Raven Press)
6. Taub *et al.* (1977). Studies of acupuncture for operative dentistry. *J. Am. Dental Assoc.*, 95, 555–561
7. Co *et al.* (1979). Acupuncture. An evaluation in the painful crises of sickle cell anaemia. *Pain*, 7, 181–185
8. Melzack *et al.* (1977). Trigger points and acupuncture points for pain. Correlation and implications. *Pain*, 3, 23
9. Ghia *et al.* (1976). Acupuncture and chronic pain mechanisms. *Pain*, 2, 285–299
10. Lewit (1979). The needle effect in the relief of myofascial pain. *Pain*, 6, 83–90
11. Viencil *et al.* (1974). Prolonged hypalgesia following "acupuncture" in monkeys. *Life Sci.*, 15, 1277–1289
12. Pomeranz *et al.* (1977). Acupuncture reduces electrophysiological and behavioural responses to noxious stimuli: pituitary is implicated. *Exp. Neurol.*, 54, 172–178
13. Sandrow *et al.* (1978). Electro-acupuncture analgesia in monkeys: a behavioural and neurophysiological assessment. *Arch. Int. Pharmacodyn. Ther.*, 231, 274–284
14. Kerr *et al.* (1978). Acupuncture reduces the trigeminal evoked response in decerebrate cats. *Exp. Neurol.*, 61, 84–95
15. Le Bars *et al.* (1979). Diffuse noxious inhibitory controls. 2. Lack of effect on non-convergent neurones. Supraspinal involvement and theoretical implications. *Pain*, 6, 307–327
16. Mayer and Price (1976). Central nervous mechanisms of analgesia. *Pain*, 2, 379–404
17. Basbaum and Fields (1978). Endogenous pain control mechanisms. Review and hypothesis. *Ann. Neurol.*, 4, 451–462
18. Watkins and Mayer (1982). Organisation of endogenous opiate and non-opiate pain control systems. *Science*, 216, 1185–1192
19. Reichmanis and Becker (1977). Relief of experimentally induced pain by stimulation at acupuncture loci. *Comp. Med. East West*, 5, 281–288
20. Fox and Melzack (1976). Transcutaneous electrical stimulation and acupuncture. Comparison of treatment for low back pain. *Pain*, 2, 141–148
21. Laitinen (1976). Acupuncture and transcutaneous electrical stimulation in the treatment of chronic sacro-lumbalgia and ischalgia. *Am. J. Chinese Med.*, 4, 169–175

Therapy 16 – needle effect

It has long been questioned whether the efficacy of local anaesthetic blocks was due to the anaesthetic agents or to the insertion of the hypodermic needles as an intense brief sensory input. "Astonishingly, the results are in favour of needling." Lewit has called this phenomenon the "needle effect"[1]. As long ago as 1952, Travell and Rinzler showed that they could obtain striking relief of myofascial pain by simply needling trigger points[2].

It was discovered in 1956 that injection of normal saline was highly effective in the relief of pain[3] and in 1958 it was reported that different kinds of anaesthetic had virtually identical effects, which were barely influenced by the amount and concentration of the material injected[4].

In 1980, a double-blind comparison was carried out of mepivacaine (a local anaesthetic) and saline, injected into trigger points for myofascial pain[5]. The group that received saline tended to have significantly more relief of pain; 80% of patients receiving saline reported pain relief, compared with 52% of those receiving mepivacaine. Furthermore, the average duration of relief was 3 hours for saline and 30 minutes for mepivacaine. Clearly, "the pain relief could not be due to the anaesthetic, but was more likely to be due to the insertion of the needles into the trigger points"[6]. They proposed that the saline was more effective because it irritated tissues which is the essential ingredient of treatment, while the mepivacaine actually blocked the irritating effect of the needles. It appears to us that this is a comparison between mepivicaine and saline, rather than an assessment of the rôle of the needle.

Lewit concluded that the effectiveness of the treatment bears little relationship to the agent injected, but that it is, "related to the intensity of the pain produced in the trigger zone and the precision with which the site of maximum tenderness was located by the needle". The results are striking relief of pain in 86% of cases and persistent relief of pain, at least for months or even permanently, in about 50% of cases.

Aim of treatment
Relief of pain.

Diagnosis
Unknown.

How it works
Unknown.

Indication
Pain of vertebral origin.

Contraindications
There are none.

Dangers
None.

Complications
Other than local sepsis, there are none.

Predictability
Outcome prediction, short-term or long-term, remains impossible.

Similar treatments
TNS, acupuncture, auriculotherapy and ice massage.

Practical clinical consequences
This seems possibly to be useful in the event of failure of other therapies.

References

1. Lewit (1979). The needle effect in the relief of myofascial pain. *Pain*, 6, 83–90
2. Travell and Rinzler (1952). The myofascial genesis of pain. *Post Grad. Med.*, 2, 425–434
3. Sola and Williams (1956). Myofascial pain syndromes. *Neurology*, 6, 91–95
4. Kibler (1958). Das Störungsfeld bei Gelenkserkrankungen inneren Krankheiten Hippo-krates, Stuttgart
5. Frost *et al.* (1980). A double blind comparison of mepivacaine injection versus saline injection for myofascial pain. *Lancet*, 8, 499–501
6. Melzack (1983). Acupuncture and related forms of folk medicine. In Wall and Melzack (eds.) *Textbook of Pain*, p.697 *et seq.* (London: Churchill Livingstone)

Therapy 17 – auriculotherapy

This is based on the claims of Nogier[1] that electrical stimulation at points of the outer ear abolishes pain, and moreover that the whole body is represented at the ear in the shape of an inverted homunculus. In a double-blind trial in 1980[2] physicians examined patients' ears for areas of enhanced skin conductivity and tenderness. They found a concordance of 75.2% between the spatial location of established medical diagnosis and the auricular diagnosis for 40 patients with musculoskeletal pains. Further work has not replicated these findings[3]. One double-blind trial failed to show any difference between simulating a designated 'Nogier point' on the ear or control spots elsewhere on the ear. A further double-blind trial showed that auriculotherapy was no more effective than placebo.

Aim of therapy
Relief of pain.

Diagnosis
Unknown.

How it works
This remains unknown, but it may be felt significant that its results have been shown to be on a level with those of placebo.

Indications
Pain of vertebral origin.

Contraindications
None.

Dangers
None.

Complications
None.

Similar treatments
Hyperstimulation therapies.

Practical clinical consequences
It seems to have little to commend it to the clinician.

References

1. Nogier (1972). Treatise of auricular therapy. *Maisonneve*, Moulin, Les Metz
2. Olsen *et al.* (1980). An experimental evaluation of auricular diagnosis. The somatotopic mapping of musculo-skeletal pain at ear acupuncture points. *Pain*, **8**, 217–229
3. Melzack and Katz (1984). Auricular therapy fails to relieve chronic pain. A controlled cross-over study. *J. Am. Med. Assoc.*, **251**(8), 1041–1043

Therapy 18 – ice massage

Ice packs and ice massage have long been used in physiotherapy. The reason for their effectiveness has not been understood until recently. Ice produces a local constriction of blood vessels, making the area feel numb, but also, because it hurts, it is a hyperstimulation treatment. In a study on patients suffering from acute dental pain, who were treated with ice massage to the back of the hand on the same side as the pain, the intensity of the dental pain was reduced by 50% or more in the majority of patients[1]. This reduction is significantly greater than that produced in control groups by tactile massage alone, or with explicit suggestion (placebo). These results suggest that ice massage has pain reducing effects comparable with those of TNS and acupuncture[2].

In a comparison of the relative effectiveness of ice massage and TNS for the relief of low back pain, the results showed that both methods were equally effective, about 65% of patients obtaining pain relief greater than 33% with each therapy. The results also revealed that ice massage is more effective than TNS for some patients, while TNS is more effective for others. Thus the methods may be regarded as alternatives, and, taken together, the results of both studies point to neuromechanisms that may be similar to those of acupuncture.

In a further comparison with ice massage for patients with dental pain, different sites were selected in four groups of patients[3]. Pain intensity was significantly decreased by 40 or 50% after ice massage of the ipsilateral hand, contralateral hand or contralateral arm. However, ice massage of the ipsilateral arm had no significant effect compared with the control procedures. These findings confirm reports in the traditional Chinese literature on acupuncture and suggest that they are based on empirical observations.

While we emphasize elsewhere the difficulties inherent in the accurate measurement of pain, we accept these figures as a crude audit.

Aim of treatment
Relief of pain.

Diagnosis
None.

How it works
Unknown.

Indications
Pain of vertebral origin.

Contraindications
None.

Dangers
None.

Complications
None.

Predictability
This is not possible, either short-term or long-term.

Similar treatments
TNS, acupuncture, needle effect and auriculotherapy.

Practical clinical consequences
It is of practical importance since this procedure is simple, and patients can easily be taught to apply ice massage themselves, and it may well be an effective treatment for low back pain. There can be little easier for the patient than to get ice from his domestic refrigerator!

References

1. Melzack *et al.* (1980). Relief of dental pain by ice massage of the hand. *Can. Med. Assoc. J.*, **122**, 189–191
2. Melzack *et al.* (1980). Ice massage and transcutaneous electrical stimulation. Comparison of treatment for low back pain. *Pain*, **9**, 209–217
3. Melzack and Bentley (1983). Relief of dental pain by ice massage of either hand or the contralateral arm. *J. Can. Dental Assoc.*, **186**, 257–260

Therapy 19 – rhizolysis and rhizotomy

Aim of treatment
Relief of pain.

Diagnosis
Supposed root pain. But see comment under this heading in Root Surgery, p.238.

How it works
This is unknown, but practitioners of 'facet denervation' hold that back pain and radicular pain are often referred from sites of degeneration or inflammation of the zygoapophyseal joints[1].

This is largely a matter of speculation. Because the procedure is performed percutaneously, with no confirmation of the nature of the lesions, there is considerable scepticism regarding the rationale of this treatment[2].
It has been reported that, in an average patient, the lumbosacral facet joint could not in fact be denervated by the Rees procedure since the blade that was used was not long enough to reach them[3]. The anatomy of the posterior primary rami and their articular branches has been studied recently. Several anatomical inaccuracies in description have been noted. The articular branches lie rostral and caudal to the zygoapophyseal joint, yet most of the reported techniques describe electrode placements lateral to the joint. It was concluded that it was probably not possible to denervate the zygoapophyseal joints selectively by a percutaneous approach[4].

Indication
Pain of vertebral origin, thought to arise in the posterior joints.

Contraindications
There are no absolute contraindications.

Dangers and complications
These are as for other injections.

Predictability
Not possible, either in the short term or in the long term.

Similar treatments
Root surgery.

Therapy time
This is not a very time-comsuming procedure, once the decision has been made to employ it.

Comment
This material illustrates two points:
1. The inadequacy of current knowledge of the physiology of root pain,
2. The importance of the basic considerations to the clinician.
It follows that, if these factors are not in the forefront of the clinician's mind, rational management of these problems is made the more difficult.

References

1. Rees (1976). Disconnective neurosurgery. Multiple bilateral percutaneous rhizolysis, (facet rhizotomy). In Morley (ed). *Current Controversies in Neurosurgery*, pp. 80–88 (Philadelphia: W.B. Saunders)
2. Dubuisson (1983). In Wall and Melzack (eds.) *Textbook of Pain*, p.595. (London: Churchill Livingstone)
3. King (1976). Randomised trial of Rees and Shealy methods for treatment of low backpain. In Morley, T.P. (ed.) *Current Controversies in Neurosurgery*, pp. 89–94. (Philadelphia: W.B. Saunders)
4. Bogduk and Long (1979). The anatomy of the so-called 'articular nerves' and their relationship to facet denervation in the treatment of low back pain. *Neurosurgery*, **51**, 172–177

Therapy 20 – root surgery

Aim of treatment
Relief of pain.

Diagnosis
Supposed root pain. But it must be remembered that this is seldom possible to prove.

How it works
As will become apparent in the discussion to follow, this is unknown.

Indication
Intractable pain of vertebral origin.

Contraindications, dangers and complications
These are the contraindications for major surgery (see Disc Surgery, p.242).

Predictability
This is not possible, either in the short term or in the long term.

Similar treatments
These include disc surgery, chemonucleolysis and rhizotomy and rhizolysis.

Therapy time
As in any major surgery, this is relatively long; not only has the patient to go through the particular techniques, but there must of necessity be a substantial period of recovery, following that of hospitalization.

General comment
This subject is, of course, outside the scope of most clinicians interested in musculoskeletal medicine, and is a matter for referral to the appropriate surgeon. There are, however, two features which are of particular interest to them.
1. The concept of treatment of the nerve root; this has frequently been used for the relief of low back pain, and therefore deserves mention and description.
2. The reasons for the variability of their results and, indeed, failure.
These problems raise issues fundamental to anyone interested in musculo-skeletal medicine.

Rationale
The basic purpose of these procedures is to denervate the the area in which pain is felt.
"It is often assumed that root section is of greatest benefit in pain due to intrinsic lesions of the sensory ganglion or the root itself, where the underlying disturbance is thought to be disordered or excessive activity of the primary afferent fibres.
"It is also commonly assumed that root section should effectively relieve pain which is peripheral and circumscribed, since the afferent territory of the adjacent spinal nerves might completely encompass the painful region.
"Judging from the long-term results of root section, however, neither of these assumptions seems entirely accurate."[15]

Some reasons for failure
The results of dorsal root section for pain associated with chronic mechanical damage and scarring of roots are poor in the long term. We know that chronic nerve and ganglion compression in animals leads to the development of mechanosensitivity of primary afferents[1]. In man, dorsal root section for post-laminectomy radicular pain might reasonably be expected to interrupt

abnormal trains of nerve impulses from the damaged sites, yet the success rate is poor[2-4]. This might be explained by spontaneous activity of chronically deafferented transmission neurones in the cord, which would not be helped by rhizotomy[5,6]. Indeed, there are reasons to suspect that further deafferentation might even aggravate the problem.

It has been known since the time of Sherrington that each cutaneous region is innervated by at least three consecutive roots[7,8]. It is now clear that the extent of dermatomal overlap is more extensive than this. Moreover, the extent of the dermatomes supplied by peripheral processes of A delta and C primary afferents has **never** been mapped significantly in **any** species, even though it is obviously relevant to root section for pain in human subjects. This raises the question as to whether enough roots may have been sectioned.

It is now known that long-ranging afferent fibres may travel for six or more segments to contact distant spinal cord neurones[9,10]. We also know that some dorsal horn neurones, deprived of their most direct primary afferent contact by multiple root section, begin to respond to these long-ranging afferents, taking on new and 'distant' receptive fields[11]. These facts partly explain the recurrence of some types of pain after section of a limited number of dorsal roots.

One surgical technique (Sindou) aims to leave intact at least some of the large proprioceptive and low threshold mechanoreceptive axones in the medial portion of the root entry zone. A more extensive lesion, involving the central and medial fibres of each rootlet, has been found useful for treating painful states of spasticity, suggesting that prolonged muscle activity could contribute to some other types of pain[12]. We do not know which populations of primary active fibres are excessively active in such conditions as chronic low back pain, painful surgical scars or amputations.

The extent of lesions affecting the cord is difficult to assess. For example, Wall (in 1962)[13] carried out physiological and anatomical studies of the dorsal horn and ascending sensory tracts following tiny lesions of the ventro-lateral cord/rootlet junction in cats. Using a dye perfusion technique, he detected a massive decrease of perfusion in the entire dorsal horn, after seemingly minor interference with the pial vessels. A variety of physiological recordings suggested the only remaining dorsal horn activity was transmission through the large group 1(a) proprioceptive afferents.

Not all authors find a distinct lateral separation of small afferents at the cord/rootlet junction. Other patterns may sometimes be present. The ultra anatomy of this region of the human cord deserves further study. Certainly, the lack of fibre subdivision within rootlets could be a cause of failure in some cases of elective surgery[14].

It is not unreasonable to think that some of the success of thermocoagulation is due to the destruction of large diameter afferents which might contribute importantly to pain in many cases treated. The pain of cranial neuralgia is known to be triggered by innocuous stimuli. In many cases pain associated with cancer, herpes zoster and other causes of deafferentation, light touch, or brushing of hairs may provoke intense, burning pain. Since the altered synaptic relationships and physiology of partially deafferentated cord and brain stem neurones are not yet understood, it seems premature to interpret the results of root or ganglion thermocoagulation solely in terms of large and small afferent fibre spectra.

There is some controversy in the use of selective nerve root blocks with local anaesthetics to predict the result of root section. Many surgeons rely on preliminary root blocks to determine the segmental level involved, to decide whether a permanent root lesion might relieve the patient's pain and to give the patient some warning of what to expect, should section be carried out. Some reports indicate that an effective root block does not reliably predict good response to subsequent root section[2,3]. We do not know how reliably such blocks, if ineffective, can identify those patients who should not have root surgery. It is difficult to eliminate the possibility that spread of the anaesthetic agent reaches adjacent roots. There is the additional possibility that many instances of apparently monoradicular pain actually involve afferents of several dorsal roots; blocking one root may reduce the total afferent drive of transmission neurones of neighbouring cord segments.

Conclusion

This material illustrates two points.
1. The reasons for failure of root surgery are largely due to the inadequacy of our knowledge of the physiology of root pain.
2. The clinical importance of the basic considerations is great.

References

1. Howe *et al.* (1977). Mechano-sensitivity of dorsal root ganglia and chronically injured axons. A physiological basis for the radicular pain of nerve root compression. *Pain*, **3**, 25–41
2. Onofrio and Campera (1972). Evaluation of rhizotomy. Review of 12 years' experience. *J. Neurosurg.*, **36**, 751–755.
3. Loeser (1972). Dorsal rhizotomy for the relief of chronic pain. *J. Neurosurg.*, **36**, 745–750
4. Bertrand (1975). The 'battered' root problem. *Orthopaed. Clin. N. Am.*, **6**, 305–310
5. Loeser and Ward (1967). Some effects of deafferentation of neurones of the cat spinal cord. *Arch. Neurology*, **17**, 629–636
6. Loeser *et al.* (1968). Chronic deafferentation of human spinal cord neurones. *J. Neurosurg.*, **29**, 48–50
7. Sherrington (1898). Experiments in the examination of the peripheral distribution of the fibres of the posterior roots of some spinal nerves. Pt II. *Phil. Trans. R. Soc. Lond. Ser. B. Biol. Sci.*, **190**, 45–186
8. Foerster (1933). The dermatomes in man. *Brain*, **56**, 1–39

9. Imai and Kusama (1969). Destruction of the dorsal root fibres in the cat. *Brain Res.*, **13**, 338–359
10. Werman (1976). The physiology and anatomy of long ranging afferent fibres within the spinal cord. *J. Physiol.*, **255**, 321–334
11. Wall (1977). The presence of ineffective synapses and the circumstances which unmask them. *Phil. Trans. R. Soc. Lond.*, **278**, 361–372
12. Sindou *et al.* (1981). Microsurgical selective posterior rhizotomes. *Pain* (Suppl. 1), 354
13. Wall (1962). The origin of a spinal cord slow potential. *J. Physiol.*, **164**, 508–526
14. Sindou (1976). Posterior spinal rhizotomy and selective posterior rhizidiotomy. *Proc. Neurol. Surg.*, **7**, 201–250
15. Dubuisson (1983). Root surgery. In Wall and Melzack (eds.) *Textbook of Pain*, p.594 *et seq.* (London: Churchill Livingstone)

Therapy 21 – disc surgery

Historical

In realistic terms, disc surgery dates from the presentation in 1933 of a series of operations for disc herniations by Mixter and Barr[1]. Following this, "the simplistic concept that low back pain, with or without sciatica, was usually caused by a disc herniation and cured by a fairly simple operation was readily and rapidly accepted all over the world, and maintained an overwhelming dominance over lay and medical minds for the next forty years."[16]

However, as time went on, surgical failures were reported, between which there appeared large variations in incidence, from 5% to 50%.

Further, the 'failed back surgery' syndrome developed a growing number of severely disabled patients presenting serious problems[2].

"Studies to identify the causes of surgical failures revealed that inaccuracy of diagnosis and poor selection of patients for the initial lumbar disc operation were more important factors than technical errors during the operation itself. The operation, discectomy, was used inappropriately on wide and loosely defined indications."[3–6]

It was proven that the single most important factor affecting success or failure of discectomy was the degree of herniation found at operation. The more herniation found, the greater the likelihood of success, and the less the more negative results were prone to be[7].

"Obviously, improvement of the surgical results was crucially dependent upon accurate pre-operative diagnosis and a strict selection of patients with high grade herniations for discectomy."

Further, it became clear that disc herniation itself was only one of a number of space-occupying lesions capable of compressing neural elements. In this connection, spinal stenosis is particularly important, because, "when stenosis is involved in a disc syndrome, the results of surgical treatment with the traditional discectomy are usually unsatisfactory or frankly disastrous." This statement needs elaboration. Stenosis most frequently involves the posterior part of the spinal canal and the lateral canals; it thus has a marked effect in lateral disc protrusions and in the presence of posterior joint osteoarthrosis, though little effect on the more central disc protrusions.

With regard to special investigations, "the diagnostic methods necessary to analyse the complicated pathological anatomy of the diseased spine have been highly amplified by the advent of:

1. Computerised tomography (CT),
2. Ultrasonic measuring techniques,
3. Epidural venography,
4. Safer water-soluble contrast agents (in particular Metrizamide) which allow functional myelography and radiculography,
5. Promising epidural contrast CT techniques.

In spite of this impressive development of the technological investigative methods, it may still be an extremely difficult task to supply the necessary diagnostic foundation for decisions about the proper surgical treatment in individual cases of lumbar pain syndromes.

"Surgical management of these conditions cannot be satisfactorily improved without a better clinical analysis and interpretation of the main symptom, i.e. pain."[16]

To this list of investigations we would add magnetic resonance imaging.

The disc operation
The surgical technique: In 1939, Love described the unilateral interlaminar approach which is still the routine technique in most quarters[8].

The extent of exposure: This is a matter of individual choice, but, "when the pre-operative diagnosis is found to be wrong, which is still unavoidable in some cases, it is wise to abstain from unplanned exploration"[16]. This is, of course, a strong argument in favour of laminectomy, as compared with more limited approaches, as the initial exposure of two discs is readily achieved.

The volume of tissue removed: Many studies have been done, and they all indicate that on average the volume of disc tissue removed at operation represents only 6–8% of the total disc volume. Moreover, it is not easy to excise disc tissue unless the disc is already in a certain condition of degeneration and fragmentation[7,9–11].

The 'combined operation': The addition of some form of fusion to discectomy adds greatly to the scale of the procedure involved. Most studies give an improvement of 5–10% in results, following a 'combined operation'.[12–14] However, the matter is controversial, and "the dominating conclusion has been that the advantage of the combined operation is too small to warrant the use of this method as a routine in patients with typical lumbar disc herniations"[16].

Re-operation after discectomy: The re-operation rate after first discectomy is usually 10–15%. The usual interval between the first and second operation is about 5 to 6 years. As Spangfort says[16], these figures do not take account of the incidence of fresh herniations, and therefore, given the natural history of this condition, there is no reason to classify the first operation as a failure.

"In patients without relief of pain for at least 6 months after the first operation, the operation has usually been an outright failure. In some cases caused by technical errors during the operation, e.g. failure to locate an offending segment or exposure at a wrong level, but in the majority of cases caused by **an incomplete or wrong pre-operative diagnosis**. Another type of operation should have been performed, or the patient should not have been exposed to surgical treatment at all."[16]

Aim of treatment
Relief of pain.

Diagnosis
Prolapse or herniation of an intervertebral disc.

How it works
Strangely enough this is unknown. In sciatica, relief of nerve root compression is often followed by relief of symptoms, but the physiology is not fully understood[15]. (See Some Reasons for Failure of Root Surgery, p.240).

Indications
Urgent: The single indication for immediate disc surgery is acute compression of nerve roots or spinal cord by a large herniation, causing a sacral syndrome, with neurological signs referred to the second and lower sacral roots, that is dysfunction of the bladder and bowel, with loss of control and loss of sensation in the sacral dermatomes. The condition is rare, probably less than 1 case per year in a population of 200,000. Immediate surgical decompression is generally considered mandatory when an acute disc herniation is identified as the cause of the syndrome.

Non-urgent: The purpose of discectomy is the relief of pain, in particular severe sciatic pain, caused by a disc herniation. As indicated above, the results are positively correlated with the degree of herniation found at operation. "Only by meticulous selection of patients with high grade herniation is it possible to improve the results of discectomy and to avoid a growing number of disastrous failures.

"The point is to establish the presence and location of an offending disc herniation, and unfortunately, surgical exposure is still the only way to do so with complete certainty."[16] Therefore, the most detailed history and examination, backed by all relevant special investigations, must be undertaken prior to surgery. In general terms it should only be contemplated if pain is unrelieved or worse after adequate trial of conservative management. This is likely to extend to 2–3 months, although this will, of course, vary with circumstances.

Contraindications
General: These are those common to all major surgery.

Specific: Inadequate evidence that disc protrusion is responsible for the patient's pain.

Dangers
The mortality rate is low, with a mean rate of 0.3%, which figure has consistently decreased over the last 35 years. The most common causes of death are pulmonary embolism and postoperative infections.

Complications
Injury to vessels and viscera
Injuries to neural structures: Injuries to nerve roots and even the cauda equina can occur, despite careful surgical techniques. Root damage is reported in 0.5–3% of all operations. Verified damage to a nerve root is not always followed by significant clinical sumptoms. Motor weakness in the leg obviously caused by the operation occurs in at least 5% of all operations, but in the majority the paresis is partial and recovers satisfactorily with time.

Dural damage: This is not uncommon and is usually harmless if detected and the lesion closed.

Thromboembolism: This is reported at around 2%.

Postoperative infection This does not exceed 2–3%, with severe infections accounting for less than 0.5%.

Postoperative discitis: The probable incidence does not exceed about 2% at present. This is characterized by the onset of extremely severe pain which lasts between 6 and 12 weeks in most cases. The prognosis is good.

Prediction of outcome

As has already been noted, the greater the size of the disc herniation, the greater the prospect of pain relief in the short term. It should be borne in mind that this is the only treatment in spinal musculoskeletal medicine in which this is the case. However, it must be remembered that quite small protrusions more laterally not only have effects equivalent to much larger more central ones, but also give results as good as do the latter, and these can be operated on most successfully.

Results permitting tentative conclusions indicate that surgical treatment does not improve the prognosis in the long term, with regard to pain or persistent neurological deficits. In a 10-year trial[17], after one year the results were significantly better after surgical treatment than after conservative treatment. After 4 years the operated patient still showed better results, but the difference was no longer significant. Only minor changes occurred throughout the last years of observation. After 10 years, no patients in the two groups complained of sciatic pain, and the rate of persistent back pain was equal in the two groups. "If the clinical situation allows a choice between conservative and surgical treatment, the patient should be informed that the benefit expected from the operation is immediate relief of sciatic pain, and not an improvement in the long-range prognosis, which is fairly good anyway."[16]

References

1. Mixter and Barr (1934). Rupture of the intervertebral disc with involvement of the spinal canal. *N Engl. J. Med.*, **211**, 210–215
2. Wilson (1967). Low back pain and sciatica. A plea for better care of the patient. *J. Am. Med. Assoc.*, **200**, 705–712
3. Macnab (1971). Negative disc exploration. *J. Bone Jt. Surg.*, **53A**, 891–903
4. Nachemson (1976). The lumbar spine. An orthopaedic challenge. *Spine*, **1**, 59–71
5. Finneson (1978). A lumbar disc surgery predictive score card. *Spine*, **3**, 186–188
6. Spengler and Freeman (1979). Patient selection of the lumbar discetomy. An objective approach. *Spine*, **4**, 129–134
7. Spangfort (1972). The lumbar disc herniation. A computer aided analysis of 2,504 operations. *Acta Orthop. Scand.*, **Suppl 142**, 1–95
8. Love (1939). Removal of protruded intervertebral discs without laminectomy. *Proceedings of the Staff Meeting of the Mayo Clinic 14*, 800 (1940). 15–4
9. Hauraets (1959). *The Degenerative Back and its Differential Diagnosis.* (Amsterdam: Elsevier)
10. O'Connell (1951). Protrusion of the lumbar intervertebral discs. *J. Bone Jt. Surg.*, **33B**, 8–30
11. Capanna *et al.* (1981). Lumbar discectomy. Percentage of disc removal and detection of anterior annulus perforations. *Spine*, **6**, 610–614

12. Nachlas (1952). End result study of the treatment of herniated nucleus pulposus by excision with fusion and without fusion. *J Bone Joint Surg.*, **34A**, 981–988
13. Hoytema and Oostrom (1961). The operation for herniation of the nucleus pulposus with invertebral body fusion. *Arch. Chirurg. Neerlandicum*, **13**, 71–80
14. White (1966). Results in surgical treatment of herniated lumbar intervertebral discs. *Clin. Neurosurg.*, **13**, 42–51
15. Nelson. Lumbar spine and low back pain. 1980 Edition. 477
16. Spangfort (1983). Disc surgery. In Wall and Melzack (eds.) *Textbook of Pain*, pp.601–606. (London: Churchill Livingstone)
17. Weber (1983). Lumbar disc herniation – a continuous prospective study. *Spine*, **8**, 131–140

Therapy 22 – chemonucleolysis

This is a controversial treatment[1].

Aim of treatment
Relief of pain.

Diagnosis
Unknown.

How it works
While its action in 'digesting' the nucleus pulposus seems clear, its mode of action in pain relief remains unknown.

Indications
Pain of vertebral origin – thought to be due to disc protrusion.

Contraindications
History of allergic reactions.

Dangers
Severe allergic reactions[2,3].

Complications
None.

Predictability
This is impossible, both in the short term and in the long term. In one series its efficacy was not significantly better than was placebo[4].

Similar treatments
None.

Practical clinical consequences
In view of its dangers and contentious results, it should be afforded low priority.

References

1. Dubuisson (1983). Root surgery. In Wall and Melzack (eds.) *Textbook of Pain*. p.595. (London: Churchill Livingstone)
2. Burnell (1974). Injection techniques in low back pain. In Twomey (Ed). *Symposium, Low Back Pain*. Western Aust. Inst. Tech. Perth. 111.
3. Kapsalis *et al.* (1974). The fate of chymopapain injections for therapy of intervertebral disc disease. *J. Lab. Clin. Med.*, 83, 532
4. Martins *et al.* (1978). Double blind evaluation of chemonucleolysis for herbiatred lumbar discs. *J. Neurosurg.*, 49, 816-827.

Therapy 23 – sclerosant therapy

Aim of treatment
Relief of pain.

Diagnosis
Unknown.

How it works
Introduced into the UK in 1975 by Barbor[1] it has been suggested that this works by improving stability through sclerosing lax ligaments of the lumbar spine. Evidence has been adduced demonstrating fibrosis and proliferation of osteophytes at the site of injection. Although lumbar instability has been clearly defined, in view of the work of Hilton[2] it is extremely difficult to identify in practice. Likewise, although success appears to follow therapy, resolution of pain may be due to a number of other agencies, and there is no clear correlation between this therapy and its apparent results.

Indication
Pain of vertebral origin.

Contraindications
None.

Similar treatments
None.

Treatment time
This is a fairly rapid treatment, both for the patient and for the doctor, usually repeated twice at about one week's interval.

Comment
This is a somewhat painful procedure, in which we find little advantage.

References

1. Barbor (1975). Presentation at Reunion sobre catalogia de la Columna Vertebral, Murcia
2. Hilton (1980). In Jayson (ed.) *The Lumbar Spine and Low Back Pain*. (London: Pitman Medical)

Therapy 24 – placebo

The use of placebo by doctors is widely misunderstood, and the degree of pain relief it can provide underestimated. Weisenberg states that, in the pain clinic, 35% of cases can be helped by this form of treatment. He also points out that this proportion is reduced to 3.2% in the laboratory. "The missing ingredient in the laboratory is the anxiety associated with the disease process and the threat of disfigurement or death."[1]

Hospital studies have shown that placebo tends to be employed in patients who:
1. Are disliked,
2. Are thought to exaggerate their pain,
3. Fail to respond to orthodox therapies,
4. Exhibit a combination of the above[2].

Under these circumstances, a positive response is assumed to show that the pain of which the patient complains has no physiological basis. However, it has been clearly shown that placebo itself does have a physiological action[3].

It has also been demonstrated that over-demanding and complaining patients are less likely to respond to placebo than are others[4]. Therefore its use, as is widespread at the present time in clinical practice, a) to assess whether the pain is 'real', b) with patients thought to be using too much medication, and c) with 'problem' patients, is quite mistaken. It is clear that the correct clinical approach needs to be positive, rather than negative.

Aim of treatment
Pain relief.

Diagnosis
Unknown.

How it works
Unknown – but . . . "thus stress, fear or hopelessness, pain intensity and duration, are all-important factors for activation of endogenous pain control mechanisms". "Suggestion in the form of either hypnosis or placebo therapy can also be remarkably effective, even for severe clinical pain."[5]

Indications
Pain of vertebral origin.

Contraindications
None.

Dangers
None.

Complications
None.

Predictability
Impossible.

Similar treatments
Hypnosis.

References

1. Weisenberg (1983). Cognitive aspects of pain. In Wall and Melzack (eds.) *Textbook of Pain*, p.167. (London: Churchill Livingstone)
2. Goodwin *et al.* (1979). Knowledge and use of placebo by house officers and nurses. *Ann. Intern. Med.*, **91**, 106–110
3. Field and Basbaum (1983). In Wall and Melzack, op. cit., p.149
4. Lasagna *et al.* (1954). A study of a placebo response. *Am. J. Med.*, **16**, 770–779
5. Field and Basbaum. (1983). op. cit., p.150

Therapy 25 – biofeedback

This subject has attracted great interest, and in the past five years almost two dozen review articles have been written on this topic[1-22]. Definition is difficult, and it has been written, "the term has come to refer to a constellation of procedures having as their only common element the use of feedback (FB) itself – presentation to an individual of a sensory signal (usually visual)."[31] Its object is to acquire voluntary control of response (vide, with regard to verbal stimuli, the Alexander technique).

Assessment difficulties
A great variety of pain syndromes has been studied. Very commonly electromyographic (EMG) feedback has been used for muscle contraction headaches. Next in frequency has been the use of vascular feedback for migraine, and for numerous other pain problems, such as Reynaud's syndrome, arthritis and low back pain.

Subject variation has been very great. In different studies, subjects have consisted of college students or public research volunteers, self-referrals or medical referrals. For this reason treatment outcome is contaminated by variability, not only in pain syndromes treated, but also in the type of subjects studied.

Overall studies are further confounded by the fact that FB practice is not a single procedure.

Subjects have received all sorts of concurrent instruction, including forms of counselling and psychotherapy, as well as relaxation training and home practice.

Various physiological and self-report measures have been used to assist the outcome of the FB intervention. All of this activity has rarely occurred within the confines of a rigorously controlled research. Poorly designed studies have far outnumbered controlled comparisons.

Aim of treatment
This is twofold: the relief of pain and the control of persistent pain.

Diagnosis
There is seldom a definitive diagnosis.

How does it work?
It is clear that, with FB treatment of headache, relaxation training and other cognitive training and behavioural interventions seem to be at least as effective. So what happens in treatment to cause improvement? In 1980 a

study compared EMG FB training for increasing, decreasing or stabilizing frontalis muscle tension with a no-treatment group[23]. The three treated groups showed equivalent, substantial improvement in tension headache at a three-month follow-up, and all three treatments were equally superior to the no-treatment group.

Built-in checks showed that FB subjects had aquired frontalis muscle control as trained, and the treatments were equally credible. "These results suggest that the learned reduction of EMG activity may play only a minor role in the outcome obtained with biofeedback."[23] The headache sufferers, when asked to list the techniques and strategies that they had aquired to control their headaches, found 11 categories, cognitive in nature, the common theme of which appeared to be an attempt at self-control. Similar findings were reported in a study on hand temperature FB for migraine. It was concluded, "dramatic therapeutic improvements in migraine headaches with hand temperature feedback is not due to a specific property of skin temperature alterations, but rather is due to non-specific effects of clinical procedures employed. The results of this double-blind study are negative, not because the treated group failed to improve, but because the two control groups improved as much as the treated group did."[24]

The results of investigations show that biofeedback does not live up to the claims of its more enthusiastic supporters. "The exact meter readouts by the knowledgeable electromyographer at the same time as he is deliberately and wisely using them as (1) a rough indicator of progress in a clinical relaxation training programme and (2) a visual placebo in reinforcing the patient's response. Any higher level of reliance on such inflated numbers is self-deception."[25]

Indications

Muscle contraction headache: FB seems clearly helpful in this application, and this is not due to spontaneous remission, regression to the mean, the passage of time or subject maturation. With regard to the actual EMG measure, so many variations have been reported that the use of EMG FB for muscle contraction headache has been questioned. If sustained frontalis tension is not the priciple cause of muscle tension headache, then why apply a treatment designed to reduce tension? "Evidence to date indicates that biofeedback is no more effective than relaxation training for headaches. Relaxation has been found to be equivalent to EEG and EMG feedback in reducing tension headaches and as efficacious as finger temperature feedback for decreasing migraine activity."[22]

Again, in a review of studies comparing EMG FB to relaxation training, it has been concluded that, "results of most of these studies indicate that either method was equally effective in producing positive results."[20]

Migraine headache: This has been treated with finger temperature FB. Overall outcome effectiveness for finger warming feedback for migraine, when objectively evaluated, has been somewhat weaker than that for EMG FB applied to tension headaches. Typical figures for migraine symptom reduction during the finger warming FB is about 30–35%, although no improvement has been reported from time to time. Virtually the same amount of improvement is found in no-treatment groups and what should be counter-therapeutic groups who attempt to decrease their finger temperature[24].

Other pain syndromes: These show similarities, in that the uncontrolled studies greatly outnumber systematic studies, and that controlled research suggests that, as with headache, generalized relaxation is as effective and may mediate improvement in a number of syndromes. FB treatments have been reported for the following:
1. Raynaud's disease.
2. Spasmodic torticollis.
3. Low back pain.
4. Chronic pain.
5. Neck injury.
6. Childbirth.
7. Menstrual distress.
8. Writer's cramp.
9. Duodenal ulcer.
10. Temporomandibular joint pain.
11. Post-traumatic headaches.

Of this group two are of particular interest to clinicians involved in musculo-skeletal medicine; chronic low back pain and post-traumatic headache.

With regard to chronic low back pain, EMG findings have varied significantly[26]. In one series significantly higher resting low back (erector spinae) EMG activity was found in low back pain sufferers, compared with 30 controls, matched for age, sex, height and weight. On the other hand, it was also found in another series that resting paralumbar muscle tension in low back pain sufferers was not significantly higher than in non-back pain volunteers, either before or after relaxation treatment[27]. It was found that paralumbar muscle activity was higher in low back pain sufferers compared with a pain-free sample during isometric tensing of muscle groups, e.g. shoulders and legs. Patients who received relaxation training with concurrent low back EMG FB did not improve more than those who received only relaxation training.

A comparison between α EMG and concurrent hypnosis in low back pain

(Melzack and Perry, 1975)[28] found that neither treatment component alone was noticeably beneficial, but that in combination they were. EMG FB seemed to be of only marginal help[29,30]. "The difficulty of obtaining improvement in this syndrome by any means other than long-term medication (with its attendant risks) recommends further investigation."[31] This statement may surprise many musculoskeletal clinicians. The fact that many post-traumatic headaches can now be proven to be the consequence of neck injury (see Clinical Presentation, p.169) and commonly to respond to local physical treatments to the neck (such as manipulation, massage, local anaesthetics and other forms of local physiotherapy) does not sit well with this statement. It seems to us to be another example of the fact that further dissemination of information across the frontiers that divide various clinical disciplines is desirable.

Contraindications
None.

Predictability
There is no known way in which either short-term or long-term outcome prediction may be made reliably.

Therapy time
From the point of view of the patient's inconvenience, this therapy has the disadvantage of needing to be conducted in the clinic, thus resulting in the loss of a substantial part of the working day at each session.

Comparison with other treatments
Cognitive therapies of various sorts. Hypnosis and relaxation techniques. The latter are as effective as feedback and simpler to administer.

Practical clinical consequences
In spite of the degree of disagreement to be found in the literature, biofeedback, in one form or another, should not be discarded as a therapeutic option, particularly in long-standing chronic pain.

References

1. Beaty and Haynes (1979). Behavioural intervention with muscle contraction headache. A Review. *Psychosom. Med.*, **41**, 165–180
2. Blanchard and Young (1974). Clinical application of biofeedback training. *Arch. Gen. Psychiatry*, **30**, 573–589
3. Carmona (1980). Biofeedback. Instrumental learning of visceral and glandular responses. *Redista Chilena Psicol.*, **3**, 43–53

4. Cox (1979). Non-pharmacological integrated treatment approach to headaches. *Behav. Med. Update*, (3), 14–19
5. Doyle (1980). Biofeedback as an adjunct to psychotherapy in the treatment of psychosomatic and physical disorders. A clinician's view. *Am J. Clin. Biofeedback*, 3 (2), 169–177
6. Ellerston (1980). Biofeedback treatment of migraine. *Tidsskrift Norsk Psykologforening*, 17, 537–541
7. Friedman (1977). Biofeedback. 1. Actual state of its clinical applications. *Acta Psychiatrica Belgica*, 77, 118–133
8. Jacobson (1978). Biofeedback. A new treatment for psychosomatic and functional disorders? *Compr. Psychiatry*, 19, 275–284
9. Jessup (1982). Psychophysiological factors in the treatment of stress of pain. Biofeedback. In Nefeld (ed.) *Psychological Stress and Psychopathology*, pp. 306–333. (New York: McGraw Hill)
10. Jessup et al. (1979). Biofeedback therapy for headache and other pain. An evaluative review. *Pain*, 7, 225–270
11. King and Montgomery (1980). Biofeedback. Induced control of human peripheral temperature. A critical review of the literature. *Psychol. Bull.*, 88 (3), 738–752
12. Miller (1978). Biofeedback and visceral learning. *Ann. Rev. Psychol.*, 29, 373–404
13. Nuechterlein and Holroyd (1980). Biofeedback in the treatment of tension headache. *Arch. Psychiatry*, 37, 866–873
14. Orne (1979). The efficacy of biofeedback therapies. *Ann. Rev. Med.*, 30, 489–583
15. Pikoff (1981). Biofeedback. A resource directory and outline of the literature. *Professional Psychol.*, 12 (2), 261–270
16. Prima et al. (1979). A review of the applications of biofeedback to migraine and tension headache. *Acta Neurol.*, 34, 510–521
17. Qualls and Sheehan (1981). Electromyograph biofeedback as a relaxation technique. A critical appraisal and reassessment. *Psychol. Bull.*, 90, 21–42
18. Sappington et al. (1979). Biofeedback as therapy in Raynaud's disease. *Biofeedback Self-regulation*, 4, 155–169
19. Surwit and Keefe (1978). Frontalis EMG feedback training. An electronic panacea? *Behav. Ther.*, 9, 779–792
20. Tarler-Benlolo (1978). The role of relaxation in biofeedback training. A critical review of the literature. *Psychol. Bull.*, 85, 727–755
21. Turk et al. (1979). Application of biofeedback for the regulation of pain. A critical review. *Psychol. Bull.*, 86, 1322–1338
22. Turner and Chapman (1982). Psychological interventions for chronic pain. A critical review. 1. Relaxation training and biofeedback. *Pain*, 12, 1–21
23. Andrasik and Holroyd (1980). A test of specific and non-specific effects in the biofeedback treatment of tension headache. *J. Consult. Clin. Psychol.*, 48, 575–586
24. Kewman and Roberts (1980). Skin temperature biofeedback and migraine headache, a double blind study. *Biofeedback Self-regulation*, 5, 327–345
25. Basmajian and DeLuca (1985). *Muscles Alive*, p.186. (Baltimore: Williams and Wilkins)
26. Grabel (1973). EMG study of low back muscle tension in subjects with and without chronic low back pain. *Dissertation Abstr. Int.*, 34(B), 2929
27. Kraitz (1978). EMG feedback and differential relaxation training to promote pain relief in chronic low back pain sufferers. *Dissertation Abstr. Int.*, 39(B), 1485–1486
28. Melzack and Perry (1975). Self regulation of pain. The use of alpha feedback and hypnotic training for the control of chronic pain. *Exp. Neurol.*, 46, 452–463
29. Nouwen and Solinger (1979). The effectiveness of EMG biofeedback training in low back pain. *Biofeedback Self-regulation*, 4, 103–111
30. Freeman et al. (1980). Biofeedback with low back pain patients. *Am. J. Clin. Biofeedback*, 3, 118–122
31. Jessup (1983). Biofeedback. In Wall and Melzack (eds.) *Textbook of Pain*, p.776 et seq (London: Churchill Livingstone)

Therapy 26 – hypnosis

"Hypnosis is amongst the oldest and best documented psychological treatments of pain."[39] Despite controversy, "hypnosis has been observed to provide almost total relief from the appreciation of pain in some individuals, in a manner not attributable to mere relaxation, stoicism or fakery."[1] Hypnosis has been extensively used and is well documented as the sole source of anaesthesia in surgery[2-5] and it is also an effective analgesic for pain arising in a variety of situations, including such illnesses as arthritis. "While the analgesic and anaesthetic effects of suggestion of pain reduction appear unequivocal for some individuals, the nature of hypnosis and the mechanisms of these effects are less certain."[39]

Hypnosis and suggestion

Despite much controversy, hypnosis may be defined as, "that state or condition which occurs when appropriate suggestions elicit distortions of perception, memory or mood."[6]

Hypnotizability

Hypnotizability is evaluated clinically by the individual's responsiveness to suggestions following induction, and may be measured by standardized tests."[7]

The hypnotic state varies considerably between individuals, some being highly responsive, others not. This responsiveness shows some changes with age, but remains a remarkably stable attribute of the person throughout adult life[8].

As a stable attribute, hypnotizability has been found to predict the efficacy of suggested analgesia in a variety of situations[9-12]. However, this is of but modest help clinically, since overall responsiveness to suggestion is not absolutely correlated with responses to a specific suggestion, such as analgesia.

Preconditions for hypnosis

The establishment of rapport, which begins the hypnotic intervention.

Case analysis, to ensure that, for physical and psychological reasons, hypnosis is not contraindicated. For example, psychologically the therapist must be certain that neither emotional disturbance, such as depression, nor psychotic problems, such as paranoia, exist.

The patient's motivation for seeking pain relief is important. For example, hypnosis has been remarkably successful in burn debridement, and this is thought to relate to the motivation resulting from the the intense pain that burn patients experience.

The establishment of the clinician's own goals and aspirations in this situation is important. For example, the decision must be made, whether or not to proceed in the face of potential side-effects.

Induction: the establishment of rapport is the sine qua non for induction, and procedures used vary enormously.

Self-hypnosis

This can be very effective, and it can be taught fairly rapidly, with the patient practising it in the absence of the therapist, thereby reducing the cost in time to both therapist and patient. Worldwide, the technique most commonly used which corresponds to self-hypnosis is autogenic training[13] but this can be unnecessarily lengthy, while with self-hypnosis a responsive patient can learn to control pain successfully within a single session. This has the additional advantage of giving the patient a sense of control over his state, and thereby conferring a cognitive advantage.

Aim of treatment

This is twofold: the relief of pain and the control of persistent pain.

Diagnosis

In musculoskeletal practice there is seldom a diagnosis which may be validated.

How does it work?

Effect on anxiety: It has been claimed that hypnosis works purely as an anxiety reducing measure, and there is certainly a component of anxiety reduction in the control of pain. However, studies do not support this claim[14-17]. "Hypnosis is apparently more than just a tranquilliser for the relief of pain – affecting both the perceptual and reactive dimensions of pain – in appropriately responsive individuals."[39]

Placebo effect: Even unhypnotizable subjects often derive some benefit from these procedures in terms of analgesia[18,19]. This effect should not be underestimated, and it can be of great help to the patient[20,21].

However, in sensitive individuals, the response does not wholly result from the placebo component, but rather from the subject's reaction to specific suggestions. These suggestions vary, but some are more effective than others[22] particularly those involving cognitive strategies antithetical to pain and by comparison with strategies emphasizing only pleasant imagery or imaginative skills. Thus, flexibility is important in tailoring procedures to the individual's ability to respond to these suggestions[16,23].

Site of action

This "appears to occur at the higher levels of the nervous system".[39] "The cognitive disassociation characteristic of successful hypno-analgesia in these individuals is illustrated by a maintenance of the involuntary physiological and behavioural responses to pain during hypnosis, despite experienced comfort and alertness[24,25]. The presence of autonomic nervous system responses to the pain in the absence of the perceived pain during hypno-analgesia clearly indicates that the response is not peripheral."[39]

Beyond this, the physiology is not understood, and therefore the mode of action is unknown.

Indications

Pain of vertebral origin: Hypnosis has been widely used, not only as a direct therapy aimed at the relief of pain, but also as an adjunct to psychotherapeutic treatment, in helping the patient not only to gain an understanding as to the meaning of the pain, thereby achieving mastery over it (cognition) but also to facilitate behavioural treatment of pain (see Behavioural Therapy, p.266).

Paradoxically, the patient's response to hypnosis does not mean that the pain has a psychological origin. On the contrary, the reverse is generally the case. This is particularly so when the pain is of uncertain organic aetiology.

Acute pain of organic aetiology: Responsiveness depends upon the nature of the pain and the context in which it occurs. For example, in dental procedures it is not uncommon to find that over 90% of patients achieve a degree of pain relief[26] compared with estimates of less than 10% who can effectively use this technique for pain control in minor surgery, and possibly fewer than 1% in major surgery[27]. When estimates are extremely high, the pain is likely to be non-threatening and not too intense or prolonged, placebo components and distraction contributing in a major way to the result.

Persistent pain of organic aetiology: This is not as straightforward as is the treatment of acute pain, because in chronic pain, illness behaviour develops. Under these circumstances, hypnosis is not only relevant to the relief of pain, but also for treating its emotional ramifications.

In conditions such as rheumatoid arthritis or persistent back pain or headache with a definite physical basis the difficulties are the same. Indeed, they may be greater, as the patient has to cope with these problems over a prolonged period. Hypnosis has proved useful particularly in the more hypnotizable individuals[28]. However, in these instances it is no more than one aspect of the overall management, and psychotherapeutic features should not be forgotten[29,30].

Chronic pain of uncertain aetiology: This group includes such syndromes as persistent tension or migraine headache and chronic low back pain. These patients will show a degree of pain behaviour greater than will those with clear organic lesions. Under these circumstances, when somatic therapy is difficult and pain behaviour is dominant, behavioural and cognitive behavioural therapy seem to be the more appropriate forms of management. In this situation, the appropriate role for hypnosis is as an adjunct to psychotherapy, that is to say, as hypnotherapy, **not** as an analgesic[31,32].

When one is dealing with a syndrome in which a major factor involves the consequences of pain behaviour – when the patient is 'rewarded' for demonstrating his sufffering – hypnosis is not likely to provide more than transient relief, with symptom substitution a distinct possibility[33,34].

Contraindications
The sole contraindication is the use of hypnosis in those patients identified as being psychologically disturbed, unless the therapist is adequately trained in psychotherapy.

Dangers
These are potentially serious. "Hypnosis may precipitate rapid development of intense transference reaction and bring to the surface psychological material with which the patient cannot cope. Experience with hypnosis per se is adequate background to give direct suggestions for relief of organic pain, but should not be confused with training in psychotherapy, which is essential to deal with the problems that can arise when uncovering techniques are employed."[39] Therefore patient selection is a matter of the first importance, as is adequate training of the therapist.

Predictability
Because there are so many variable factors, and because hypnosis is so closely involved with many other forms of treatment, firm conclusions as to its value are difficult to draw.

Similar therapies
The factors involved in pain control include the following.
1. Specific reductions in perceived pain and suffering in hypnotically responsive individuals.
2. Reduced suffering due to non-specific placebo effects on relaxation and anxiety.
3. Moderation of pain perception through suggestions that involve distraction and other cognitive strategies that are not an essential part of hypnosis, but which nevertheless contribute to the attenuation of pain.

Thus it may be seen that hypnosis is closely associated with many other forms of psychotherapy.

Acupuncture: This has been compared with hypnosis. While these two therapies are substantially different, when compared for efficacy hypnotic suggestion appears to produce greater relief in both experimental and clinical subjects than does acupuncture or placebo acupuncture[35,36].

Psychotherapeutic comparison: In a variety of studies, all treatments are superior to drug placebo, hypnosis is somewhat more effective than psychotherapy and as effective as biofeedback, although the latter is more difficult for the patient to transfer from the clinic to the real world. Hypnosis has been reported to be more effective than EEG α biofeedback for pain relief in some chronic pain patients, but the two procedures combined were the most effective[37].

Treatment time

From the pont of view of the patient's convenience, except in the case of self-hypnosis, this treatment has the disadvantage of needing to be carried out in the clinic, thus necessitating a fairly prolonged absence from work or home.

Practical clinical consequences

Clearly, hypnosis has a role to play in acute pain of organic aetiology. However, there are many alternative therapies available.

In persistent pain of proven organic aetiology it may have a useful role to play, depending upon the hypnotizability of the patient.

With regard to persistent pain of uncertain aetiology, so commonly found in musculoskeletal practice, it is sadly of little help, and may itself present dangers.

References

1. Hilgard *et al.* (1974). The psychophysics of cold pressor pain and its modification through hypnotic suggestion. *Am. J. Psychol.*, 87, 17–31
2. Tinterow (1969). The use of hypnotic anaesthia for major surgical procedures. *Am. Surgeon*, 26, 732–737
3. Scott (1973). Hypno-analgesia for major surgery. A psychodynamic process. *Am. J. Clin. Hypnosis*, 16, 84–91
4. Hilgard and Hilgard (1975). *Hypnosis in the Relief of Pain.* (Los Alton, CA: William Kaufmann)
5. Finer (1980). Hypnosis and anaesthia. In Burrows and Dennerstein (eds.) *Handbook of Hypnosis and Psychosomatic Medicine.*, Vol.16, p.293 (Amsterdam: Elsevier North Holland)
6. Orne (1980). On the construct of hypnosis. How its definition affects research and its clinical application. In Burrows and Dennerstein (eds.) *Handbook of Hypnosis and Psychosomatic Medicine.* Vol.3, p.29 (Amsterdam: Elsevier North Holland)

INDIVIDUAL THERAPIES

7. Hilgard (1982). Hypnotic susceptability and implications for measurement. *Int. J. Clin. Exp. Hypnosis*, **30**, 394–403
8. Morgan *et al.* (1974). The stability of hypnotic susceptibility. A longitudinal study. *Int. J. Clin. Exp. Hypnosis*, **22**, 249–257
10. Spanos *et al.* (1979). The effects of hypnotic susceptability, suggestions for analgesia, and the utilisation of cognitive strategies on the reduction of pain. *J. Abnorm. Psychol.*, **88**, 282–292
11. Hilgard and Le Baron (1982). Relief of anxiety and pain in children and adolescents with cancer. Quantitative measures and clinical observations. *Int. J. Clin. Exp. Hypnosis*, **30**, 417–442
12. Schafer (1975). Hypnosis use on a burn unit. *Int. J. Clin. Exp. Hypnosis*, **23**, 1–14
13. Luthe (1965). *Autogenic Training: Correlationes Psychosomaticae*. (New York: Grune and Stratton)
14. Chapman and Feather (1973). Effects of diazepam on human pain tolerance and pain sensitivity. *Psychosom. Med.*, **35**, 330–340
15. Johnson (1974). Suggestions for pain reduction and response to cold induced pain. *Psychol. Rec.*, **24**, 161–169
16. Greene and Reyher (1972). Pain tolerance in hypnotic analgesic and imagination states. *J. Abnorm. Psychol.*, **79**, 29–38
17. Knox *et al.* (1974). Pain and suffering in ischemia. *Arch. Gen. Psychiatry*, **30**, 840–847
18. Hilgard *et al.* (1978). The reality of hypnotic analgesia. A comparison of highly hypnotizables with simulators. *J. Abnorm. Psychol.*, **87**, 239–246
19. McGlashan *et al.* (1969). The nature of hypnotic analgesia and placebo response to experimental pain. *Psychosom. Med.*, **31**, 227–246
20. Crasilneck and Hall (1975). *Clinical Hypnosis. Principles and Applications.* ((New York: Grune and Stratton)
21. Kroger (1977). *Clinical and Experimental Hypnosis*, 2nd edn. (Philadelphia: J.B. Lippincott)
22. Spanos *et al.* (1975). The effects of two cognitive strategies on pain thresholds. *J. Abnorm. Psychol.*, **84**, 677–681
23. Greene and Reyher (1972). Pain tolerance in hypnotic analgesic and imagination states. *J. Abnorm. Psychol.*, **79**, 29–38
24. Piccione (1980). The effects jof structured hypnotic imagery on the perception and reduction of ischaemic pain by hypnotizable female students grouped as high or low imagers. *Dissertation*, University Microfilms International, Ann Arbor, Michigan
25. Shor (1959). Explorations in hypnosis. A theoretical and experimental study. *Dissertation*, Brandeis University
26. Bowers (1976). *Hypnosis for the Seriously Curious.* (Monterey, Calif.:Brook/Cole)
27. Barber (1977). Rapid induction analgesia. A clinical report. *Am. J. Clin. Hypnosis*, **19**, 138–157
28. Marmer (1963). Hypnosis in anaesthiology and surgery. In Schneck (ed.) *Hypnosis in Modern Medicine.* (Springfield, Illinois: Charles C Thomas)
29. Cedercruetz *et al.* (1976). Hypnotic treatment of headache and vertigo in skull injured patients. *Int. J. Clin. Exp. Hypnosis*, **24**, 195–201.
30. Cioppa and Thal (1975). Hypnotherapy in a case of juvenile rheumatoid arthritis. *Am. J. Clin. Hypnosis*, **18**, 105–110.
31. Crasilneck (1979). Hypnosis in the control of chronic low back pain. *Am. J. Clin. Hypnosis*, **22**, 71–78.
32. Elton *et al.* (1980). Chronic pain and hypnosis. In Burrows and Dennerstein (eds.) *Handbook of Hypnosis and Psychosomatic Medicine*, Vol.15, p.269. (Amsterdam: Elsevier North Holland)
33. Howard *et al.* (1982). Modifying migraine headache through rational state directed hypnotherapy. A cognitive experimental perspective. *Int. J. Clin. Exp. Hypnosis*, **30**, 257–269.
34. Block *et al.* (1980). Behavioural treatment of chronic pain. Variables effecting treatment efficacy. *Pain*, **8**, 367–375.
35. Wadden and Anderton (1982). The clinical use of hypnosis. *Psychol. Bull.*, **91**, 215–243.

261

36. Stern *et al.* (1977). A comparison of hypnosis, acupuncture, morphine, valium, aspirin and placebo in the management of experimentally induced pain. *Ann. N. York Acad. Sci.*, **296**, 175–193.
37. Ulett *et al.* (1978). Acupuncture, hypnosis and experimental pain. 2. Study with patients. *Acupuncture Electrother. Res. Int. J.*, 3, 191–201
38. Melzack and Perry (1975). Self-regulation of pain. The use of alpha feedback and hypnotic training for the control of chronic pain. *Exp. Neurol.*, 46, 452–469
39. Orne and Pincus (1983) Hypnosis. In Wall and Melzack (eds.) *Textbook of Pain*, p.806 *et seq.* (London: Churchill Livingstone)

Therapy 27 – relaxation therapy

Relaxation techniques are commonly used in the form of relaxation training, hypnosis or cognitive behavioural therapy[1]. "The wide use of relaxation type interventions in the treatment of chronic pain is in contrast to their poorly understood mechanisms of action."[14] They have, however, a common underlying feature, the relaxation response.

The relaxation response and subjective experiences
These constitute an altered state of consciousness and have been described as peace of mind, feeling at ease with the world and as a sense of well-being. Such a state of mind, and the techniques used to achieve it, have been known throughout history in every culture, and have been associated with religious practices. Meditation and Yoga utilize such techniques, as do many repetitive prayers. For example, the instructions given in the fourteenth century by Gregory of Sinai for the "prayer of the heart" or "prayer of Jesus"; "Sit down alone and in silence. Lower your head, shut your eyes, breathe out gently and imagine yourself looking into your own heart. Carry your mind, that is your thoughts, from your head to your heart. As you breathe out say Lord Jesus Christ have mercy upon me. Say it moving your lips gently, or simply say it in your mind. Try to put all other thoughts aside. Be calm, be patient, and repeat the process very frequently."[2]

Such practices are also common in secular circumstances. For example, the late Alfred Lord Tennyson experienced visions of ecstasy that were the foundation for his deepest belief in, "the unity of all things, the reality of the unseen, and the persistence of life."[3] For him, the state was achieved through the repetition of his own name. Readers, we are sure, will be able to bring to mind persons of their acquaintance who would find such a technique congenial!

Secular technique
A simple secular technique involves the following instructions: Sit quietly in a comfortable position, and close your eyes. Deeply relax all your muscles, beginning at your feet and progressing up to your face. Keep them deeply relaxed. . . Breathe through your nose and become aware of your breathing. As you breathe out, say the word 'one' silently to yourself. Continue this for twenty minutes. When you have finished, sit quietly for several minutes more, at first with your eyes closed, then with them opened. Do not worry about whether you are successful in achieving a deep level of relaxation, maintain a passive attitude, and permit relaxation to occur at its own pace. With practice, the response should come with little effort.

In a responsive patient, self-hypnosis may be more readily learned and more conveniently deployed.

Other secular techniques that elicit the relaxation response
Autogenic training: The purpose of autogenic training is to elicit the relaxation response[4]. There are six standard exercises.
1. This focuses on feelings of heaviness in the limbs.
2. This involves cultivation of a sense of warmth in the limbs.
3. This concentrates on cardiac regulation.
4. This involves passive concentration on breathing.
5. This cultivates a sense of warmth in the upper abdomen.
6. This is directed to a sense of coolness of the forehead.

"The subject's attitude during the exercises must not be intense and compulsive, but rather of a quiet, 'let it happen' nature, which is referred to as 'passive concentration' and deemed absolutely essential."[14]

Progressive relaxation
This is a technique aimed at gaining control over skeletal muscle until very low levels of muscle tone are achieved in the major muscle groups[5].

It is practised in a supine position in a quiet room, and a passive attitude is essential. The subject is taught to recognize even a slight muscle contraction, so that he can avoid it and achieve the deepest degree of relaxation possible.

Hypnosis
This is an artificially induced state, characterized by increased suggestibility. The hypnotic induction procedure (autosuggestion in the case of self-hypnosis) usually includes suggestion of relaxation and drowsiness, closed eyes and a recumbent or semisupine position (used as a relaxation technique)[6,7].

Validation for the use of relaxation in pain relief
Clinical: In a series recently published, a control group of 'medically physically' treated patients showed no significant pain relief over 10 weeks (i.e. a placebo was controlled) while a 'mindfulness meditation' group partaking in a 10-week programme showed marked pain alleviation. Using the McGill Pain Questionnaire, it was reported that the pain rating index was reduced by more than 33% in 72% of patients who elicited the relaxation response, and 61% had a reduction of more than 50%[8]. Other measures, such as pain drawings and psychiatric scores, yielded similar results.

While the real medications in the control group were not placebos in the strict sense, their attendant explicit suggestion constitutes an essential element of the placebo effect. The failure of this group to demonstrate pain relief indicates that the placebo effect itself is inadequate to explain the pain reduction observed in the meditational group[9,10]. Duration of benefit was prolonged, as shown in the 15-month follow-up, in which the psychiatric scores remained remarkably improved, although the pain rating index had returned to pretreatment levels. The 15-month follow-up also demonstrated that the aquired skills were effective for many months. The procedure was obviously transferable to the home environment, where the relaxation response was elicited on a daily basis.

In studies in chronic headache syndromes, various forms of progressive relaxation and hypnosis have all caused a decrease in pain in both tension and migraine headache. There is no clear evidence that one technique is inferior to the others[11–13].

Aim of treatment
This is twofold: first as a means of pain relief, but further (in conjunction with other therapies) as a means of pain control.

Diagnosis
Precisely what is being treated is usually unknown.

How does it work?
The way in which this operates remains unknown.

Indication
Pain of vertebral origin.

Contraindications
There are none.

Dangers
None

Complications
None.

Predictability
This is not possible, either in the short term or in the long term.

Similar treatments
These are hypnosis, biofeedback and placebo.

Treatment time
Clearly. wherever practised, this may be a fairly time-consuming therapy.

References

1. Turner and Chapman (1982). Psychological interventions for chronic pain. A critical review. 1. Relaxation training and biofeedback. *Pain*, 12 3–21
2. French (1968). *The Way of a Pilgrim*. (New York: Seebury Press)
3. Spurgeon (1970). *Mysticism in English Literature*. (Port Washington: Kennikat Press)
4. Luthe (1969). *Autogenic Therapy*, Vols. 1–5. (New York: Grune and Stratton)
5. Jacobson (1938). *Progressive relaxation*. (Chicago: University of Chicago Press)
6. Gorton (1949). Physiology of hypnosis. *Psychiatr. Q.*, 23, 317–343, 457–485
7. Barber (1970). Physiological effects of hypnosis and suggestion. In *Biofeedback and Self-control*. 1970. (Chicago: Aldine-Atherton)
8. Kabat-Zinn (1982). An outpatient programme in behavioural medicine for chronic pain based on the practice of mindfulness meditation. Theoretical considerations and preliminary results. *Gen. Hosp. Psychiatry*, 4, 33–48
9. Benson and Epstein (1975). The placebo effect. A neglected asset in the care of patients. *J. Am. Med. Assoc.*.232, 1225–1227
10. Benson and McCallie (1979). Angina pectoris and the placebo effect. *N. Engl. J. Med.*. 300, 1424–1429
11. Mullinix *et al.* (1978). Skin temperature biofeedback and migraine. *Headache*, 17, 242–244
12. Cox *et al.* (1975). Differential effectiveness of electromyographic feedback, verbal relaxation and instructions and medication placebo with tension headaches. *J. Consul. Clin. Psychol.*. 43. 892–898
13. Haynes *et al.* (1975). Electromyographic biofeedback and relaxation instructions in the treatment of muscle contraction headaches. *Behav. Ther.*, 6, 672–679
14. Benson *et al.* (1983). The relaxation responses and pain. In Wall and Melzack (eds.) *Textbook of Pain*, p.817 *et seq.* (London: Churchill Livingstone)

Therapy 28 – behavioural therapy

Evaluation of pain behaviours

Pain behaviours include such activities as limping, groaning and taking to bed. Pain behaviour reinforcement includes attention from others, avoidance of disagreeable tasks and situations, drug use, income related to disability etc.

Inadvertent reinforcement of pain behaviour

Recent work on pain behaviour in terminal cancer patients has shown, "inadvertent social reinforcement by hospital staff and family members causing the frequency of the behaviours to increase. Those persons present at the time of the behaviours themselves become cues which elicit the behaviours. By withdrawing social attention from the unwanted behaviours with patient's and families' approval and making the attention contingent upon socially acceptable behaviour, the symptoms disappear, and the patient (as well as family and staff) becomes much more comfortable and content."[1,2]

It has also been shown that patients' self-medication prior to hospital admission is less than they receive in hospital[3]. Thus medical and nursing personnel are shown to play a role in the reinforcement of pain behaviour. This should surely be borne in mind by all those managing such patients.

Assessment

A number of endeavours has been made in this context, the most systematic being the development of a psychological pain inventory (PSPI) a structured interview with rating assigned to 25 items[4]. Items which were most highly correlated with total scores on the PSPI are:

1. Pain behaviours at home.
2. The number of surgical operations for pain.
3. The time in hospital for pain and any change in work status.
4. Pain-contingent financial gain.
5. Rest periods.
6. Social reinforcement for pain behaviour.
7. Drug and alcohol use.
8. Avoidance of performance demands.
9. Stressful life events.
10. Previous exposure to the chronic invalid role[5].

PSPI scores

High total scores, in a small pilot study, predicted poor response to medical or surgical treatment for pain.

The PSPI scores have no significant correlation with the Minnesota

Multiphasic Personality Inventory and only slight correlation with the McGill Pain Questionnaire. This "suggests that the extent to which pain behaviours come under environmental influence may have little to do with either personality variables or with pain description, but rather with the laws of learning according to which behaviour is governed by its consequence"[16].

PSPI scores have been used in some centres as a means of patient selection[6]. For example, patients involved in active litigation and those whose families refused to co-operate are sometimes excluded from behavioural treatment. This raises the ethical issue as to how proper it is to exclude patients on the grounds that it is likely they will prove difficult to treat.

Methods of behavioural pain treatment

In most centres an explicit or written contract is established with: (a) realistic goals, (b) what the patient can do to achieve them, and (c) how the staff will help them to do so[7].

Patients and others concerned are given an explanation of the rationale of the course of treatment, so that they and the staff share a common concept and a common vocabulary.

Almost always a chart of daily activities is kept[5].

As far as possible, medication is withdrawn. This is because: a) drug takers, by comparison with those from whom drugs have been withdrawn make few therapeutic gains, and b) often patients take drugs on an as-required basis (that is to say that they wait until pain is severe and then take the analgesic) which reduces the pain severity, but which reinforces drug taking as a behaviour. (See Behavioural Assessment, p.112). This emphasizes once again one of the consequences of over-medication.

Physiotherapy and other activities are employed. These are usually set well within the patient's capabilities, and are gradually increased. The staff regularly appraise the attainment of the particular therapeutic objectives.

Pain behaviours are ignored, with no attention being paid to moaning, limping, falling and requests for drugs or other help.

Healthy behaviours are praised; for example the attainment of various subgoals.

Relaxation procedures and biofeedback are often used. These are, of course, 'contaminants' of pure behavioural therapy. In practice there is unlikely to be any such thing as pure behavioural therapy.

Aims of treatment

"The extinction through negative reinforcement of pain behaviour and a simultaneous shaping and development through positive reinforcement of healthy and adaptive behaviours."[16] As has been seen above, there is some contamination with other forms of treatment, but, "the core of the programme is the reinforcement by staff and by the patient's record keeping and graphs of the acquisition of skills desired by the patient."[8]

Spouse and family training are also provided. This is extremely important to prevent relapse and to maintain healthy behaviour, and to make a successful translation from the clinic to the home environment.

In essence behavioural therapy is directed to eliminating pain disability.

Diagnosis
This is unknown.

How it works
This remains largely a mystery.

Indications
Pain of vertebral origin.

Contraindications
There are none.

Dangers
None.

Complications
None.

Predictability
Many studies have been described. "Although significant improvement in functioning over baseline levels is reported and maintained over follow-up periods of varying lengths, the multiple independent variables and lack of control groups makes these reports difficult to evaluate."[7,9-13]

Pure behavioural therapy
The first report that can be so described concerned 36 patients with varying pain syndromes who were treated as indicated above, with a mean period of follow-up of nearly two years. There were significant improvements in pain and activity levels from admission to discharge, and these were maintained at the follow-up[14].

A more recent and controlled study involved 34 patients in a similar behavioural programme, consisting of an in-patient programme of 6-8 weeks duration, and involving physical and occupational therapy, gradual reduction of drugs, staff inattention to pain behaviours and family instruction. In the follow-up periods, ranging from 1 to 8 years, 20 of 26 patients available for evaluation (77%) were leading lives essentially no different from normal (the criterion for success). As controls, only 1 of 20 patients rejected the treatment, and 0 out of 12 who refused treatment met such stringent criteria for success. This, compared with any other form of treatment for chronic pain, alone or in combination, must be regarded as being remarkably successful[15].

Similar treatments
Behavioural therapy has similarities to cognitive behavioural therapy.

Treatment time
Behavioural therapy is one which must involve a substantial commitment of time by the patient. It is clinic orientated, cannot be practised in a hurry, and probably requires a number of sessions, each of necessity disrupting the life of the patient.

Practical clinical consequences
In general it is felt that if patients on long-term follow-up are performing at a level indistinguishable from age and sex matched normals, whereas before treatment they were nearly totally disabled, then the behavioural intervention is largely successful.

However, it remains impossible to predict outcome with any certainty, so that this is yet another form of therapy which must be approached with empiricism.

References

1. Redd (1982). Treatment of excessive crying in a terminal cancer patient. A time series analysis. *J. Behav. Med.*, **5**, 225–235
2. Redd (1982). Behavioural analysis and control of psychosomatic symptoms with patients receiving intensive cancer treatment. *Br. J. Clin. Psychol.*, **21**, 351–358
3. Ready *et al.* (1982). Self reported versus actual use of medication in chronic pain patients. *Pain*, **12**, 285–295
4. Heaton *et al.* (1982). A standardized evaluation of psychosocial factors in chronic pain. *Pain*, **12**, 165–174
5. Fordyce (1976). *Behavioural Methods for Chronic Pain and Illness*. (St Louis: C.B. Mosby)
6. Maruta *et al.* (1979). Chronic pain. Which patients may a pain management programme help? *Pain*, **7**, 321–329
7. Sternbach (1974). *Pain Patients. Traits and Treatments*. (New York: Academic Press)
8. Fordyce (1978). Learning processes in pain. In Sternbach (ed.) *Psychology of Pain*, pp. 49–72. (New York: Raven Press)
9. Igenelzi *et al.* (1977). The pain ward. Follow-up analyses. *Pain*, **3**, 277–280
10. Khatami and Rush (1978). A pilot study of the treatment of outpatients with chronic pain. Symptom control, stimulus control and social system intervention. *Pain*, **5**, 163–172
11. Seres and Newman (1976). Results of treatment of chronic low back pain at the Portland Pain Centre. *J. Neurosurg.*, **45**, 32–36
12. Seres *et al.* (1977). Evaluation and management of chronic pain by non-surgical means. In Lee (ed.) *Pain Management Symposium on the Neurosurgical Treatment of Pain*, pp. 33–53.

(Baltimore: Williams and Wilkins)
13. Swanson *et al.* (1979). Results of behaviour modification in the treatment of chronic pain. *Psychosom. Med.*, **41**, 55–61
14. Fordyce *et al.* (1973). Operant conditioning in the treatment of chronic clinical pain. *Arch. Phys. Med. Rehabil.*, **54**, 399–408
15. Roberts and Reinhardt (1980). The behavioural management of chronic pain. Long term follow-up of comparison groups. *Pain*, **8**, 151–162
16. Sternbach (1983). Behaviour therapy. In Wall and Melzack (eds.) *Textbook of Pain*, p.802 *et seq.* (London: Churchill Livingstone)

Therapy 29 – cognitive behavioural therapies

Following the worldwide growth of pain clinics, there has developed a broad range of psychological and somatic treatments. These are multidimensional in concept, based on the gate control theory[1,2]. Thus, "the surgical and pharmacological attacks on pain might well profit from redirecting thinking towards the neglected and almost forgotten contribution of motivational and cognitional processes. Pain can be treated not only by trying to cut down sensory input by anaesthetic blocks, surgical interventions and the like, but also by influencing the motivational, affective and cognitive factors as well."[3]

With regard to decreasing sensory input, this is only one factor in the inevitably complex manner in which these therapies work. Out of many suggested comprehensive pain management programmes, two of particular interest have evolved.
1. The operant conditioning approach.
2. The cognitive behavioural approach described here.
The common denominators are as follows:
1. Interest in the nature and modification of a patient's thoughts, feelings and beliefs, as well as behaviour.
2. Some commitment to behavioural therapy procedures in promoting change. In this context, such procedures represent informational feedback that provides an opportunity for the patient to question, reappraise and acquire self-control over harmful thoughts feelings and behaviour[4-8].

Treatment
This is flexible and is applicable to both groups of patients and to individuals.

Treatment objectives
1. To identify and correct distorted ideas and beliefs.
2. To be aware of the impact of distorted ideas and beliefs in maintaining harmful behaviours.

3. To link affect, cognition and behaviour and to appreciate their joint consequences. (See Relevant Psychology, p.88 *et seq.*)
4. To translate all this into practice, so as to modify behaviour in its various forms, as also the patient's perception of the role he plays in his treatment.

Practical application
In brief, this involves fourteen one hour sessions, in six overlapping stages: an initial assessment, requiring two sessions; modification of the patient's ideas about his pain, requiring another two sessions; acquisition of skills and consolidation, requiring another two sessions; cognitive and behavioural 'rehearsals', sessions eight to ten; relapse prevention (throughout, but especially in sessions ten to twelve); a follow-up of at least two sessions, following the end of initial treatment[2].

Comments
The stages overlap, are flexible and are tailored to the individual. The objective is not to eliminate pain, but to lead to a more effective and satisfying life. A further objective is to reduce dependence on doctors and drugs.

This system of management fits in readily with other forms of treatment, both psychological and somatic. It aims to lead to a sense of control.

Stages 1 and 2 – Assessment and rethinking (interdependent)
The functions of these stages are: to provide baseline material for the assessment of progress; to obtain details of the patient's circumstances and attitudes; to establish realistic goals; to inform the patient of the complexity of the pain experience; to inspect the role of 'significant others'; to provide new ideas; for example that pain is not a general, overwhelming experience, but that it contains specific difficulties to be dealt with (these new ideas include patient preparation for future management, and are designed to anticipate and to minimize patient resistance and treatment non-compliance); to develop further the idea of the complexity of the pain experience, so that the patient can be educated to think in terms of a treatment that will be effective in enhancing their lives, even if pain cannot be eliminated.

First contact with the patient: The patient must play an active role in the proceedings. He must be encouraged to see pain as episodic and thereby subject to modification, if not control.

The pain behaviour of patients and 'significant others' must be identified and explained; in particular with regard to moaning, inactivity, lying down etc.

A card intensity rating system should be provided, designed: (a) to show fluctuations in pain, and (b) to establish whether there is a pattern in the pain – whether it is predictable.

Preliminary formulation of treatment goals: This should not be general (e.g. to feel better) but specifically addressed to drug reduction, household work, etc. It should encompass the establishment of short-, medium- and long-term goals.

Exercise: The life style of chronic pain behaviour is often sedentary. Any exercise programme, of course, has to be carefully graded and must be appropriate to the patient's physical status, age and gender. The programme of exercise activity has two objectives:
1. That of physical exercise itself, since physical activity has physiological consequences that may exacerbate pain,
2. That of providing a competing interest with pain, for both the patient and those about him. In this way, pain competes for attention with other life demands. This is a use of exercise not always appreciated by physiotherapists and doctors interested in musculoskeletal medicine.

Medication: This is frequently excessive, and the programme is aimed at reducing medication to the minimum necessary, if not to achieve its complete withdrawal. Of course, this requires careful monitoring, because of the possibility of side-effects in reducing medication. Overmedication can be seen to be harmful on psychological grounds.

Patient education: An elementary explanation of the gate control theory is offered, and emphasis is placed on the roles of stress, cognition and anxiety, and their relationships to pain.

Pain intensity rating cards are used to illustrate their relationship to pain.

The point is emphasized that pain is manageable; that it comes in phases, and is not a prolonged, unvarying experience.

A pessimistic approach is discussed and its desired reversal is emphasized. A positive approach is offered to the patient, to try to persuade him to adopt it in his particular circumstance, as a means of his gaining control.

Stage 3 – Acquisition and consolidation of skills
These vary, but all are aimed at control and self-sufficiency.

Stage 4 – Role reversal
In this the patient is asked to reverse roles with the therapist. This induces an

attitude of flexibility in the patient, which involves improvization and thereby engenders a more imaginative attitude towards his situation.

Stage 5 – Generalization and maintainance
This is fostered throughout the treatment and is aimed at 'inoculating' any difficulties the patient may experience.

Stage 6 – Follow-up
This is normally applied at intervals of three months, six months and one year.

Relaxation and controlled breathing
There are many relaxation procedures, but controlled breathing is the one most commonly used in this type of management programme. First, it can be easily learned, and second, it can be readily used in stressful situations. Similar treatments, such as biofeedback and hypnosis seem rather more laborious in application.

Attentional training
This is given great importance in this programme. It can be presented to the patient by analogy with the simultaneous availability of all channels on television, whereas only one channel can be fully attended to at any one time. Imagery and no-imagery can be used, depending upon the individual patient's skills.

Aim of treatment
Reduction of pain disability.

Diagnosis
Unknown.

How it works
Unknown.

Indications
Pain of vertebral origin.

Contraindications
None.

Dangers
None.

Predictability
Outcome studies have been conducted in the laboratory and with a variety of pain syndromes, including headaches[9-11], arthritis[12], low back pain[13,14] and a combination of the varied set of chronic, intractable, benign pain syndromes[15-17]. It has also been used in combination with a variety of other therapies, such as biofeedback[18-20].

"In summary, the cognitive behavioural approach offers promise for use in a variety of chronic pain symdromes."[21] However, much further research needs to be done. For example, comparing this management with a purely operant orientated treatment approach: "We know almost nothing about which of the two major psychologically based treatments would be effective and for what type of patient."[21] "Moreover, there is little research to determine how best to combine psychologically based interventions, somatically based interventions (medications, transcutaneous nerve stimulation,) and so forth."[21]

It is apparent that predictability, short-term or long-term, currently remains beyond our reach.

Similar treatments
Behavioural therapy.

Treatment time
As with all psychological therapies, time is of the essence, and they all require to be unhurried. The patient must therefore be prepared to devote an appreciable period to each session, possibly at the expense of the demands of his work, and this may mount in aggregate to a substantial total treatment time.

Practical clinical consequences of the psychological therapies
Clinicians interested in musculoskeletal medicine may feel that these treatments have little to do with their work.

However, in the event of failure to obtain relief by other means, the doctor should know to whom to refer his patient, the kind of procedures that are likely to be applied to him, and their aim. This, which should be clearly understood, is not 'cure' of the patient, but is twofold:
1. Pain control for the patient, bringing its level within acceptable limits.
2. Attenuation of the patient's disability (even its abolition, from the point of view of his being re-enabled to earn his living).

In addition, from the point of view of the chronic pain patient, there are certain basic principles which are relevant to every clinician involved with these problems.

1. He needs to find out what are the patient's ideas with regard to his diagnosis and prognosis. Has he been told to "learn to live with it"? He needs to correct any false concepts, replacing these with more adequate and accurate information.
2. Under current health care systems, worldwide, patients tend to be allocated a passive role. Chronic pain patients must be encouraged to play a much more involved role and as far as possible to participate in their therapy.
3. The establishment of realistic goals is paramount. These should not be too optimistic, so as to avoid further disappointment, with which the patient may be only too familiar.
4. This is particularly important to remember in respect of patients in whom all previous therapies have failed. It is reasonable to reassure them that they are not "at the end of the line", and that, if need be, referral to appropriate regimes is available, and to tell them what these may achieve for them.
5. The clinician needs to remember that the family of the chronic pain patient who are, after all, closely involved, should also be enlisted, so as to ensure:
   a. That they also are fully informed as to the situation, together with appropriate counselling.
   b. That they may be advised as to how they may best be of assistance to the patient.

References

1. Ng (1981). New approaches to treatment of chronic pain. A review of multidisciplinary pain clinics and pain centres. DHSS Publication No. 81. 1089. United States Government Printing Office, Washington, D.C
2. Turk *et al.* (1983). *Pain and Behavioural Medicine. A Cognitive Behavioural Perspective.* (New York: Guilford Press
3. Melzack and Casey (1968). Sensory, motivational and central control determinants of pain. A new conceptual model. In Kenshalo (ed.) *The Skin Senses.* (Springfield, Illinois: Charles C. Thomas)
4. Beck *et al.* (1979). *Cognitive Therapy of Depression.* (New York: Guilford Press)
5. Foreyt and Rathjen (1978). *Cognitive Behavioural Therapies. Research and Application.* (New York: Plenum Press)
6. Kendall and Hollon (1979). *Cognitive Behavioural Interventions. Theory, Research and Procedures.* (New York: Academic Press)
7. Kendall (1982). *Advances in Cognitive Behavioural Research Therapy 1.* (New York: Academic Press)
8. Meichenbaum (1977). *Cognitive Behaviour Modification. An Integrative Approach.* (New York: Plenum Press)
9. Bakal *et al.* (1981). Cognitive behavioural treatment of chronic headache. *Headache*, **21**, 81–86
10. Figueroa (1982). Group treatment of chronic tension headaches. A comparative treatment study. *Behav. Modification*, **6**, 229–239

11. Holroyd *et al.* (1977). Cognitive control of tension headache. *Cognitive Ther. Res.*, **1**, 129–134
12. Randich (1982). Evaluation of stress inoculation training as a pain management programme for rheumatoid arthritis. Unpublished doctoral thesis dissertation. Washington University, St. Louis
13. Redden and Braddom (1980). Chronic low back pain. Self control cognitive modification techniques. Paper presented at the 57th annual session of the American Congress of Rehabilitation and Medicine, Washington, D.C., October
14. Turner (1979). Evaluation of two behavioural interventions for chronic low back pain. Unpublished doctoral disssertation. University of California, Los Angeles
15. Herman and Baptiste (1981). Pain control. Mastery through group experience. *Pain*, **10**, 79–86
16. Rybstein-Blinchik and Grzesiak (1979). Re-interpretive cognitive strategies in chronic pain management. *Arch. Phys. Med. Rehabil.*, **60**, 609–612
17. Turk and Kerns (1981). Efficacy of a cognitive behavioural group outpatients approach for the treatment of chronic pain. A paper presented at the third annual meeting at the Society of Behavioural Medicine, Chicago, March
18. Brena *et al.* (1981). Chronic pain as a learned experience. In Ng (ed.) *New Approaches to Treatment of Chronic Pain. A Review of Multidiciplinary Pain Clinics and Pain Centres.* (Emory University Pain Control Centre)
19. Gottlieb *et al.* (1977). Comprehensive rehabilitation with patients having chronic low back pain. *Arch. Phys. Med. Rehabil.*, **58**, 101–108
20. Khatami and Rush (1978). A pilot study of the treatment of outpatients with chronic pain. Symptom control, stimulus control, and social system intervention. *Pain*, **5**, 163–172
21. Turk and Meichenbaum (1983). A cognitive–behavioural approach to pain management. In Wall and Melzack (eds.) *Textbook of Pain*, p.793 *et seq.* (London: Churchill Livingstone)

Therapy 30 – Exercises

It will be noted that this form of treatment is not included in the management chart we present. The reason for this is that exercises are not in fact a means of relieving pain. Rather are they commonly used in behavioural and cognitive behavioural regimes, as an adjunct to pain control. We make this distinction deliberately, pain control being directed at the reduction of disability, whereas pain relief is aimed at the reduction of pain severity.

Exercises are used in the management of back pain for three purposes.
1. To strengthen muscles.
2. To correct faulty motor patterns (by those who believe in them).
3. To increase mobility.
They are primarily designed for the prophylaxis of back pain.

Although exercises are the most widely used of therapies, worldwide[1] their efficacy remains unproven, and there exists some confusion regarding their mode of action.

Mode of action
It is commonly believed that exercises strengthen muscles. However, this is difficult to demonstrate because of the phenomenon of muscle substitution[2]. The difficulties lie in the available means of testing muscle strength.
a. Measurement by using trunk movements against a chest harness connected to a force measuring load cell (for example) can only provide the crudest of measurements, in that many muscles are inevitably involved, and this unpredictably[3].
b. Assessment is most commonly practised manually[2].
c. Some clinicians make this assessment visually, but this is, of course, difficult to quantify[4].
With regard to (b) and (c), "these tests are subjective and their accuracy depends on the training, skill, and experience of the clinician performing the examination."[4] "There are no quantitative methods for measuring muscle function in clinical use today for the diagnosis and management of patients complaining of weakness."[5]

Fibre composition
An issue frequently raised is whether or not exercises alter muscle fibres. "The effects of athletic training and exercise on muscle fibre metabolism and architecture are currently an issue of considerable discussion. Numerous studies have been reported, with a variety of conflicting results."[6]

Control strategy
It is clear that exercises do not alter control strategies. It has been shown that the control strategy for activating the individual motor units in a given muscle does NOT alter with training[7].
Thus it may be concluded that it is the interaction of muscles that must be altered with training. Otherwise, individuals would not be able to improve their performance with practice. As a result of study of EMG activity, what really happens with training is that movements get progressively more efficient. "Before the training, the rhythmical flexion and extension of the elbow were effected by exuberant, apparently wasteful activity of the antagonist which is overcome by the greater activity of the agonist. With training, there is a progressive inhibition of the antagonist during the movements of flexion and extension until, with advanced training, the inhibition becomes complete."[8]
In the training stages, coactivation is common, apparently as a result of excitation radiation. Later it is extinguished[9].
It has been noted that subjects who were requested to practise flexion/extension exercises of the knee daily demonstrated a continual rise in the torque output in the first six days, followed by a plateau. Biopsies of the

277

vastus lateralis revealed no signicficant alteration in fibre area or type. Kamen also found that the net force measured at the joint he studied increased daily for six days[10].

"It is surprising how often one finds that modification in the interaction of the agonist/antagonist musculature explains the results of numerous biomechanical studies reported in the literature."[11]

Isometric exercises
Recent work has altered attitudes as to which exercises are appropriate.

Professor Jayson wrote, "In my view, the right sort of exercises for most back pain patients are isometric exercises, aimed at strengthening the paraspinal and abdominal muscles."[12]

Nachemson, over twenty years' measuring intradiscal pressures in the lumbar spine, has shown that some exercises increase the load on the lumbar spine to such an extent that the intradiscal pressures reach levels as high as those measured in standing, and leaning forwards with weights in the hands. Particularly marked is the rise in sitting up exercises, with the knees either flexed or extended. Therefore it must be accepted that these exercises should be avoided, which is one of the reasons why isometric exercises are currently in favour[13].

Nachemson's figures for intradiscal pressures at L3/4 show a load of 70 kg on standing; of 120 kg on bilateral straight leg raising; of 180 kg and 175 kg on sitting up exercises, knees flexed or extended; and of 110 kg on isometric abdominal muscle exercises[13].

Moreover, it is known that, when lifting or carrying very heavy objects, the increase of intra-abdominal pressure resulting from the concommitant contraction of the abdominal, pelvic and costal muscles and the diaphragm, will relieve some of the load on the lumbar spine. Therefore it is "reasonable" (Nachemson) to perform exercises aimed at strengthening these muscles[1].

Comment
Exercises are employed for many purposes. They are an essential part of behavioural and cognitive behavioural regimes, aimed at diminution of disability. They are also used, as stated above, to strengthen muscles, to correct faulty motor patterns and to increase mobility. As has been shown, the increase in joint mobility and the increase in muscular strength have not yet been scientifically demonstrated.

Changes in EMG activity have been demonstrated in muscles subserving simple functions in peripheral joints. Such changes have NOT been demonstrated in relation to spinal movements, for the reasons given elsewhere.

In the light of these facts, the prescription of **isometric** exercises aimed at the abdominal and chest muscles is rational, may be helpful and, above all, is harmless. In this respect exercises are seen to have much in common with other modalities of back pain management, and it will be appreciated that harmlessness is a very important consideration.

References

1. Nachemson (1980). *The Lumbar Spine and Low Back Pain*, p.459. (London: Pitman Medical)
2. Basmajian and DeLuca (1985). *Muscles Alive*. 5th Edn., p.220. (Baltimore: Williams and Wilkins)
3. Schultz (1982). Biomechanics of the spine. In Colt Symposium, pp. 20–24 (London: National Back Pain Association)
4. Kendall *et al.* (1971). *Muscles. Testing and Function* (Baltimore: Williams and Wilkins)
5. Edwards and Hyde (1977). Methods of measuring muscle strength and fatigue. *Physiotherapy*, **63**, 51–55
6. Basmajian and DeLuca (1985). op. cit., p.219
7. DeLuca *et al.* (1982). Controls scheme governing concurrently active human motor units in voluntary contraction. *J. Physiol.*, **329**, 129–142
8. Person (1958). Electromyographic investigation of coordinated activity of antagonistic muscles in movements of fingers of the human hand (Russian Text). *J. Physiol. USSR*, **94**, 455–462
9. Bratanova (1966). On bioelectric activity of muscle antagonists in the course of elaboration of a motor habit (Russian text). *Zh. Vyssh. Nerv. Diat. Pavlov*, **16**, 411–416
10. Kamen (1983). The aquisition of maximal isometric plantar flexor/strength. A force/time curve analysis. *J. Motor Behav.*, **15**, 63–73
11. Basmajian and DeLuca (1985). op. cit., p.230
12. Jayson (1982). Rheumatology. In Colt Symposium, pp.87–89. (London: National Back Pain Association)
13. Nachemson (1980). *The Lumbar Spine and Low Back Pain*. (London: Pitman Medical)

13
MANAGEMENT CHART

Notes to management chart

a. In the great majority of cases clinical diagnosis is not attainable.
b. This is intended as an index of inconvenience for the patient, and is defined as the overall time he is likely to need to interrupt his domestic/work activities for each treatment. It is recorded, perhaps rather crudely, as requiring minutes (A), hours (B), days (C) or weeks (D).
c. PVO = pain of vertebral origin.
d. These drugs must not be considered solely from an analgesic point of view, as they also may modify the psychology of the pain state under consideration in an unpredictable manner. (See Relevant Psychology, p.108).
e. Overdosage may prove fatal.
f. While the inhibitory action of A-fibres on C-fibres is the only mechanism known to operate, there may well be others involved, e.g. "In the cat both noxious stimuli and light tapping of the skin consistently excite many raphe spinal fields." (See Endogenous Pain Control Mechanisms, p.58.)
g. Manipulation is thought by some to result in the correction of previously identified bony displacement, by others in the restoration of 'normal' ranges of movements in joints previously restricted. While either may be the case, we have found no sound evidence to support these views.
h. It is possible that extreme sensitivity may cause death - we have not come across this in the literature in respect of local block.
i. Arachnoiditis and local sepsis.
j. Lumbar, thoracic and cervical epidurals.
k. At sufficiently high frequencies, TNS becomes stimulation therapy.
m. This is unique, in that it is the only occasion upon which a valid diagnosis is made before treatment. However, it must be stressed that this diagnosis can only be finally confirmed at operation itself.
n. This is the only treatment in which prediction of short-term outcome is possible. It is correlated with the degree of herniation of the disc found at operation.
p. "Pain disability" means relief of impairment of function due to the pain suffered.
q. Pure behavioural therapy has no cognitive contaminants – it is rarely used.

TABLE 13.1 - COMPARISON OF THERAPIES FOR PAIN OF VERTEBRAL ORIGIN

Treatment	Aim of treatment	Diagnosis[a]	How does it work?	Indications	Contra-indications
1. Non-narcotic analgesics	Pain relief	Unknown	Unknown	PVO[c]	No
2. NSAIDs	" A/inflamm.	"	"	"	Yes
3. Anti-depressants	Pain relief[d]	"	"	"	No
4. Neuroleptics	"[d]	"	"	"	"
5. Tranquillizers	"	"	"	"	"
6. Bedrest	"	"	"	"	"
7. Heat and cold	"	"	"	"	Yes
8. Collars/corsets	"	"	"	"	"
9. Traction	"	"	A on C[f]	"	"
10. Massage	"	"	"	"	No
11. Manipulation[g]	"	"	"	"	Yes
12. Local block	"	"	Unknown	"	"
13. Caudal epidural	"	"	"	"	"
14. TNS	"	"	A on C[f]	"	"
15. Acupuncture	"	"	Unknown	"	No

Dangers	Complic-ations	Predictability short-term	Predictability long-term	Similar therapies	Therapy time[b]
Yes	No	No	No	2	A
"	Yes	"	"	1	A
"e	"	"	"	4/5	A
"e	"	"	"	3/5	A
"e	"	"	"	3/4	A
No	"	"	"	No	D
Yes	"	"	"	18	B
"	No	"	"	No	A
No	Yes	"	"	11	B
"	No	"	"	11/15	B
Yes	Yes	"	"	10/15	B
No[h]	"	"	"	No	B
"[h]	"[i]	"	"	Yes[j]	B
No[h]	No	"	"	15/16/17/18[k]	A/B
"	"	"	"	14/16/17/18	B

Treatment	Aim of treatment	Diagnosis	How does it work?	Indications	Contra-indication
16. Needle effect	Pain relief	Unknown	Unknown	PVO	No
17. Auriculotherapy	"	"	"	"	"
18. Ice massage	"	"	"	"	"
19. Rhizolysis	"	"	"	"	"
20. Root surgery	"	"	"	"	Yes
21. Disc surgery	"	PID^m	"	PID^m	"
22. Chemonucleolysis	"	Unknown	"	PVO	"
23. Sclerosants	"	"	"	"	No
24. Placebo	"	"	"	"	"
25. Biofeedback	Pain relief Pain control	"	"	"	"
26. Hypnosis	Pain relief Pain control	"	"	"	Yes
27. Relaxation response	Pain relief Pain control	"	"	"	No
28. Behavioural therapy	Pain disability^p	"	"	"	"
29. Cognitive behavioural therapy	Pain disability	"	"	"	"

Dangers	Complications	Predictability short-term	Predictability long-term	Similar therapies	Therapy time[b]
No	Yes	No	No	14/15/17/18	B
"	"	"	"	14/15/16/18	B
"	"	"	"	14/15/16/17	B
"	"	"	"	20	C
Yes	"	"	"	19	D
"	"	"ⁿ	"	No	D
"	"	"	"	"	D
No	No	"	"	"	B
"	"	"	"	25/26/27	–
"	"	"	"	24/26/27	B
Yes	"	"	"	24/25/27	B
No	"	"	"	24/25/26	B
"	"	"	"	q 29	B
"	"	"	"	28	B

Conclusions

Because the mode of action of all these treatments is unknown and the outcome of their use unpredictable, there can be no scientific basis for their deployment, save for the negative factors of their individual contra-indications, dangers and complications.

Thus the reality of management differs radically from the current assumption that they do have a scientific basis.

For this reason, empiricism is inevitable, and pragmatism must be the dominant consideration in selection of therapy; i.e. safety, simplicity[1] and such factors as the time involved in their deployment and their cost.

This leads to a point of fundamental importance. The current medical practice, common world-wide, of assuring the patient after the failure of one or two treatments that nothing can be done for him, with frequently devastating consequences, is clearly mistaken. "C'est pire qu'un crime, c'est une faute." (Talleyrand).

Reference

1. Mehta (1984). Pain clinic treatments. Presentation at BAMM Symposium, London, April 1984.

14
TIERS OF MANAGEMENT

With so wide a range of therapies from which to choose, it seems to us reasonable to offer a tier system, presenting the majority of the therapies discussed in a working sequence. This is summarized in Table 14.1 on p.290.

Tier 1

This includes those therapies suitable as first choices, and it will be noted that they are suitable for use in both acute and chronic cases. There are major differences between these two states; indeed chronic pain is very much more complex and unpredictable. The same therapies may be used in either state, but in dealing with chronic pain the clinician must be prepared to identify additional clinical features that are themselves a functional disability (e.g. pain behaviours, neuroticism and the problems associated with the family. If it is the case that 10% of pain clinic patients have clinical depression, these patients should be identified and treated accordingly.)

Some clinicians favour bedrest. We discuss this under Therapy 6 (p.202). It involves the clinician minimally, but it is of substantial inconvenience to the patient. For this reason we try to avoid this mode of management. It is of no proven value in back pain.

There are those who deploy acupuncture as a first choice therapy. This is perfectly reasonable, its chief disadvantages being that it is relatively time consuming for both the clinician and the patient, and that it needs appropriate training. It is discussed under Therapy 15 (p.228).

Injection of trigger points or other tender areas, while it is to a degree invasive, is an excellent and rapid form of treatment, which we have found particularly useful in cases where manipulation is contraindicated. This we discuss under Therapy 12 (p.215).

Analgesics and NSAIDs again are perfectly legitimate treatments for first choice use. Their prescription is rapid for the clinician, and taking them is of minimal inconvenience to the patient. As detailed under Therapies 1 and 2 (pp.183 and 186) they have certain potential disadvantages.

Manipulation, discussed under Therapy 11 (p.213), is our treatment of first choice, in the absence of any contraindication. This is chiefly because of its extreme safety and rapidity of action (when it works!). It is no more unpredictable than is any other treatment. Of course, its usefulness is restricted to those clinicians who have developed a competence in these techniques. (See *An Introduction to Medical Manipulation*[1].)

Ice massage (Therapy 8, p.235) is a therapy we do not currently employ but, in view of its simplicity, safety and convenience for the patient, it should be considered in the first tier. Its ease of prescription in general practice is obvious.

Tier 2

This includes those therapies suitable as second choices; choices made necessary by virtue of failure of one or other of the tier 1 therapies or by their contraindication, or by the clinician not having adequate competence in manipulative techniques or acupuncture.

We have deliberately included the tranquillizers in this tier, as we feel that they are best used where there are clear signs of neuroticism.

To these may be added TNS, discussed under Therapy 14 (p.223). Although time consuming for the clinician in the first place, in teaching its use to the patient, the subsequent inconvenience to the patient is minimal in its domiciliary application.

To the local injections, which may be the first choice of some clinicians, but are commonly second choice (particularly for the practised manipulator,) we add the caudal epidural, discussed under Therapy 13 (p.220). This is a simple, safe procedure, well suited to deployment in general practice in addition to the out-patient clinic, which is not very time consuming for the clinician or the patient.

Some of the relaxation techniques may be included here (Therapies 25, 26 and 27, pp.251, 256 and 262) either as a therapeutic second choice, or as an adjunct to other therapeutic modalities. Again, there will be some who favour this approach, on the basis of suitable experience or aptitude. This also applies to counselling, which we discuss under Therapy 29, p.270. More often, however, these will be 'relegated' to tier 4.

Tier 3

This comprises a few 'reserve therapies: those quite readily available, but not customarily used with any great frequency.

We include TNS again, though we have already discussed this under tier 2. TNS is probably mostly to be found in intractable pain clinics, and so might be classified under tier 4.

The neuroleptics, particularly the phenothiazine derivatives, must be included under tier 3. These are discussed under Therapy 5, and they are not suitable for early use (see p.199). On the other hand, they do represent a valuable addition to the doctor's therapeutic 'armoury, particularly for the general practitioner with rather remote hospital resources.

Physiotherapy referral is included in this tier, although some may think of this as having a place in either tier 2 or tier 3. These treatments are grouped together under Therapy 7 (p.204). The same comment is aplicable to traction, discussed under Therapy 9 (p.211).

Tier 4

This comprises a hotchpotch of therapies, linked chiefly by their common demand for referral. Once more, we are here primarily concerned with the general practitioner.

We have included sclerosant therapy here, not because it requires referral, but rather because (although we have both used it in the past) we regard it as a last resort. It is discussed under Therapy 23 (p.248).

The psychotherapies (discussed under Therapies 28 and 29, pp.266 and 270) are included in this tier on account of their being a very specialised form of treatment, suitable for the intractable pain problem and for use by highly skilled therapists.

There remain the rather more invasive approaches: rhizolysis and rhizotomy, discussed under Therapy 19 (p.237), and chemonucleolysis (Therapy 22, p.247) and lastly surgery (Therapies 20 and 21, pp.238 and 242). In mounting degree, these must be regarded as really last resorts, as they share a common invasive feature and involve the clinician in considerable expenditure of time, as also the patient, and are none of them without their dangers.

Comment

It will be noted that, in all tiers, our choice seems somewhat restricted. This is because we are more familiar with these treatments than others, and therefore tend to make more use of them. It does not imply that they are necessarily better than the alternatives, our decisions being based on the criteria already detailed (see p.287 *et seq.*).

Reference

1. Paterson and Burn (1983). *An Introduction to Medical Manipulation* (Lancaster: MTP Press)

Table 14.1 Tiers of management

Therapy   *Therapy number*

TIER 1 Therapies suitable as first choices, in acute or chronic cases, dependent on personal inclination and absent contraindications.

Manipulation	11
Analgesics	1
NSAIDs	2
Acupuncture	15
Injections	12
Bedrest	6
Ice massage	18

TIER 2 Therapies suitable as second choices, following failure or because of contraindication of first choice therapy.

Injections – including caudal epidurals	12 and 13
Acupuncture	15
TNS	14
Relaxation techniques	25, 26 and 27
Counselling	29

TIER 3 Therapies readily available – suitable in case of recurrent therapeutic failure.

TNS	14
Neuroleptic drugs	4
Physiotherapy referral	7

TIER 4 Therapies demanding referral – suitable in difficult chronic pain situations.

Traction	9
Sclerosant therapy	23
Psychotherapies	28 and 29
Rhizolysis	19
Chemonucleolysis	22
Surgery	20 and 21

15
PATIENT ADVICE

Patients frequently seek advice with regard to pain of vertebral origin, already confused by the plethora of conflicting material available to them. It is often difficult for the clinician to find the time to offer adequate, individual explanations. To meet this demand, we are publishing (in Spring 1991) a short book for the public, based on this text.

16
ENVOI

In our introduction to this book, we mentioned how neglected a field was musculoskeletal medicine within current medical education. We are sure that the reader will be surprised to learn, for example, that the mode of action and predictability of outcome of all treatments is at best but marginally understood. It is reasonable to suggest that this educational neglect is one of the causes of the current public demand for non-medical practitioners.

The scale of musculoskeletal problems is indisputable, but their manifestations are protean, in that they intrude into so many clinical areas of medical practice. Yet this is a fact many doctors would feel to be currently insufficiently appreciated.

Review of the relevant literature reveals that the scientific bases of epidemiology, anatomy, physiology, psychology and pathology are applicable to basic case analysis and management, in that the identification of the unknown is as important as the establishment of facts. We feel that the employment of such scientific bases, limited as it clearly now is, is sufficient for the physician to practice rationally, without the necessity for him to rely upon hypotheses. These, sadly, are at present no more than allegories of supposition.

This further implies that any doctor may safely bypass such literature (of which there is an abundance and which bedevils this difficult field of medicine) without prejudice to his patient. This approach has the additional merit of being subject to and welcoming constant modification in the light of fresh scientific evidence.

Those doctors with a deeper interest in this field naturally review such hypotheses and adopt what they find helpful in their individual practices, and this is right and proper, provided that the basic considerations are respected. Many schools of thought exist, lay and medical, and all should be carefully and critically evaluated. None should be embraced in its entirety.

"Each school of thought and training has reasonably tended to approach pain problems from a particular bias and to write articles and textbooks expressing that emphasis. It now seems apparent that all those biases are both right and wrong, and that the problem and the patients benefit from a multiple approach."[1] With regard to management, the importance of this approach cannot be over-emphasized.

292

"The brain specialises in dynamic, homeostatic controls. Unfortunately, those controls may change to a pain producing pathological setting. A single therapy may temporarily tilt the control back towards normal, followed by a central nervous system reaction to reconstruct the former levels. Many therapies are plagued with effects which are given different names; adaptation, habituation, tolerance, fading and long term failure. Combination, alternation and circulation of therapies may well be the best tactic to defeat the homeostatic abilities of the nervous mechanisms to restore pathological states."[1]

The two most significant features to emerge from the study of musculoskeletal medicine are the breadth of scientific background required for adequate case analysis (see Introduction to Case Analysis, p.151), and the need for the potentially most effective doctor to have knowledge of and access to as great a variety of treatments as possible.

At the present time, as a result of the current inadequacy of medical education, the patient with persistent pain is compelled to seek treatment from an extraordinary variety of practitioners of widely differing educational background and training.

If, in the light of existing knowledge, the medical profession were better aquainted with therapies of potential, if unpredictable, value, this compulsion would be diminished.

Reference

1.   Wall (1983). In Wall and Melzack (eds.) *Textbook of Pain*. (London: Churchill Livingstone)

INDEX